CARMEN STURDY'S
every last bite

a deliciously
clean approach to
**THE SPECIFIC
CARBOHYDRATE DIET**
———— with ————
over 150 grain-free,
dairy-free & allergy-
friendly recipes

VICTORY BELT PUBLISHING INC.

Las Vegas

First published in 2020 by Victory Belt Publishing Inc.

ISBN-13: 978-1-628604-04-7

The information included in this book is for educational purposes only. It is not intended or implied to be a substitute for professional medical advice. The reader should always consult his or her health-care provider to determine the appropriateness of the information for his or her own situation or if he or she has any questions regarding a medical condition or treatment plan. Reading the information in this book does not constitute a physician-patient relationship. The statements in this book have not been evaluated by the Food and Drug Administration. The products or supplements in this book are not intended to diagnose, treat, cure, or prevent any disease. The author and publisher expressly disclaim responsibility for any adverse effects that may result from the use or application of the information contained in this book.

Author photos by Nicole Engelmann

Cover design by Justin-Aaron Velasco

Interior design by Yordan Terziev and Boryana Yordanova

Printed in Canada

TC 0120

This book is dedicated to my mom, who always inspired me with the creativity and enthusiasm she had for everything she did. She taught me everything I know about cooking, to live life to the fullest, and to always follow my passion. She is the inspiration behind every recipe I create.

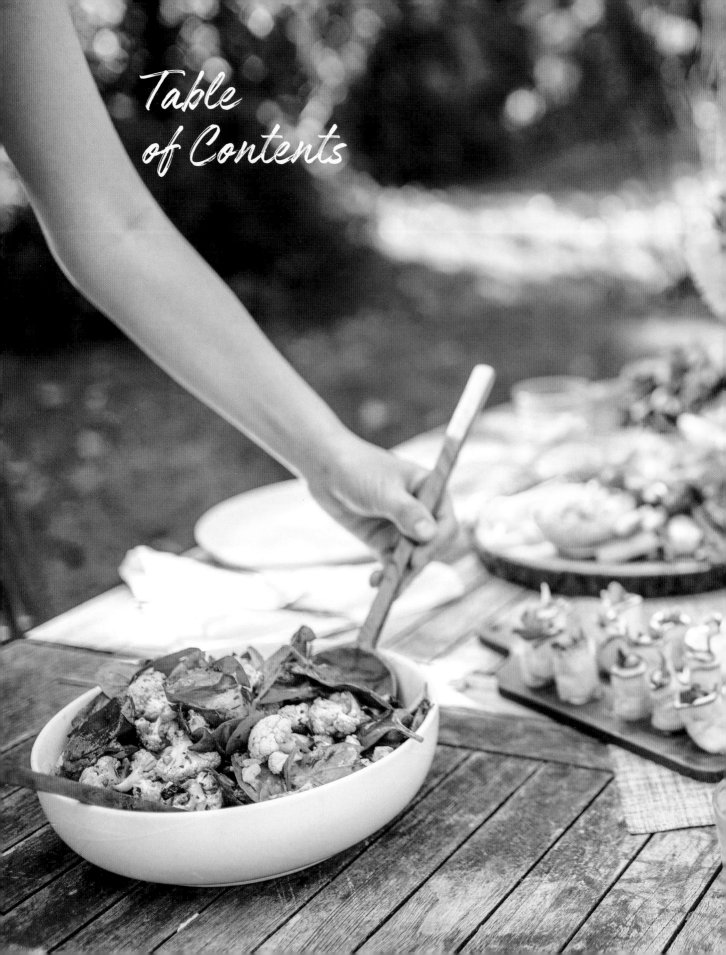

Table of Contents

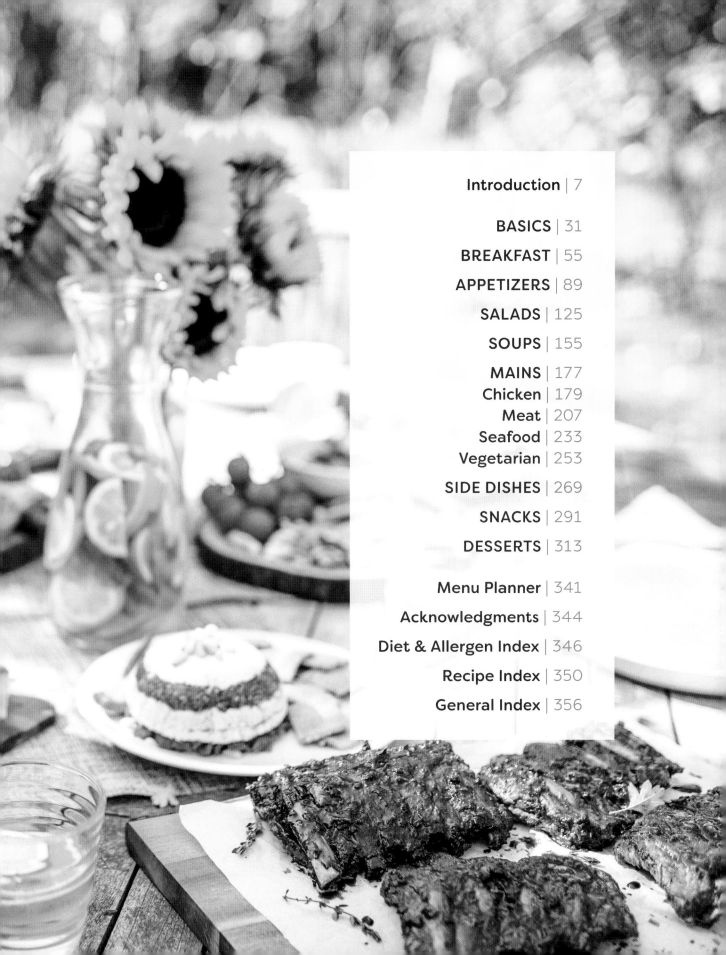

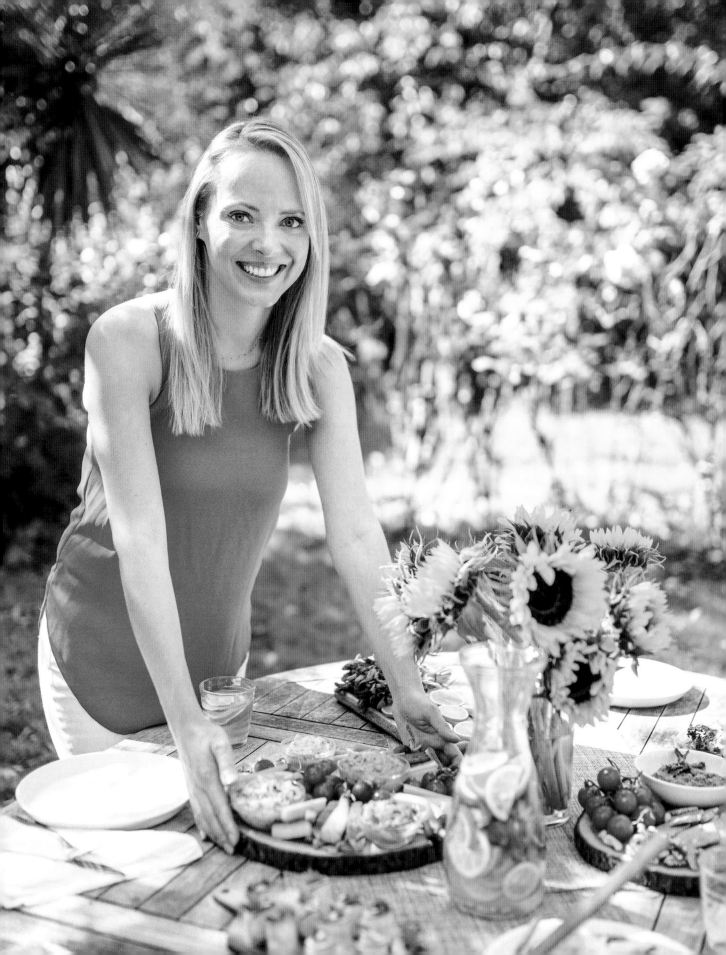

Introduction

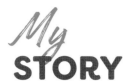

My STORY

Food has always been a big part of my life and so much more than just fuel for my body. I love the experience of food, both cooking and eating, and how meals bring together family and friends. My fondest food memories from my childhood are the times when I would sit at the dinner table with my family, discussing the day's events or watching my mom cook in the kitchen. She was always so creative, reinventing old dishes and teaching me what secret ingredients to add to elevate the flavors of every meal.

I was always in my happy place in the kitchen with my mom, learning everything I could about cooking and entertaining and helping her prepare for dinner parties and big gatherings. My love for cooking carried on into high school and university, where I loved preparing big feasts for friends and learned that a stick of butter, 1 cup of Parmesan, or ½ cup of cream makes anything taste good. *Healthy* wasn't a word in my vocabulary.

Fast-forward to 2012. I had moved to London, England, and was working at an investment bank and living a relatively unhealthy lifestyle. I started experiencing gastrointestinal issues (with symptoms similar to ones that my mom had before being diagnosed with colon cancer), and I completely freaked out. I went to a specialist who did extensive testing and diagnosed me with ulcerative colitis (UC), an autoimmune disease that attacks the intestines. My doctor immediately put me on a long list of strong medications and told me that the disease was incurable; I would have to get used to the new norm. Months later, my symptoms persisted, and I was taking thirty-two pills a day with side effects that included a swollen "moon face," insomnia, hair loss, and a foggy head. The side effects of the drugs became worse than the symptoms of the disease, and my doctor's only response was to continue to prescribe me more medication.

Six months later, I finally hit a breaking point and began to research nonmedicinal treatment options. The Specific Carbohydrate Diet (SCD) appeared in every search, so I ordered *Breaking the Vicious Cycle* by Elaine Gottschall and learned everything I could about the diet. The science behind the diet was very convincing, but the long list of restricted foods was hard for me to come to terms with. As a self-proclaimed foodie, a life without pasta, bread, rice, or ice cream seemed impossible, but I was desperate and willing to try anything.

After two weeks on the diet and a year with the disease, my symptoms had improved. I spent a lot of time on the internet looking for SCD recipes and was disheartened by how simple and unimaginative the dishes looked. The diet was making me better, but eating the same soups, bland meat, and steamed vegetables was crushing my spirit and making me lose the love I once had for cooking and eating. As my health improved, I began to experiment more in the kitchen, trying to create some of the dishes I craved using SCD-approved ingredients. It took some imagination, but soon I was using cauliflower to make ice cream and zucchini for enchiladas, and my passion for cooking had returned. I loved creating dishes that friends and family (including my picky husband, SA) could enjoy without having any idea that they were Specific Carbohydrate Diet legal.

In 2014, I started the Every Last Bite blog (everylastbite.com) as a way to share my kitchen creations with other people who were following the Specific Carbohydrate Diet. My hope was it would show others that no matter how restrictive a diet you are on, you can still make delicious food that won't leave you feeling deprived.

After two-and-a-half years strictly following the diet and two years of medication-free remission, I began to reintroduce foods into my diet. I started slowly, always testing just one food at a time to determine its effect before trying another. Now, five years later, I am much more flexible with the foods I eat, and I am still in remission.

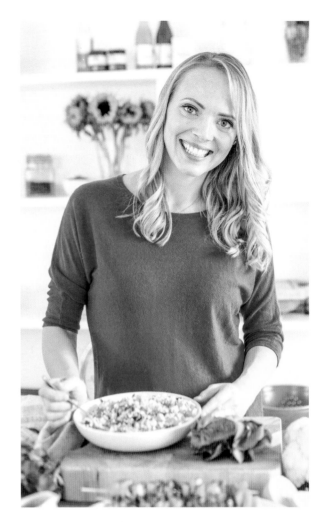

Over the years, I have connected with hundreds of people who suffer from a variety of autoimmune diseases and follow the Specific Carbohydrate Diet. As my blog has grown, I've realized that my audience is no longer an SCD-only group; it also includes those following other restrictive diets, including Paleo, keto, and low-FODMAP, and each diet has a lot in common with the others. Because of this, I've begun to include ingredient variations for some of the recipes so that as many people as possible can make and enjoy them.

As you will see in this book, my recipes don't require fancy cooking skills or lots of expensive equipment. Every recipe is easy to prepare and, most important, delicious. Whether you're on a dairy-free diet, following the Specific Carbohydrate Diet, or just like eating healthily, these dishes are sure to satisfy you. I've included reinvented twists on classic comfort foods, 30-minute meals, foolproof recipes for brand-new chefs, and lots of dishes inspired by my travels around the world. I hope that the recipes in this book can bring joy to each meal, and I encourage you to gather family and friends to share delicious food that everyone can enjoy, no matter their dietary restrictions.

SCD 101

If you're planning on starting the Specific Carbohydrate Diet, I highly recommend that you read Elaine Gottschall's *Breaking the Vicious Cycle,* which thoroughly explains the diet. I believe that knowing what is and is not allowed on the diet is important, but understanding the science behind the Specific Carbohydrate Diet is what makes sticking to it a lot easier.

I'm not a nutritionist, a dietitian, or a doctor; I'm just a girl who loves to eat. So please humor me with my very basic description of the Specific Carbohydrate Diet; I'm providing a simplified summary for anyone who wants to get a general gist of the diet.

Where Did the Specific Carbohydrate Diet Come From?

Dr. Sidney Haas originally developed the SCD in the 1920s to treat celiac disease. The diet gained wider recognition in the 1980s when Elaine Gottschall wrote *Breaking the Vicious Cycle* after she'd used the diet to treat her daughter's ulcerative colitis. The book is incredibly thorough, and I recommend it for anyone new to the diet.

Who Can the Specific Carbohydrate Diet Help?

The SCD is designed to help anyone suffering from inflammatory bowel disease (Crohn's disease and ulcerative colitis), diverticulitis, celiac disease, and irritable bowel syndrome, but it's also been shown to help those with autism, cystic fibrosis, and other autoimmune diseases.

How Does the Specific Carbohydrate Diet Work?

The SCD is based on the idea that not everyone's digestive system can optimally digest all carbohydrates. Carbohydrates are restricted to monosaccharides (or single-molecule carbohydrates), which are the quickest and easiest-to-digest form of carbohydrates, whereas complex carbohydrates (polysaccharides, disaccharides, etc.) take longer to digest and aren't immediately absorbed. When these undigested carbohydrates remain in your gut, harmful bacteria feed on it and grow, causing your intestines to become inflamed and triggering a flare. Limiting your consumption of carbohydrates to those that are easiest to digest kills off the bad bacteria by starving them. Consequently, your gut can heal.

What Can You Eat on the SCD?

The SCD breaks food down into different categories: legal, illegal, and foods that you can reintroduce after you've been in remission for six months to one year. The illegal list includes all grain, gluten, lactose (but not all dairy), refined sugar, soy, and starchy vegetables. The following is a general summary of the legal and illegal foods, but I suggest that you visit breakingtheviciouscycle.info for a much more detailed list.

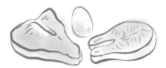

MEATS/PROTEIN

✓ **LEGAL:** Bacon (nitrate and sugar-free), beef, chicken, duck, eggs, fish (canned fish in water is allowed), lamb, pork, seafood, turkey

✗ **ILLEGAL:** Processed meats such as ham, hot dogs, smoked meats

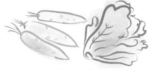

VEGETABLES

✓ **LEGAL:** All fresh and frozen vegetables except the vegetables in the illegal category

✗ **ILLEGAL:** Corn, jicama, okra, parsnips, potatoes, sweet potatoes, yams, all canned vegetables

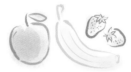

FRUITS

✓ **LEGAL:** All fresh, frozen, cooked, and dried fruit as long as there is no added sugar

✗ **ILLEGAL:** Canned fruit or juices with added sugar or preservatives

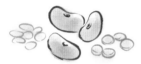

LEGUMES/GRAINS

✓ **LEGAL:** Dried black beans, lentils, lima beans, navy beans, split peas

✗ **ILLEGAL:** Barley, buckwheat, canned beans, couscous, flours, garbanzo beans (chickpeas), millet, oats, pinto beans, rice, spelt, wheat

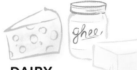

DAIRY

✓ **LEGAL:** Butter; ghee; hard aged cheeses such as cheddar, Gouda, and Parmesan; homemade SCD yogurt (which I don't use in this book but you can find in online recipes)

✗ **ILLEGAL:** Milk; cream; soft cheeses such as cottage cheese, cream cheese, mascarpone, mozzarella, processed cheese, ricotta; sour cream; store-bought yogurt, ice cream

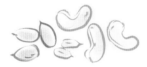

NUTS/SEEDS

✓ **LEGAL:** All unsalted nuts including peanuts (which are actually a legume), natural nut butters, almond flour, pumpkin seeds, sesame seeds, sunflower seeds

✗ **ILLEGAL:** Chia seeds, flax seeds, hemp seeds, mixed nuts, nuts with a starchy/sugary coating

Things I've Learned After Following the SCD

Although the legal and illegal food lists for the diet are a good place to start, everyone tolerates foods differently. To be as inclusive as possible, I do not include some SCD-legal ingredients in the recipes in this book, including beans and SCD yogurt, and I use only a minimal amount of cheese. Listen to your body; if you notice that you have a bad reaction every time you eat a particular food, even if it's SCD legal, try removing it from your diet for a few weeks to see if your symptoms improve.

Unfortunately, Elaine Gottschall passed away in 2005, and although research has been done on the diet since that time, the lists of legal and illegal foods on the website have not been updated. In my opinion, food production and labeling have greatly improved in the past fifteen years, so although you should still take great precaution when checking labels, a lot more SCD-legal products are available now.

The Specific Carbohydrate Diet
VERSUS THE PALEO DIET

The Paleo diet and Specific Carbohydrate Diet are both commonly used to help treat autoimmune diseases. The two diets are free of grain, gluten, refined sugar, and soy and share a lot of similarities in the allowable foods. Here is a summary of the similarities and differences between the two diets.

Specific Carbohydrate Diet

The SCD eliminates anything hard for your body to digest to prevent the overgrowth of bad bacteria and give your gut time to heal. It was created to treat UC, Crohn's, and a variety of other autoimmune diseases.

Paleo Diet

The Paleo diet is based on the concept that our bodies haven't evolved to digest our modern diet of grains, processed foods, etc. Paleo is short for Paleolithic and refers to the idea of eating like the hunter-gatherers of the Paleolithic era.

	Specific Carbohydrate Diet		Paleo Diet	
GRAINS		None		None
DAIRY	✓ Homemade SCD yogurt ✓ Aged hard cheeses that are virtually lactose-free (cheddar, Gouda, Havarti, Parmesan, etc.) ✓ Butter/ghee	✗ Soft cheeses (mozzarella, ricotta, etc.) ✗ All other milk/cream-based products	✓ Ghee (clarified butter)	✗ All cheeses (both soft and hard) ✗ All milk/cream-based products (ice cream, yogurt, sour cream, etc.)
VEGETABLES	✓ Most vegetables	✗ Sweet potatoes ✗ Potatoes ✗ Okra ✗ Turnips ✗ Parsnips ✗ Corn ✗ Plantains	✓ Most vegetables	✗ Corn
FRUIT	✓ All fruit		✓ All fruit	
LEGUMES, SEEDS, AND NUTS	✓ All nuts ✓ Peanuts ✓ Some beans, including dried black beans, lima beans, navy beans, lentils, split peas	✗ Chickpeas ✗ Butter beans ✗ Cannellini beans ✗ Flax seeds ✗ Chia seeds ✗ Hemp seeds	✓ All nuts ✓ Flax seeds ✓ Chia seeds ✓ Hemp seeds	✗ Peanuts ✗ All beans
BAKING INGREDIENTS AND SWEETENERS	✓ Almond flour ✓ Coconut flour ✓ Baking soda ✓ Honey	✗ Cocoa powder ✗ Cassava flour ✗ Arrowroot flour ✗ Baking powder ✗ Tapioca starch ✗ Maple syrup ✗ Coconut sugar	✓ Cocoa powder ✓ Cassava flour ✓ Arrowroot flour ✓ Baking powder ✓ Maple syrup ✓ Tapioca starch ✓ Coconut sugar ✓ Almond flour ✓ Coconut flour ✓ Baking soda ✓ Honey	

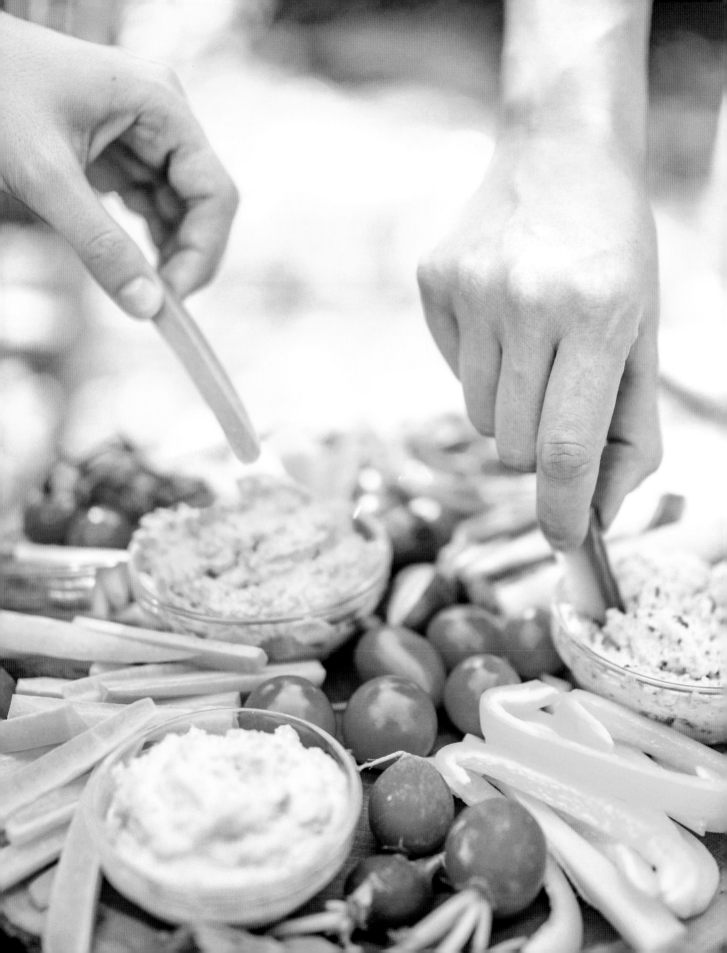

SCD Pantry/Fridge STAPLES

Having a well-stocked pantry, fridge, and freezer helps make healthy cooking and eating easy. Following is a list of the products that I use in recipes throughout the book. I recommend having them stocked in your kitchen.

The brands that are SCD legal differ from region to region, which is why I haven't included many specific brands. There are lots of great websites that provide lists of SCD-legal products and where you can find them.

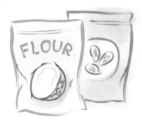

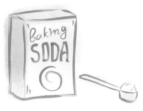

ALMOND FLOUR AND COCONUT FLOUR

Almond flour and coconut flour are the only two flours allowed on the SCD. Finely ground blanched almond flour produces the best baked goods. Coconut flour is more difficult to bake with; it's so absorbent that batters can dry out too much during baking. Unfortunately, these flours cannot be substituted for one another in recipes.

BAKING SODA

Store-bought baking powder is not allowed on the SCD because it contains starch, and homemade baking powder is also illegal if it includes cream of tartar. Consequently, baking soda is the best leavening agent for SCD baking. Adding an acidic liquid such as vinegar or lemon or lime juice activates the baking soda and causes the batter to rise when baking.

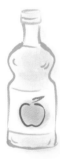

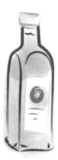

APPLE CIDER VINEGAR

Only apple cider vinegar without mother is allowed on SCD. Mother is a bacteria that helps the vinegar to ferment. If the bottle is not clearly labeled "without mother," look for apple cider vinegar that is completely clear with no sediment floating in the bottle.

BALSAMIC VINEGAR

Cheap balsamic vinegar has added sugar, but balsamic vinegar that has been aged for fifteen years is allowed on the SCD; the downside is that it's more expensive. I have included a recipe for an easy-to-make aged balsamic vinegar substitute on page 46.

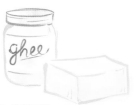

BUTTER AND GHEE

Ghee is a type of clarified butter, which means that it has been simmered until the milk solids rise to the top so you can skim them off. Although ghee isn't technically dairy-free, it's used in dairy-free diets such as Whole30 and Paleo because all of the milk solids have been removed, making it lactose free. Ghee and butter can be used interchangeably in recipes. If you can't tolerate ghee or butter, use an equal amount of melted coconut oil in recipes where ghee or butter is used.

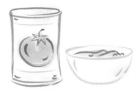

CANNED DICED TOMATOES AND TOMATO PASTE

Italian law requires that manufacturers list all ingredients (even trace amounts) on product labels. Because of this, I recommend looking for Italian brands, such as Pomi, that contain only tomatoes and salt. Alternatively, tomato paste and sauce are easy to make at home (see pages 35 and 36).

CASHEWS

I use cashews in a lot of recipes throughout this book. When soaked, drained, and then blended with water or unsweetened almond milk, they develop a smooth and creamy consistency that makes a great replacement for thick dairy products, including cream, ricotta, and goat cheese. If you're allergic to cashews, you can substitute an equal amount of macadamia nuts or blanched almonds to get a similar result.

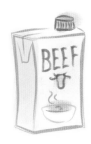

CHICKEN/VEGETABLE/BEEF STOCK

I use stocks in a lot of the recipes in this book. Although it's easy to make homemade stocks (see pages 52 and 53), I also like to keep store-bought stock in my pantry for times when a recipe calls for less than a cup. Pacific and Imagine both have SCD-legal stock.

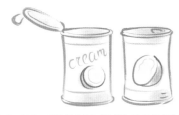

COCONUT CREAM AND COCONUT MILK

Be sure to check the labels to ensure that the cream/milk contains only coconut and no gums (guar or xanthan) or stabilizers. Also, make sure the cans are BPA-free. Many recipes in this book call for coconut cream; if you're unable to find canned coconut cream, use full-fat canned coconut milk that's been in the refrigerator for at least 12 hours. The cream and water separate in the can, and you can easily scoop out the thick coconut cream.

DIJON MUSTARD

There are a few brands of SCD-legal Dijon. You also can use dry mustard; simply mix 1 teaspoon of dry mustard with 2 teaspoons of water as a substitute for 1 tablespoon of Dijon mustard.

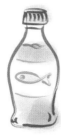

FISH SAUCE

Fish sauce adds a great saltiness and umami flavor to Asian dishes. I use Red Boat brand, which is SCD legal and contains only anchovies and salt.

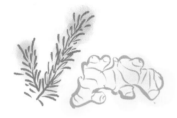

HERBS AND SPICES

The items I list here are the basics I always have in my pantry. When using fresh herbs in place of dried, use three times the amount because dried have a more concentrated flavor. In general, ⅓ teaspoon dried equals 1 teaspoon fresh.

- Cayenne pepper
- Chipotle powder
- Ground cinnamon
- Ground coriander
- Ground cumin
- Garam masala
- Ginger
- Nutmeg
- Oregano leaves
- Paprika
- Rosemary leaves
- Thyme leaves
- Turmeric

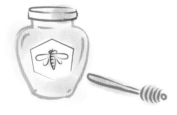

HONEY

Honey is the only liquid sweetener allowed on the SCD. For Paleo, you can swap the honey for maple syrup in recipes throughout the book to make them vegan or low-FODMAP, although they will no longer be SCD legal.

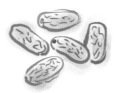

MEDJOOL DATES

You can use Medjool dates as a sweetener in recipes to make them vegan. Soak the dates in hot water for ten minutes before blending them into a paste with a splash of water. You can substitute date paste one-for-one in place of honey in sauces and dressings.

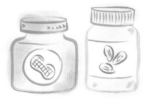

NUT BUTTERS

Almond, cashew, hazelnut, and peanut butter are interchangeable in baking recipes; you can pick your desired flavor. Although peanut butter is SCD legal (but not Paleo), many people report having problems with it, so you can use almond butter in its place. You can find some SCD-legal nut butters that contain just nuts, oil, and salt; alternatively, you can make your own by blending 2 to 3 cups of raw nuts in a food processor or blender until smooth.

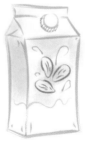

NUT MILKS

I use unsweetened almond milk frequently in recipes. Although homemade nut milk is relatively easy to make, there are brands, such as MALK, that make SCD-legal nut milk without sweeteners.

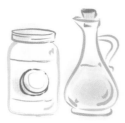

OILS

My pantry is always stocked with the following five oils, which each have a place in my daily cooking:

- Avocado oil is a mild-flavored oil that's good in dressings or sauces (such as mayonnaise). You also can use it for sautéing and frying.

- Coconut oil is a good replacement for butter or ghee in baking recipes. I prefer refined coconut oil, which is both tasteless and odorless. Extra-virgin coconut oil has a more prominent coconut flavor, which can be hard to mask. You also can use coconut oil for cooking or frying at a high temperature.

- Extra-virgin olive oil is best used for cold foods or foods that you cook at moderate heat.

- Light olive oil has a milder flavor than extra-virgin olive oil. You can use it for cooking foods at a higher heat than you would use with extra-virgin olive oil.

- Toasted sesame oil is my favorite oil to use in Asian recipes. It has a strong flavor, and it works in a variety of applications, such as in dressings and sauces or for sautéing and frying.

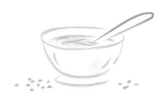

TAHINI

Tahini is a paste made from ground sesame seeds that is often used in Middle Eastern cuisine. I use it in a lot of dressings and dips to make them creamy. You also can use it in place of nut butter to make a recipe nut-free.

You can find it in most grocery stores, but you also can make it yourself:

Place 1 cup hulled sesame seeds in a dry large pan and toast them on medium heat for 4 to 5 minutes, until they start to turn golden. Transfer the toasted seeds to a food processor and add 3 tablespoons of light olive oil; blend until you have a smooth and creamy paste. Store in the fridge for up to 1 month.

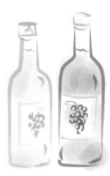

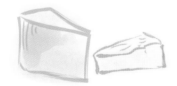

SEMIHARD AND HARD CHEESES

Semihard and hard cheeses that have been aged a minimum of 30 days are allowed on the Specific Carbohydrate Diet because they're lactose-free, but I have included cheeses in only a few recipes in this book. For any SCD recipes that list Parmesan or cheddar cheese as an ingredient, I have also included instructions for using nutritional yeast, which will make the recipe dairy-free, Paleo, and sometimes vegan (but not SCD).

WHITE WINE AND RED WINE VINEGARS

Make sure that the vinegars you buy have no added sugar.

Gizmos
AND GADGETS

Living in a small apartment in London with a kitchen no bigger than a closet means that I have room for only the most essential cooking tools. In fact, beyond the basics with which most kitchens are stocked (stove, microwave, kettle, measuring spoons and cups, and sharp knives), you could make every recipe in this book with just a few pieces of relatively inexpensive equipment.

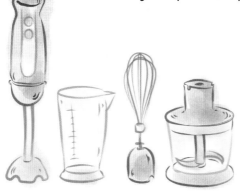

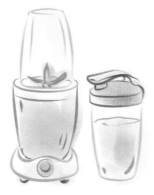

HAND BLENDER WITH ATTACHMENTS

This little gadget is a jack-of-all-trades. The immersion blender and whisk attachments are handy for pureeing soups or making coconut whip, but the mini processor attachment is my favorite. I use it daily for finely dicing onions and garlic, but it's also great for making energy balls, ricing cauliflower, or making chunkier sauces like chimichurri or salsa that would become too pureed in a high-powered blender. If you have storage space concerns, I recommend this tool rather than a large food processor.

HIGH-POWERED BLENDER

It wasn't until I bought my high-powered blender—a NutriBullet—that I fully understood the appeal and versatility of blended cashews. Some less powerful blenders will create a gritty cashew mixture, but when you use a NutriBullet, you get a velvety smooth cream that is used in recipes throughout the book. My NutriBullet is one of my most-used kitchen appliances for making everything from smoothies, sauces, and marinades to the smoothest cashew cream. I like that, unlike with a big blender, it's easy to blend small portions of things using a small container.

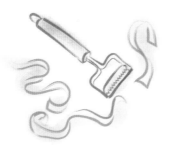

JULIENNE PEELER, VEGETABLE PEELER, OR SPIRAL SLICER

You need a tool to cut thin strips of zucchini for the Chicken Enchiladas (page 196) and to make butternut squash noodles and zucchini noodles. For making vegetable noodles, I prefer using a julienne peeler to using a spiral slicer.

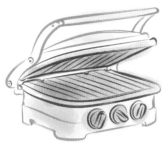

PANINI PRESS

My apartment has no outdoor space, so a panini press has become my go-to for making "grilled" food that I'd otherwise cook on a barbecue. The top of the grill adds pressure and heat to the food, which causes it to cook faster than it would on either a grill pan or a barbecue. A bonus is the dark grill marks you get on both sides of the food. You can use a panini press for cooking grilled vegetables, chicken skewers, Celery Root Tortillas (page 44), steak, hamburgers, or anything else you would otherwise cook on a barbecue. Of course, if you already have a barbecue or grill pan, you don't have to invest in a panini press.

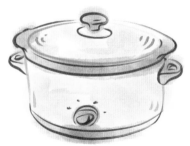

SLOW COOKER

I love coming home after a busy day to the smells of something that I've left to cook all day in the slow cooker. In terms of ease, it's hard to beat a slow cooker, but don't stress if you don't have one; you can achieve similar results by cooking at a low temperature in the oven for two-plus hours.

FOUR ESSENTIAL POTS AND PANS

You can get by with just four pots and pans in your kitchen if cost or space is an issue:

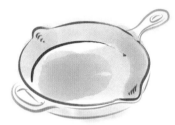

- **An 8- to 10-inch nonstick skillet** is handy for making things that run a high risk of sticking in a cast-iron skillet, such as omelets or frittatas.

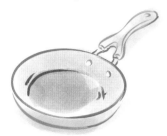

- **A 10- to 12-inch cast-iron skillet** is great for searing and stove-to-oven recipes. It requires slightly more maintenance than nonstick cookware, but a well-cared-for cast-iron skillet will last for generations.

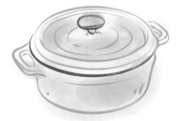

- **A 4- to 5-quart Dutch oven** works on the stove for making soups and stews or in the oven for slow braising meat.

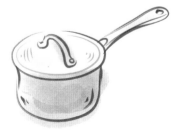

- **A 2- to 3-quart saucepan** is ideal for making sauces and smaller portions of soup, steaming vegetables, and poaching or boiling eggs.

Make the Recipes
WORK FOR YOU

With more and more people being diagnosed with food intolerances and allergies, it can be hard to prepare meals to accommodate everyone. Every recipe in this book is Specific Carbohydrate Diet legal, meaning they are all free from grain, gluten, refined sugar, and soy. I have also included variations whenever possible to make recipes AIP, keto, low-FODMAP, Paleo, vegan, vegetarian, dairy-free, and nut-free. Use the diet and allergen chart that starts on page 346 to easily navigate through the book and find the recipes that best suit your dietary requirements. If a recipe is not compliant with your diet, there are often one or two simple adjustments you can easily make so that it's suitable for you; I list these alternatives in the "Substitutions" section of each recipe.

Although I like to steer clear of making the focus of a recipe the calories, carbs, and so on and instead want to create a delicious dish made from clean ingredients, I understand that nutritional information is important to many people. If you're interested in those details, you can find a downloadable file on my site (www.everylastbite.com/cookbook) that lists the nutritional information for every recipe. On this page, you can also find a guide to which recipes in the book are Whole30.

I've included a section called "SCD Basics" (page 31) for those people who are on the Specific Carbohydrate Diet; these recipes include an aged balsamic vinegar substitute, coconut aminos, pastes, stocks, and condiments so you can make a homemade version if you're unable to find SCD-legal products. Try to keep a batch of these basics in your fridge or freezer to make meal prep quick and fuss-free.

The following table describes substitutions you can make in recipes to accommodate various dietary restrictions.

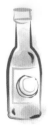

CASHEWS
In place of blended cashews, use blanched almonds or macadamia nuts.

HONEY
You can replace honey with maple syrup (although this substitution means the recipe is no longer SCD legal).

COCONUT AMINOS
Coconut aminos is a soy sauce and gluten-free soy sauce (tamari) substitute. If you are following the SCD, use my homemade recipe on page 47. If you are Paleo/keto/Whole30/gluten- or grain-free, you can use store-bought coconut aminos. Those on a gluten-free diet can use tamari, and if you have no food intolerances, you can use soy sauce.

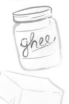

PEANUT BUTTER
You can replace peanut butter with almond butter in baking recipes throughout the book.

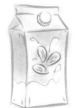

ALMOND MILK
If you have a nut allergy, you can use coconut milk or any other nondairy milk of choice in place of almond milk throughout the book to make recipes nut-free.

BUTTER/GHEE
For baking recipes, you can use melted coconut oil in place of butter or ghee.

For recipes that use butter or ghee for frying or sautéing, you can replace them with extra-virgin olive oil.

Ten Freezer Tips

I would not be able to succeed on the Specific Carbohydrate Diet without my freezer, which is packed with food. I fill it with everything from extra batches of soups and sauces to overripe produce, cooking staples, and leftovers that I can reheat when I don't feel like cooking. These are a few freezer tips I have learned over the years that I hope you find useful.

1. Measure 1 tablespoon of ingredients like tomato paste, chipotle paste, and harissa, and place the scoops into an ice cube tray. After the paste has frozen, put the cubes in a zip-top freezer bag and store it in the freezer; that way, it's easy to grab the premeasured cubes to add to sauces, soups, and other recipes.

2. Measure other basics such as tomato sauce and chicken/beef/vegetable stock in ½-cup quantities into silicone muffin pans. Once frozen, pop the blocks out of the muffin pan and transfer to a zip-top freezer bag for more space-efficient storage.

3. Have a carton of eggs that are about to go bad? Crack the eggs into an ice cube tray and freeze them. Then allow them to thaw in the fridge before adding them to recipes. They will last for up to 10 months in the freezer.

4. Put overripe fruit in zip-top freezer bags to use in smoothies. You can also freeze steamed cauliflower or broccoli, shredded zucchini, and raw spinach or kale. Toss the frozen veggies and fruit from the bag into a blender with some almond milk or juice for a quick-and-easy smoothie.

5. To preserve freezer space, I recommend freezing sauces, soups, stews, and so on in zip-top freezer bags that you've laid flat and squeezed to expel excess air. This technique makes them ready for space-efficient stacking in the freezer.

6. Ginger is easier to grate when frozen. Peel pieces of fresh ginger and store them in the freezer in a zip-top freezer bag.

7. Have leftover coconut cream/milk or nut milk? Freeze it in ice cube trays. You can add the cubes to soups, sauces, or smoothies or even top them with hot coffee or tea to make a refreshing iced drink.

8. Freeze individual portions of cauliflower mash in a silicone muffin pan. The portions of mash are great to have on hand whenever you need a side dish for a weeknight dinner.

9. Always allow foods to cool completely before you put them in the freezer. Putting food in the freezer when it's still warm will increase the temperature in the freezer and may cause other foods to defrost.

10. Store nuts in the freezer to prevent them from going stale.

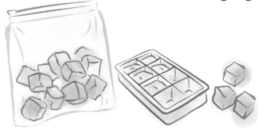

HOW LONG DO THINGS LAST IN THE FREEZER?

Always use your best judgment to determine whether you've stored something for too long. For example, is the food freezer burned? Throw it out! This table shows the general timelines that I try to stick to.

Raw chicken	9 months
Raw ground meat	4 months
Raw fish	3 to 4 months
Raw beef/pork	8 to 10 months
Cooked chicken	4 to 6 months
Raw fruits/vegetables	1 year
Soup/stew	3 to 4 months
Cooked meat	3 months

The following recipes freeze well. After I thaw the food, I reheat it the way I originally cooked it to get the best texture and consistency. For example, you should reheat soups in a pot on the stove, reheat anything you cooked in a skillet on the stove, and reheat anything you baked in the oven (lasagna, enchiladas, etc.) in the oven.

 ## BREAKFAST

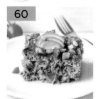
60
Mexican Breakfast Casserole

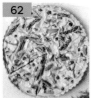
62
Salmon, Asparagus & Caper Quiche

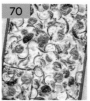
70
Roasted Vegetable Sheet Pan Frittata

74
Broccoli & Bacon Egg Muffins

76
Chunky Banana & Pecan Muffins

78
Apple Cinnamon Breakfast Cookies

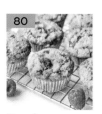
80
Raspberry Orange Muffins

To reheat any of the breakfast items, I recommend transferring them from the freezer to the fridge the night before to allow them to thaw. Then you can reheat egg-based recipes in the oven for ten minutes at 350°F or in the microwave.

APPETIZERS

90
Muhammara

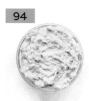
92
Jalapeño Cashew Dip

94
Roasted Cauliflower Hummus

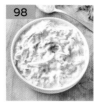
98
Tzatziki

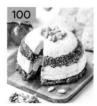
100
"Goat Cheese," Sun-Dried Tomato & Pesto Tower

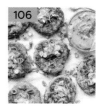
106
Bacon & Scallion Spaghetti Squash Fritters

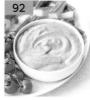
114
Spicy Orange Chicken Wings

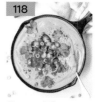
118
Queso Dip

❄ SOUPS

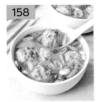
158
Wonton Meatball Soup

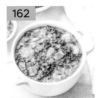
160
Hot & Sour Soup

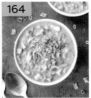
162
Zuppa Toscana

164
Southwest Chicken & Bacon Chowder Soup

Unlike other dishes, soup can go directly from the freezer to the stove for reheating. When you're heating from frozen, place the frozen soup in a pot with a splash of water and set over medium heat until warmed through.

166
Mom's Feel-Better Chicken & Rice Soup

168
Chicken Pot Pie Soup

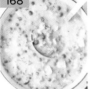
172
Cheesy Broccoli Soup

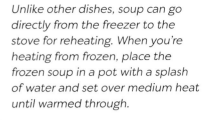
174
Butternut Squash, Leek & Apple Soup

❄ MAINS

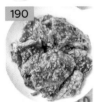
190
Spicy Honey Un-Fried Chicken

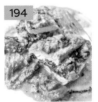
192
Italian Chicken Burgers

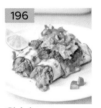
194
Sun-Dried Tomato, Basil & "Goat Cheese" Stuffed Chicken Breasts

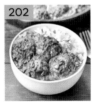
196
Chicken Enchiladas

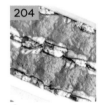
202
Butter Chicken Meatballs

204
Creamy Chicken & Spinach Cannelloni

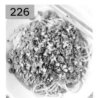
210
The Most Epic Grain-Free Beef Lasagna

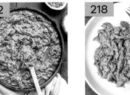
212
Shredded Beef Ragu

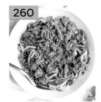
218
Beef Stroganoff

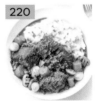
220
Short Rib Beef Bourguignonne

222
Greek 7-Layer Lamb Dip*

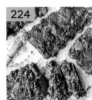
224
Slow Cooker Honey Balsamic Ribs

226
Dan Dan Noodles**

228
BBQ Pulled Pork

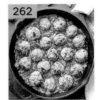
238
Easy Canned Tuna Cakes

260
Eggplant Ragu

262
Eggplant Meatless Meatballs

* Only the minced lamb
** Without the cucumber noodles

SIDES

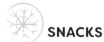 ## SNACKS

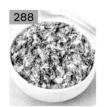
282

The BEST
Cauliflower
Mash

288

Creamed
Spinach & Kale

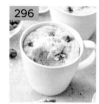
294

Jalapeño, Bacon
& Cauliflower
Muffins

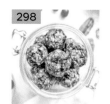
296

Lemon
Blueberry Mug
Cake

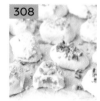
298

Orange,
Cranberry &
Pecan Energy
Balls

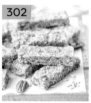
299

Hazelnut &
Coffee Energy
Balls

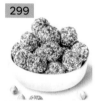
302

Crunchy Nut
Bars

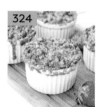
308

Vanilla-Coated
Frozen Banana
Bites

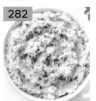 ## DESSERTS

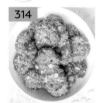
314

Chewy Almond
& Orange
Cookies

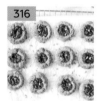
316

Peanut Butter &
Jam Thumbprint
Cookies

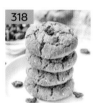
318

N'oatmeal
Raisin Cookies

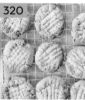
320

Nut Butter
Cookies

322

Pecan & Salted
Caramel
Shortbread Bars

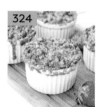
324

Individual
Strawberry
Rhubarb
Crumbles

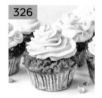
326

Carrot
Cupcakes

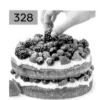
328

Lemon & Berry
Layer Cake

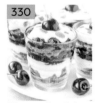
330

Cherry Parfait
Cups

332

Caramelized
Peach Skillet
Crisp

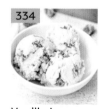
334

Vanilla Ice
Cream with
Crunchy
Caramel Pecans

336

Blackberry,
Lemon, or
Coconut & Lime
Granita

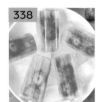
338

Strawberry
Lemonade
Ice Pops

Five Common Concerns About Sticking to a Restrictive Diet

Over the past five years of blogging, I have received thousands of emails from people with questions and concerns about how to follow a restrictive diet long term. Below is a list of the most common questions that I've been asked and my advice on how to handle each situation.

1) What should I do on days when I'm exhausted and don't feel like cooking?

It's 8:00 p.m. You just got home after a busy day, and you have zero desire to start cooking. Let me introduce you to your new best friend: the freezer. Other than a bit of extra chopping, doubling or tripling a recipe usually requires no more effort than making a single batch, so make extra to freeze. I like to pack my freezer full of food—hearty soups, rich stews, comforting bowls of shredded meat, and even sweet treats—that I can thaw and have on the table in less than fifteen minutes.

2) I hate spending so much time in the kitchen; how can I enjoy it more?

Set aside blocks of time each week to cook large batches of food for the freezer and the week ahead. Pop in some headphones and listen to your favorite podcast or playlist, or set up a laptop or tablet nearby to watch your favorite shows while you cook. One of my friends hates cooking but loves the *Real Housewives*, so I told her to watch it only when she does her weekly meal prepping. She now says that she enjoys her weekly cooking sessions and manages to get a lot done while indulging in her guilty pleasure.

3) My partner/family doesn't want to eat this way; what do I do?

There is no need to create two separate meals. Many of these recipes can be modified slightly to accommodate everyone. Prepare something like the Spicy Fish Tacos (page 240) or Korean Beef Tacos (page 214) and serve with both Celery Root Tortillas (page 44) and regular tortillas. Enjoy your ragu on zucchini noodles while others enjoy theirs on pasta, or serve the Butter Chicken Meatballs (page 202) with both cauliflower rice (for you) and white or brown rice (for them). By preparing a simple starch or grain side for other people and including extra vegetables for you, everyone is happy.

4) I'm craving cake, chips, and candy soooo badly. One bite wouldn't be the end of the world, right?

The SCD isn't like a low-calorie diet where a bite of cake might slow your progress but do little harm. With the SCD, each passing month on the diet helps to heal your gut. Eating illegal foods such as candy, chips, or cake reintroduces bad bacteria into your system, but you've spent months on the diet trying to kill off that bacteria. Cheating could potentially interfere with months of healing progress. When a craving hits, try making an SCD-legal snack or sweet from this book. You would be amazed at how well an SCD-legal treat can satisfy a craving.

5) What's the best way to dine out when on SCD?

When I first started the SCD, I avoided eating out at all costs. As I became more comfortable with the diet and what I could and could not eat, the idea of going to a restaurant became less daunting. Because food allergies have become much more common over the past ten years, waiters and chefs at many restaurants are trained to deal with special requests. I've also found that slightly more expensive restaurants are accommodating of dietary requests and ensuring that they provide a meal you can enjoy. Here are a few tips for dining out:

- Seafood and steak restaurants are usually good choices because they don't tend to use a lot of sauces (or they serve them on the side), and it can be quite easy to find a dish to modify on the menu.

- Take a look at the menu online before going so that you have an idea of what you will order. My go-tos are always grilled fish, scallops, or shrimp with olive oil and lemon or a grilled steak. Usually, if they have fish or steak on the menu, you can ask them to modify the dish for you so it's grilled without sauce; just be sure to ask if the steak is marinated or brined. Good side dishes include steamed carrots, sautéed spinach or broccoli with butter or olive oil and lemon juice, or grilled asparagus, zucchini, or peppers. A simple side salad with olive oil and lemon juice dressing is also a good option, but be sure to ask what they include in the salad. (You don't want any croutons or candied nuts.)

- Call ahead and ask if the restaurant will be able to accommodate your requests. They will often put a chef on the phone to discuss appropriate options for you. Trust me; this happens a lot more often than you may think.

- If you're worried that the restaurant might not offer food that you can have, eat at home before you go out. Ideally, the kitchen will end up being able to make a meal you can enjoy, but if that's not possible, you can have a salad or steamed vegetables without feeling ravenous.

- Going out for breakfast? Stick to poached or fried eggs, smashed avocado (without the toast), or grilled tomatoes, or ask for an omelet with a vegetable filling. (Make sure that the cook doesn't use milk in the omelet, though.)

- Invited for a meal at someone else's house? Don't make a big deal out of telling them everything you can and cannot eat. Instead, explain that you are on a restrictive diet and would love to bring a few side dishes or salads to share with everyone. This removes any pressure the hosts feel about trying to accommodate you, plus they will likely be happy that you are offering to help.

Tips for Traveling

Over the past ten years, I have spent a lot of time on long-haul flights as I've traveled between the UK, Canada, and South Africa. As someone who loves to snack, I've learned a few tricks to make eating on flights of ten-plus hours less daunting.

- Eat a large high-protein meal before leaving for the airport.

- Measure 3.4 ounces (to comply with airline requirements) of hummus (like the one on page 94) into a zip-top bag and freeze it. Fill another zip-top bag with veggies and place the frozen hummus alongside to act as an "ice pack" to keep them cold. By the time you're on the plane, it will be thawed and perfect for dipping. You can also do this with nut butter and sliced apples.

- Energy balls (such as those on pages 298 and 299) are a great high-protein snack to have stashed in the bottom of your bag all throughout your travels. They are relatively indestructible. Granola is also a great option.

- Baking an entire batch of muffins can seem like quite an undertaking when you're packing for a trip, so I like to make a mug cake (page 296) and remove it from the mug. Alternatively, bake a batch of cookies or muffins a few weeks in advance and store them in the freezer. Right before leaving on your trip, pull them from the freezer to take with you.

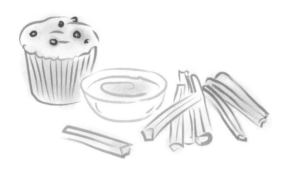

Key to THE RECIPES

1 The yield (the number of servings or a total quantity), prep time, and cook time.

2 Applicable diets and allergens for each recipe. The diets and allergens listed in gray text are those for which the recipe works if you make modifications to the base recipe.

3 I provide storage information so you know how long you can keep leftovers in the fridge or freezer. If a meal can be fully or partially prepared in advance, I include those directions, too.

4 Special icons indicate which recipes are freezer-friendly, take 30 minutes or less to make, or can be made ahead.

5 In the Substitutions section, you can find various alternatives to make a recipe comply with a particular diet or allergen option.

6 I offer handy tips and general cooking tricks with some recipes.

(2)

(4) <30 min

Avocado, Bacon & Egg
BREAKFAST SANDWICHES

(1) **Yield:** 2 servings   **Prep Time:** 10 minutes   **Cook Time:** 20 minutes

All it takes is a bit of creativity to turn your typical breakfast ingredients into a delicious sandwich that's fun to eat. When you make these sandwiches, grill extra portobello mushrooms to use for burger or sandwich buns.

4 large portobello mushrooms

1 tablespoon extra-virgin olive oil

Salt

4 strips thick-cut bacon, cut in half lengthwise

2 medium eggs

1 avocado, peeled and pitted

4 slices tomato (about ½ tomato)

2 pinches of red pepper flakes (optional)

Ground black pepper

1. Remove the stem from each of the portobello mushrooms and scoop out the gills using a spoon. Brush the mushrooms on both sides with the oil and sprinkle with the salt.

2. Heat a grill pan over medium heat and cook the mushrooms for 5 minutes per side or until tender. Place the cooked mushrooms on a plate and set aside. Note: If you don't have a grill pan, you can cook the mushrooms in a panini press or bake them in a preheated 400°F oven for 15 minutes.

3. Cook the bacon in a medium-sized skillet over medium heat for 6 minutes, or until crisp. Set the bacon on a paper towel–lined plate, leaving the grease in the skillet.

4. Reduce the heat to medium-low. Crack the eggs into the skillet and cook for 4 minutes, or until the whites are set but the yolks are still runny.

5. While the eggs are cooking, place the avocado in a bowl and smash it with a fork until it has a chunky consistency. Sprinkle with a pinch of salt.

6. To assemble: Evenly spread the smashed avocado on 2 of the portobello mushroom caps, then top each with 4 pieces of bacon, 2 slices of tomato, and a fried egg. Sprinkle each with a pinch of red pepper flakes, if desired, and season to taste with salt and pepper. Top with the other 2 portobello mushrooms and serve.

(6) **Ripe Avocado Test**
Rather than squeeze (and bruise) an avocado to test ripeness, flick off the little nub at the top. If it doesn't come off easily, the avocado isn't ripe enough to eat. If you see brown under the nub, the avocado is likely overripe, and you will find brown spots inside. The perfect avocado will still be green under the nub.

(5) **SUBSTITUTIONS:** *Use 2 slices of eggplant in place of the portobello mushrooms as buns and omit the avocado to make the sandwiches low-FODMAP. Skip the bacon to make these sandwiches vegetarian.*

(3) **STORAGE:** *The cooked portobello mushrooms will last in the fridge for up to 4 days.*

58   *Breakfast*

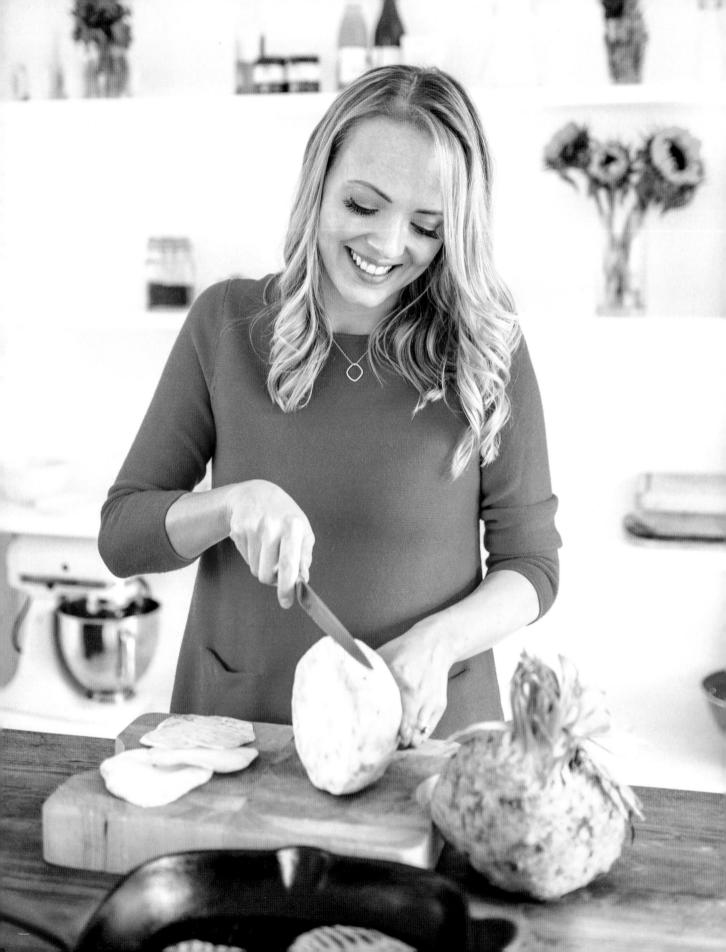

Basics

Pastes

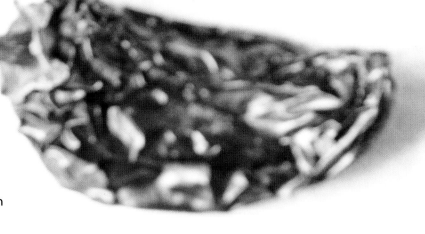

You will see the following three pastes listed as ingredients in recipes throughout the book. I highly recommend making all three pastes and having them on hand to quickly add to dishes.

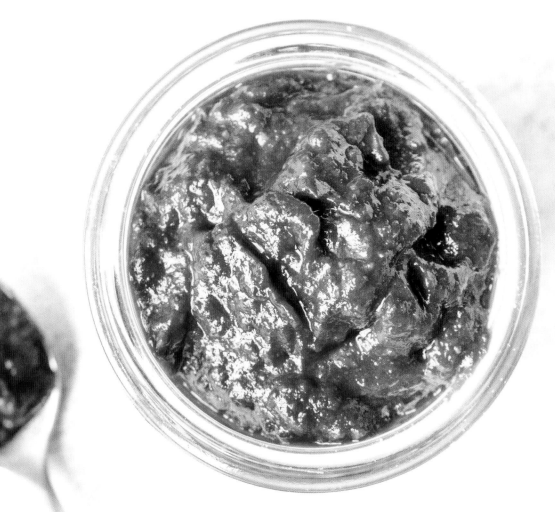

STORAGE: *Allow the pastes to cool before putting them in an airtight container and storing them in the fridge for up to a week. Alternatively, spoon about 1 tablespoon into the wells of an ice cube tray or onto a parchment paper–lined sheet pan and freeze. Transfer the frozen portions into a zip-top bag to store in the freezer for up to 3 months. Add the frozen paste directly to sauces and soups or thaw the cubes in the microwave for 30 seconds.*

HARISSA

KETO
PALEO
VEGAN
VEGETARIAN
DAIRY-FREE
EGG-FREE
NUT-FREE

Yield: ⅔ cup **Prep Time:** 15 minutes **Cook Time:** 20 minutes

1 red bell pepper

1 tablespoon extra-virgin olive oil, divided

½ medium red onion, roughly chopped

3 cloves garlic, peeled

2 red chili peppers, such as Fresno, roughly chopped

1 tablespoon freshly squeezed lemon juice

1½ teaspoons tomato paste

½ teaspoon ground cumin

½ teaspoon ground coriander

½ teaspoon paprika

¼ teaspoon salt

1. Preheat the oven to 425°F.

2. Put the bell pepper on a sheet pan and drizzle with 1½ teaspoons of the oil. Roast for 20 minutes, flipping halfway through to ensure it chars on both sides.

3. Meanwhile, place the onion, garlic, and chili peppers in a food processor and blend until finely chopped.

4. Heat the remaining 1½ teaspoons of oil in a medium-sized skillet over medium heat. Transfer the finely chopped vegetables to the skillet and sauté for 10 minutes, or until golden brown.

5. Remove the sheet pan from the oven and invert a bowl over the charred bell pepper to trap the steam and let it rest for 10 minutes. (This will make it much easier to peel.) Remove the bowl and peel the skin from the pepper, discarding the stem and seeds.

6. Put the peeled bell pepper, sautéed mixture, lemon juice, tomato paste, spices, and salt into a food processor and blend into a smooth paste.

SCD BASICS
Tomato Paste (page 35)

USE IN
Butternut Squash Toast Four Ways (page 56)
Eggplant & Harissa Shakshuka (page 64)
Harissa & Orange Spatchcock Roast Chicken (page 186)

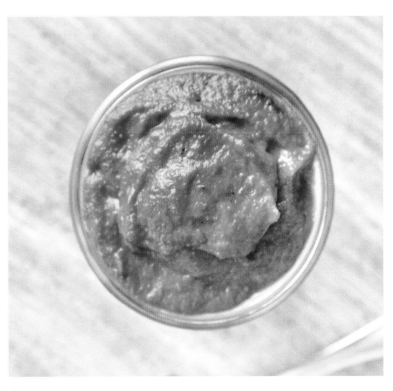

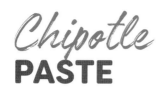

Chipotle
PASTE

Yield: About ½ cup   **Prep Time:** 25 minutes   **Cook Time:** 15 minutes

½ ounce dried chipotle chili peppers

½ cup boiling water

1 teaspoon extra-virgin olive oil

½ medium yellow onion, finely diced

2 cloves garlic, minced

⅓ cup chopped tomatoes

1. Place the dried chipotle chili peppers in a small bowl and cover with the boiling water; allow to soak for 15 minutes, or until they have softened.

2. While the peppers soak, heat the oil in a medium-sized skillet over medium heat. Add the onion and garlic and sauté for 5 minutes, or until the onion is translucent.

3. Once the peppers have softened, remove from the bowl, reserving the water. Cut off the stems and chop the peppers into small pieces. Add them to the skillet along with the tomatoes and 4 tablespoons of the soaking water. Let simmer for 10 minutes, or until the tomatoes have softened.

4. Transfer the mixture to a blender and blend until completely smooth.

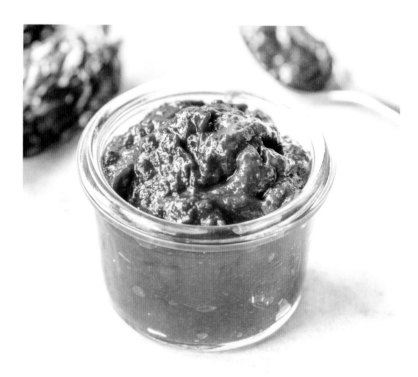

USE IN

Queso Dip (page 118)

Chipotle Butternut Squash Salad
(page 146)

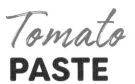

Tomato
PASTE

KETO

LOW-FODMAP

PALEO

VEGAN

VEGETARIAN

DAIRY-FREE

EGG-FREE

NUT-FREE

Yield: 2 cups   **Prep Time:** 10 minutes   **Cook Time:** 4 hours

10 pounds ripe tomatoes, such as Roma or San Marzano

½ teaspoon salt

1. Cut the tomatoes in half lengthwise and use your fingers to remove the seeds.

2. Place the tomatoes in a large pot over medium-high heat. Stir in the salt and cook, uncovered, for about an hour or until the tomatoes have reduced to approximately 4 cups of sauce. At this point, you can pour the sauce into a sieve placed over a bowl to remove any of the tomato skins, but I find that they mostly break down into the sauce and that step isn't necessary.

3. Preheat the oven to 200°F and line a large sheet pan with parchment paper.

4. Pour the tomato sauce onto the prepared sheet pan and use a rubber spatula to spread it in an even layer.

5. Bake for 30 minutes. Remove from the oven and stir the mixture with a spoon, spread it in an even layer, and return to the oven. Continue to bake for 2½ hours, stirring every 30 to 45 minutes, until the paste has reduced by half and has the consistency of a thick puree.

USE IN

Butter Chicken Meatballs (page 202)

The Most Epic Grain-Free Beef Lasagna (page 210)

Shredded Beef Ragu (page 212)

Eggplant Ragu (page 260)

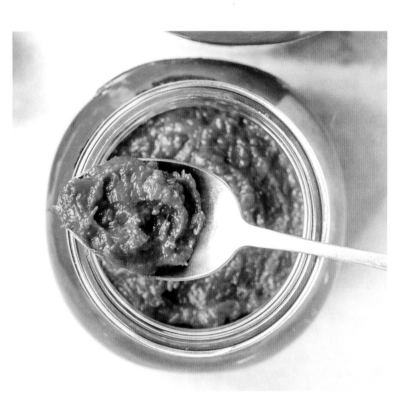

KETO
LOW-FODMAP
PALEO
VEGAN
VEGETARIAN
DAIRY-FREE
EGG-FREE
NUT-FREE

Tomato SAUCE

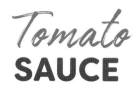

Yield: About 8 cups **Prep Time:** 15 minutes **Cook Time:** 13 minutes

This chunky tomato sauce is to be used in place of canned diced tomatoes, which are a base for sauces throughout the book. As I discuss in the "SCD Pantry/Fridge Staples" section (page 14), there are some SCD-legal brands of canned tomatoes, but if you aren't able to find them, this sauce is a good substitute. If it's a smooth sauce you're after, use an immersion blender to blend the sauce into a smooth puree.

5 pounds ripe tomatoes, such as Roma or San Marzano

1 teaspoon salt

4 cups boiling water

1. Use a knife to score an X on the bottom of each tomato, then place in a large bowl.

2. Pour the boiling water over the tomatoes and let them sit for 3 minutes. The skin around the Xs should begin to pull back. Use a slotted spoon to remove the tomatoes from the bowl and allow them to cool slightly before peeling off the skins and cutting out the cores.

3. Roughly chop the tomatoes and place them in a pot over medium heat. Season with the salt and simmer for 10 minutes, or until they have softened into a chunky sauce. Use as it is or, to make a smooth sauce, puree in a blender or with an immersion blender.

4. Allow the sauce to cool before storing.

STORAGE: *Pour the sauce into sterilized mason jars and keep in the fridge for up to 1 week. Alternatively, pour ½-cup portions into a 12-well silicone muffin pan and place in the freezer. Once frozen, transfer to a zip-top bag and store in the freezer for up to 4 months.*

USE IN

The Most Epic Grain-Free Beef Lasagna (page 210)

Shredded Beef Ragu (page 212)

Eggplant Ragu (page 260)

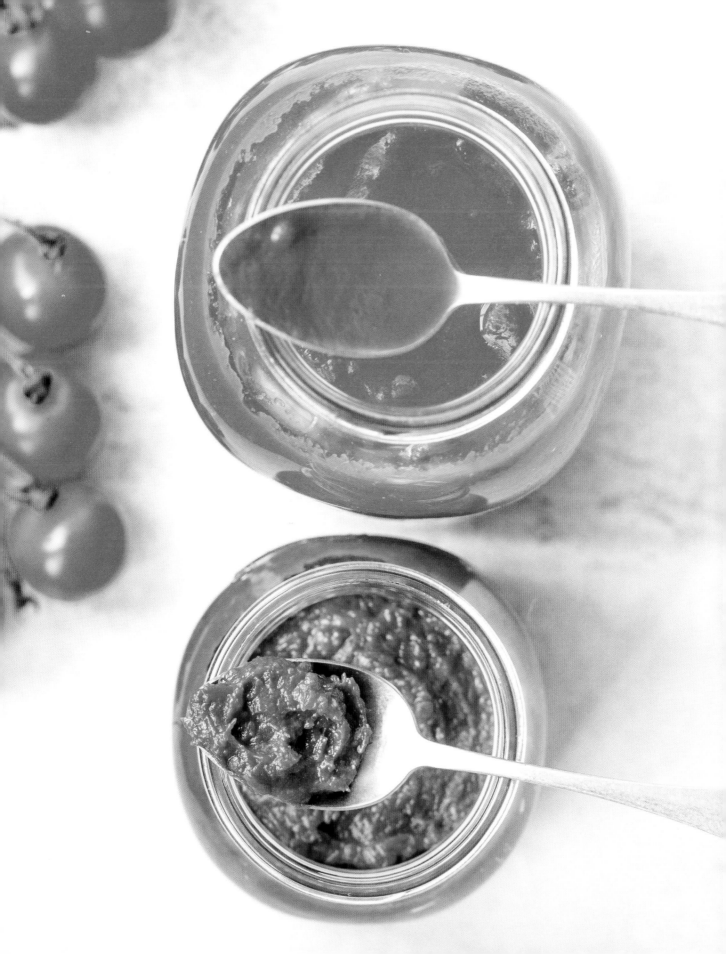

KETO
LOW-FODMAP
PALEO
VEGAN
VEGETARIAN
DAIRY-FREE
EGG-FREE
NUT-FREE

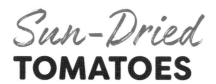

Sun-Dried
TOMATOES

Yield: 2 cups **Prep Time:** 10 minutes **Cook Time:** 2 hours

Sun-dried tomatoes often contain sneaky additives like sulfites. If you struggle to find some that are SCD legal, this recipe is a great make-at-home option. Alternatively, you can buy packaged sun-dried tomatoes (not packed in oil and jarred), place them in a mason jar, and follow Step 4 to make your own oil-packed tomatoes, which are easier to chop up to use in recipes.

1 pound cherry tomatoes

2 tablespoons extra-virgin olive oil

½ teaspoon salt

For Oil-Packed Dried Tomatoes (Optional)

¾ cup extra-virgin olive oil, plus more if needed

Sprigs of fresh rosemary or thyme (optional)

Thinly sliced garlic (optional)

¼ teaspoon black peppercorns (optional)

1. Preheat the oven to 275°F and line a sheet pan with parchment paper.

2. Cut the cherry tomatoes in half, spread them evenly on the prepared pan, gently brush them with 2 tablespoons of oil, and season them with the salt.

3. Bake for 2 hours, checking every 30 minutes or so to ensure that the tomatoes don't burn. Allow the dried tomatoes to cool before packing them into a sterilized 8-ounce mason jar.

4. To make oil-packed dried tomatoes, pour in ¾ cup oil to cover the dried tomatoes; if desired, add sprigs of rosemary or thyme, sliced garlic, or peppercorns to the jar for flavor.

STORAGE: *The tomatoes will keep in the fridge for up to 1 month.*

USE IN

"Goat Cheese," Sun-Dried Tomato & Pesto Tower (page 100)

Sun-Dried Tomato, Chicken & Cauliflower Salad with Creamy Balsamic Dressing (page 134)

Italian Chicken Burgers (page 192)

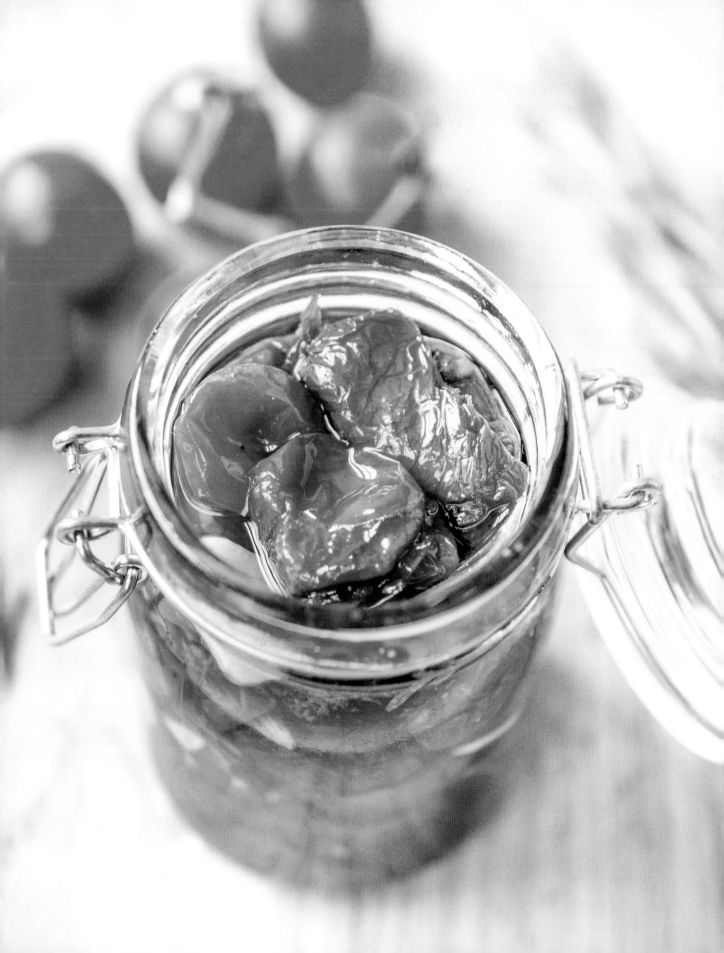

AIP
KETO
PALEO
VEGAN
VEGETARIAN
DAIRY-FREE
EGG-FREE
NUT-FREE

Egg-Free
MAYONNAISE (TOUM)

Yield: 1 cup **Prep Time:** 10 minutes **Cook Time:** —

Toum is a great vegan substitute for mayonnaise. But be warned—it packs a serious garlicky punch, so keep your toothbrush on standby. Also, when you use this in place of mayonnaise in dips, salad dressings, etc., I recommend leaving out any garlic that is in the recipe ingredients.

6 large cloves garlic (about 1½ ounces), peeled

2 tablespoons freshly squeezed lemon juice

1 tablespoon apple cider vinegar

1 teaspoon Dijon mustard

¼ teaspoon salt

1¼ cups light olive oil or avocado oil, divided

SPECIAL EQUIPMENT
Immersion blender

1. Place the garlic cloves in a wide-mouth 16-ounce mason jar. Place an immersion blender into the jar and break up the cloves, then add the lemon juice, vinegar, mustard, and salt and blend into a smooth paste.

2. With the blender running, slowly pour in ¼ cup of the oil and blend for 20 seconds before slowly adding another ¼ cup. Remove the immersion blender and use a rubber spatula to scrape down the sides before continuing to add the remainder of the oil, in ¼-cup amounts, and blending.

3. Once all of the oil has been added, the mixture should be thick and creamy. Cover the jar with the lid before storing.

SUBSTITUTIONS: *I prefer using light olive oil because of its mild flavor and light color, but you also can use avocado oil (but the result will be a yellow-colored mayonnaise). For AIP, omit the mustard.*

STORAGE: *The toum will last in the fridge for up to 3 weeks.*

TIP: *Adding the oil very slowly helps ensure that the mixture emulsifies into a thick and creamy consistency. From time to time, the garlic doesn't emulsify, and the mixture is too runny to use in place of mayonnaise. However, it still makes a great marinade or salad dressing.*

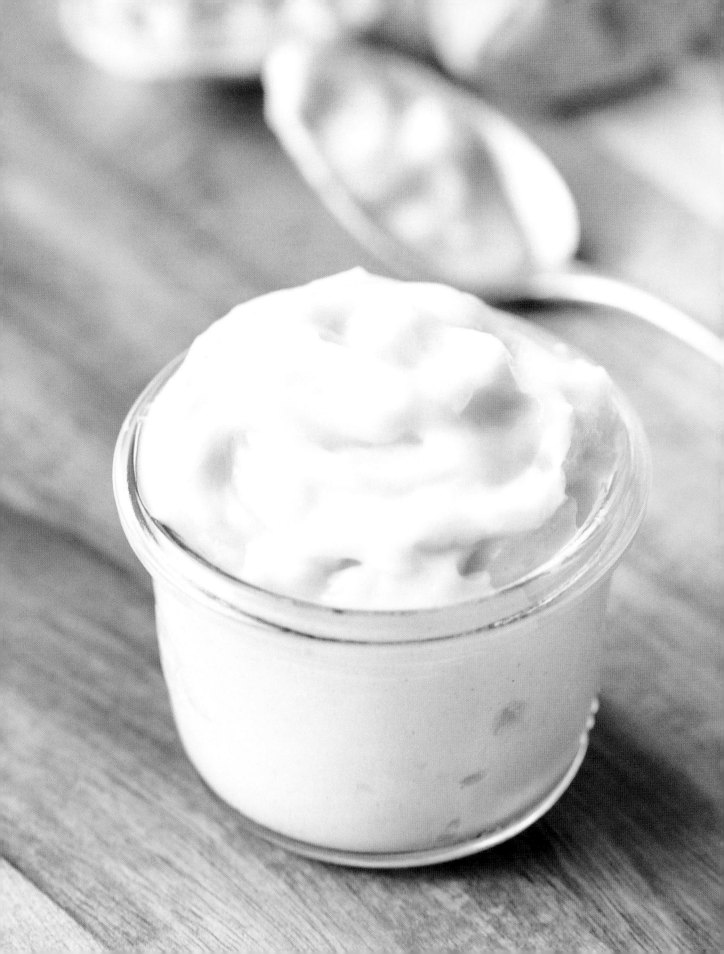

KETO
LOW-FODMAP
PALEO
VEGETARIAN
DAIRY-FREE
NUT-FREE

Easy 3-Minute
MAYONNAISE

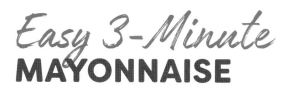

Yield: 1 cup **Prep Time:** 3 minutes **Cook Time:** —

Mayonnaise is one of my most used condiments, and I always have some in my fridge. I love adding it to salad dressings and dips and using it to help bind things together. It really couldn't be any easier to make; you just need 3 minutes, which is less time than it used to take me to get the lid off a jar of store-bought mayonnaise. I've included some flavor variations that you can use as sauces to spice up meals.

1 medium egg, at room temperature

½ teaspoon dry mustard, or 1 teaspoon Dijon mustard

2 teaspoons freshly squeezed lemon juice

¼ teaspoon salt

1 cup light olive oil or avocado oil

SPECIAL EQUIPMENT
Immersion blender

STORAGE: *This mayonnaise will last in the fridge for up to a week.*

1. Put all of the ingredients, in the order they are listed, in a wide-mouth 16-ounce mason jar.

2. Place an immersion blender into the jar, ensuring that it touches the bottom of the jar and the egg is trapped between the blades.

3. Turn on the blender and let it run at the bottom of the container for 30 seconds before very slowly lifting it and continuing to blend for another 20 seconds. Continue blending until the mixture has thickened.

4. Cover the jar with the lid and store in the fridge.

Mayo Flavor Variations

In a bowl, combine ½ cup of the mayonnaise with the ingredients for one of the following flavor variations:

GARLIC CHIVE

1 clove garlic, minced

⅓ cup fresh chopped chives

½ teaspoon ground black pepper

CILANTRO LIME

2 tablespoons chopped fresh cilantro

1 teaspoon freshly squeezed lime juice

1 clove garlic, minced

HONEY MUSTARD

1 tablespoon honey

1 tablespoon Dijon mustard

½ teaspoon freshly squeezed lemon juice

TARTAR SAUCE

2 tablespoons chopped pickles (page 48)

1 tablespoon freshly squeezed lemon juice

1 tablespoon chopped fresh Italian parsley

1 tablespoon chopped fresh dill

½ teaspoon dry mustard

CHIPOTLE LIME

1½ teaspoons chipotle paste (page 34) or chipotle chili powder

1 teaspoon freshly squeezed lime juice

1 clove garlic, minced

½ teaspoon salt

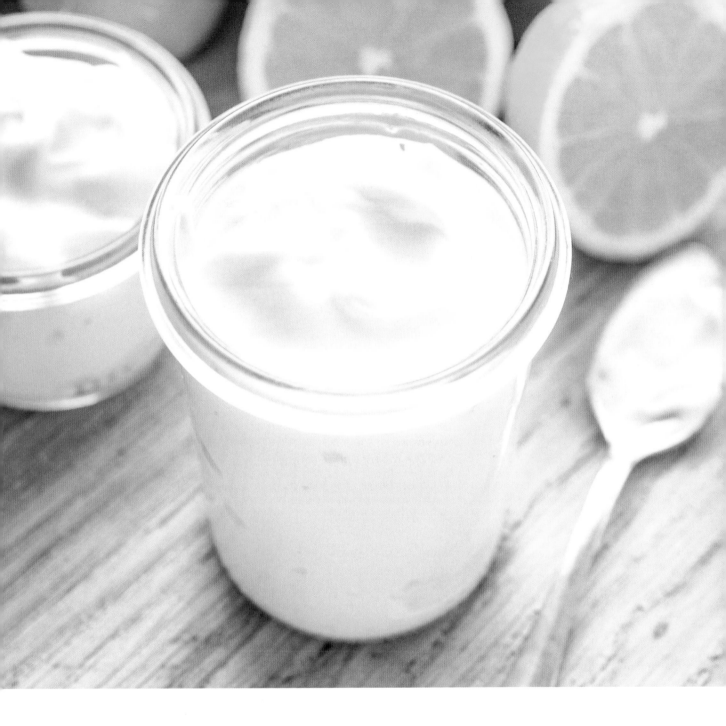

The Fresh Egg Test

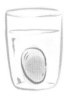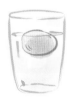

Fill a bowl with cold water and gently place an egg into the bowl. If the egg rests on its side at the bottom, it is very fresh. If one end of the egg rises while the other end rests on the bottom, the egg is 2 to 3 weeks old, and you should eat it soon. If the egg floats to the surface, it's gone bad, and you should throw it out. Because eggs are consumed raw in mayonnaise, I recommend using only the freshest eggs for this recipe.

AIP
KETO
LOW-FODMAP
PALEO
VEGAN
VEGETARIAN
DAIRY-FREE
EGG-FREE
NUT-FREE

Celery Root
TORTILLAS

Yield: 6 to 8 tortillas *Prep Time:* 10 minutes *Cook Time:* 4 minutes

These tortillas are a complete game-changer! Out of everything I have ever created in the kitchen, nothing has made me more excited than these celery root tortillas. As a former taco addict, I was really missing tortillas, and lettuce cups just weren't filling the void. It turns out that when you grill thin slices of celery root, they become pliable, can withstand the weight of a lot of filling, and are easy to pick up with your hands to eat. Look for the largest celery root you can find, and buy in bulk when you find them because they last at least a month in the fridge. You can use these tortillas for the Korean Beef Tacos (page 214) or Spicy Fish Tacos (page 240), or try them filled with scrambled eggs, bacon, guacamole, and salsa for a delicious breakfast taco.

1 large celery root (2½ to 3 pounds)

1. Cut both ends off of the celery root, then set it down on one of the cut ends so that it sits flat. Then, use a sharp knife to cut off the entire outer peel.

2. Cut the celery root into slices as thinly as possible. Lay each slice flat on a cutting board and run your knife over the surface to shave down any of the thicker parts so that it is very thin.

3. Grill following one of the two methods below or store uncooked slices in the fridge.

What does celery root taste like?

This is a question people often ask me, and my answer is, "Not much." Celery root has a very mild celery taste that is completely undetectable when the tortillas are grilled and topped with filling.

Using a Panini Press
Preheat a panini press. Once the panini press is warm, place a celery root slice on the grill, close the lid, and cook for 3 to 4 minutes, until grill marks form and the celery root is tender and pliable. Set aside and repeat with the remaining slices.

Using a Grill Pan
Heat a grill pan over medium-high heat. Place a celery root slice onto the pan and place a sheet pan or metal bowl on top of the slice to create some pressure. (This will make the tortilla more pliable.) After 2 minutes of cooking, flip the slice over and continue cooking for another 2 minutes on the other side. Set aside and repeat with the remaining slices.

STORAGE: *Place grilled celery root tortillas in a zip-top bag with a paper towel between each tortilla. They'll last in the fridge for 2 days. Cooked tortillas can be reheated in a grill pan for just a minute per side or alternatively warmed in the microwave for 20 seconds. You can store uncooked celery root slices in an airtight container in the fridge for 5 days so you can quickly grill them as needed.*

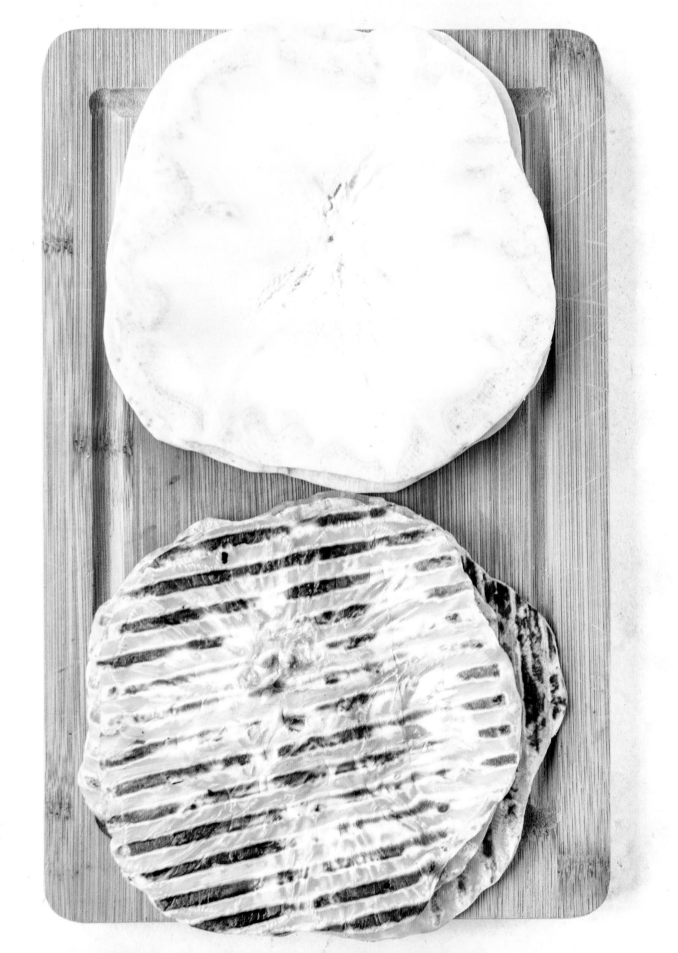

AIP
LOW-FODMAP
PALEO
VEGAN
VEGETARIAN
DAIRY-FREE
EGG-FREE
NUT-FREE

SCD Balsamic
VINEGAR

Yield: 1 cup **Prep Time:** 1 minute **Cook Time:** 10 minutes

The book *Breaking the Vicious Cycle* explains that most inexpensive balsamic vinegars have sugar added to them. However, traditional balsamic vinegar, which is aged fifteen-plus years, is allowable on the Specific Carbohydrate Diet because it doesn't include added sugar. Unfortunately, aged balsamic vinegar can be quite expensive, so this quick-and-easy homemade alternative is great to have on hand to add to salad dressings, sauces, and marinades.

1 cup red wine vinegar

1 cup no-sugar-added grape juice

Combine the vinegar and grape juice in a small saucepan over medium-high heat and boil for 10 minutes, or until the liquid has reduced by half. Allow to cool before transferring to a mason jar.

STORAGE: *This vinegar will last in the fridge for up to 2 weeks.*

TIP: *Use Welch's Grape Juice because it is SCD legal.*

USE IN

Roasted Cauliflower, Date, Red Onion & Parsley Salad (page 142)

Slow Cooker Honey Balsamic Ribs (page 224)

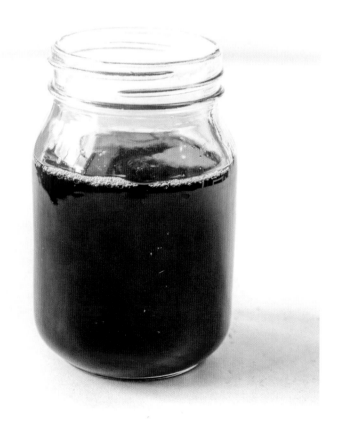

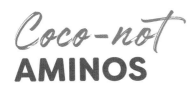

Coco-not AMINOS

PALEO
DAIRY-FREE
EGG-FREE
NUT-FREE

Yield: 1½ cups   **Prep Time:** 2 minutes   **Cook Time:** 15 minutes

Coconut aminos is a soy- and gluten-free substitute for soy sauce. When I started on SCD, coconut aminos was a relatively unknown product, and many people assumed that it was allowed on the diet. It wasn't until I'd been in remission for a few years that I learned that it is not allowed on the diet because of the uncertainty about whether all the sugar is broken down during manufacturing. If you strictly follow SCD, use this homemade substitute to add a salty umami flavor to sauces and dressings.

2 cups beef stock

¼ cup aged balsamic vinegar

1½ tablespoons apple cider vinegar

½ teaspoon salt

¼ teaspoon ground white pepper

¼ teaspoon ginger powder

1. In a small saucepan over medium-high heat, bring all of the ingredients to a boil. Reduce the heat to medium and simmer for 15 minutes, or until it has reduced by half.

2. Allow to cool before transferring to a container and storing in the fridge.

STORAGE: *This condiment will last in the fridge for up to 3 weeks.*

SCD BASICS
Beef Stock (page 52)
SCD Balsamic Vinegar (page 46)

USE IN
Spicy Orange Chicken Wings (page 114)
Crunchy Asian Slaw (page 152)
Wonton Meatball Soup (page 158)
Hot & Sour Soup (page 160)
Kung Pao Chicken (page 180)
Grilled Skirt Steak with Asian Salsa Verde (page 208)

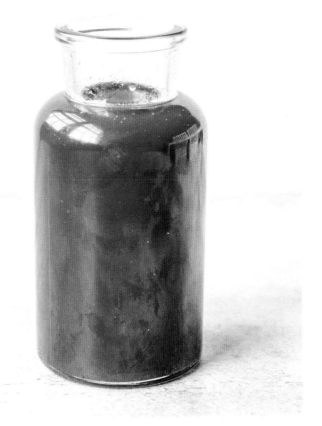

KETO
PALEO
VEGAN
VEGETARIAN
DAIRY-FREE
EGG-FREE
NUT-FREE

Quick PICKLED VEGGIES

Yield: 2 (16-ounce) jars   **Prep Time:** 10 minutes, plus 24 hours for pickling   **Cook Time:** 5 minutes

I always have a few jars of pickled vegetables in my fridge to snack on or add to salads for a vinegary kick of flavor. My favorite vegetables to pickle are green beans, pearl onions, jalapeños, and sliced cucumbers, but other great options include sliced carrots, whole cherry tomatoes, beets, red onions, or bell peppers.

1 pound vegetables such as Persian cucumber, green beans, pearl onions, red onions, or peeled carrots

1 clove garlic, thinly sliced, or 2 cloves garlic, peeled

1 teaspoon black peppercorns

1 teaspoon coriander seeds

1 red chili pepper, such as Fresno, thinly sliced (optional)

1 cup water

1 cup apple cider vinegar

2 teaspoons kosher salt

1. Wash and dry the vegetables; if necessary, cut them into uniform size. The smaller you cut the vegetables, the quicker they will pickle.

2. Divide the vegetables between two 16-ounce sterilized mason jars, making sure to pack them in tightly. Divide the garlic, peppercorns, coriander, and red chili evenly between the jars.

3. In a small saucepan over medium-high heat, bring the water, vinegar, and salt to a boil. Reduce the heat to medium and simmer for 3 minutes, or until the salt dissolves, then pour the liquid into the jars, filling them to ½ inch below the rim. Allow the liquid to cool to room temperature, and then cover the jars with the lids and put the jars in the fridge for 1 day before opening and eating.

STORAGE: *The pickles will last in the fridge for up to 2 months.*

TIP: *If you prefer a strong garlicky flavor then use sliced garlic; for a much milder hint of garlic flavor, use whole peeled cloves of garlic.*

USE IN
Salmon Gravlax & "Cream Cheese" Platter (page 120)
Italian Chicken Burgers (page 192)
Spicy Fish Tacos (page 240)

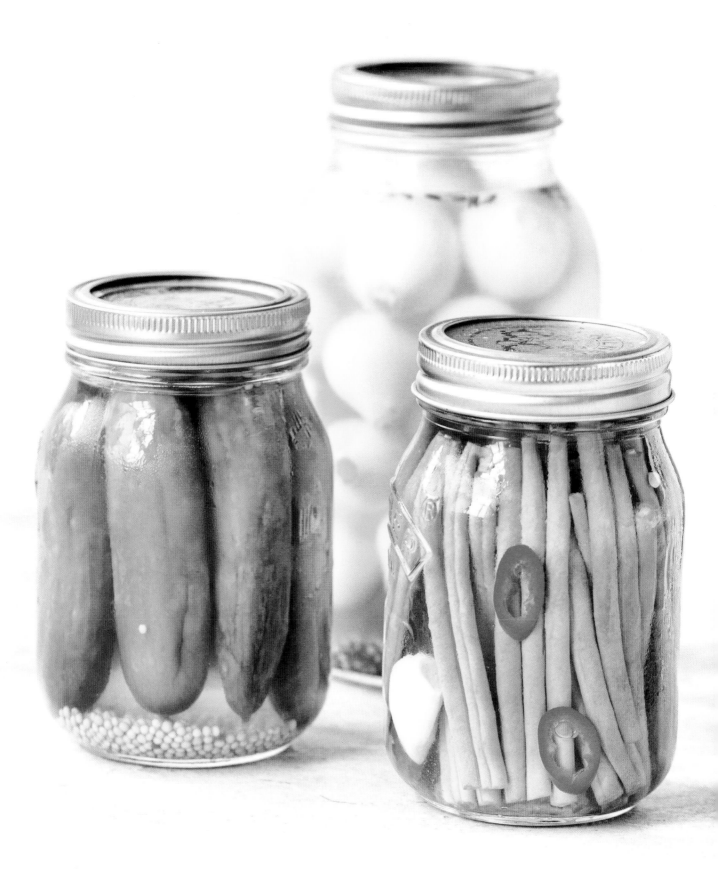

KETO
LOW-FODMAP
PALEO
DAIRY-FREE
EGG-FREE
NUT-FREE

CHORIZO

Yield: 1½ pounds (8 servings)   **Prep Time:** 20 minutes, plus at least 4 hours to refrigerate   **Cook Time:** 10 minutes

I love chorizo, but finding any that is SCD-legal and doesn't contain fillers and additives can be difficult. This spicy ground pork and bacon mince can be formed into patties and served with eggs for breakfast or used as a crumbly mixture on Mexican Eggs Benedict (page 72) or stirred into One-Pan Spanish Chicken & Rice (page 198).

8 ounces bacon

1 pound ground pork (see tip)

2 tablespoons apple cider vinegar

1½ teaspoons paprika

2 teaspoons ancho or chipotle chili powder

1 teaspoon dried oregano leaves

1 teaspoon ground cumin

½ teaspoon red pepper flakes

½ teaspoon ground black pepper

½ teaspoon ground coriander

½ teaspoon salt

1½ teaspoons extra-virgin olive oil, for frying

1. Place the bacon in a food processor and pulse until it's minced, then add the ground pork and pulse for a few seconds.

2. Transfer the mixture to a bowl and add all of the remaining ingredients, except the oil. Using your hands, mix thoroughly to ensure that everything is well combined and the spices are evenly dispersed. Cover with plastic wrap and store in the fridge for at least 4 hours but ideally overnight.

3. To cook as ground chorizo, heat the oil in a medium-sized skillet over medium heat. Add the chorizo and cook for 8 to 10 minutes, or until it's no longer pink, using a wooden spoon to break the meat into crumbles as it cooks. To cook as patties, divide the chorizo into eight portions, approximately 2 tablespoons each, and flatten each portion into a 1-inch-thick patty. Heat the oil in a medium-sized skillet over medium heat. Add the patties and cook for 4 minutes on each side, or until completely cooked through.

STORAGE: *The meat will last in the freezer (before or after cooking) for up to 4 months.*

TIP: *For the best flavor and texture, use ground pork with a high fat content, ideally 10 percent or higher.*

USE IN
Mexican Eggs Benedict (page 72)
One-Pan Spanish Chicken & Rice (page 198)

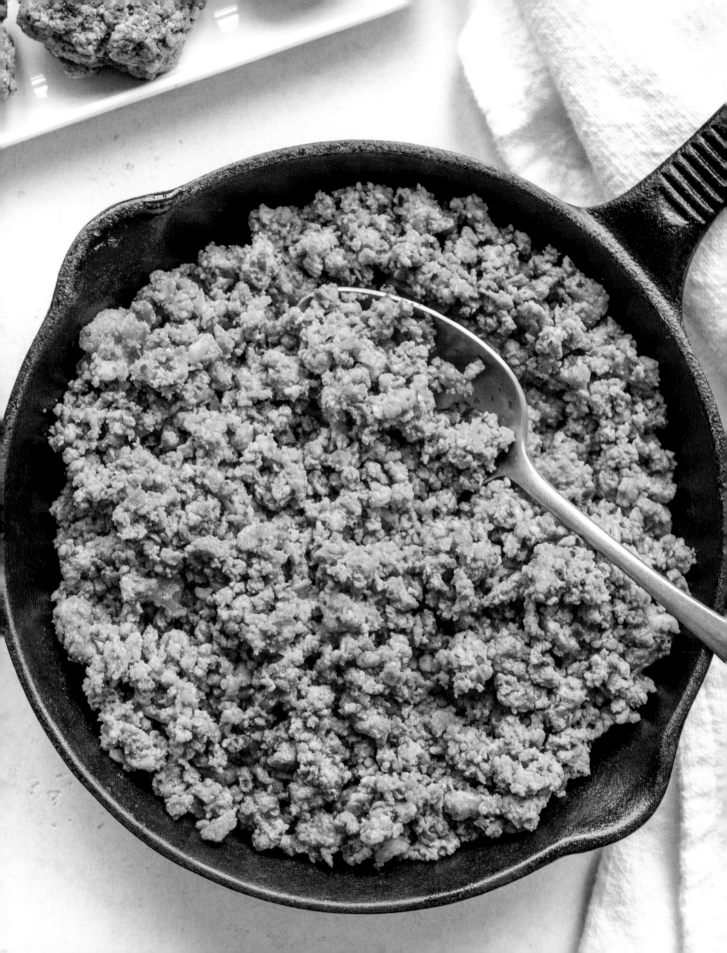

KETO
PALEO
VEGAN
VEGETARIAN
DAIRY-FREE
EGG-FREE
NUT-FREE

STOCKS

Yield: 10 cups **Prep Time:** 15 minutes **Cook Time:** 2 to 7 hours

Although you can find SCD-legal stocks in stores, making your own at home is easy and a great way to use kitchen scraps. Many recipes in this book include stocks, so I recommend keeping portions of all three of the following stocks in the freezer to add to dishes or use as a base for a quick soup.

Stock Up for Stocks

Keep three individual bags in the freezer for vegetable scraps (peels, ends, etc.), chicken scraps (bones/skin), and beef scraps (bones/fat) to use when you've accumulated enough scraps to make a stock.

STORAGE: *Allow the strained stocks to cool before storing. They will last in an airtight container in the fridge for up to 5 days. Alternatively, pour ½-cup portions into a 12-well muffin pan and place in freezer. Once frozen, transfer to a zip-top bag and store in the freezer for up to 3 months.*

Beef Stock

4 pounds beef bones

2 medium yellow onions, quartered

2 carrots, cut into 2-inch pieces

2 stalks celery, cut into 2-inch pieces

4 cloves garlic, peeled

1 teaspoon salt

3 quarts water

2 tablespoons apple cider vinegar

2 bay leaves

2 sprigs fresh thyme

1. Preheat the oven to 400°F.

2. Place the bones, onions, carrots, celery, and garlic on a sheet pan. Sprinkle with the salt and bake for 40 minutes.

3. Remove from the oven and transfer the bones and vegetables to a large pot along with the water, vinegar, and herbs. Bring to a boil over medium-high heat, then reduce the heat to low and simmer for 5 hours; skim the foam from the top of the pot every hour or so. Alternatively, you can use a 6-quart slow cooker set on high for 7 hours.

4. After cooking, pour the stock through a mesh strainer. Let it cool, skim any fat off the top, and transfer the stock to a container to store in the fridge or freezer.

Chicken Stock

4 pounds chicken pieces (legs, thighs, neck, wings, etc.), or 2 chicken carcasses

3 carrots, cut in 2-inch pieces

3 stalks celery, cut in 2-inch pieces

2 yellow onions, quartered

5 cloves garlic, peeled

2 bay leaves

2 sprigs fresh thyme

1 teaspoon salt

¼ cup freshly squeezed lemon juice

4 quarts water

1. Place all of the ingredients in a large pot over medium-high heat. Bring to a boil, reduce the heat to low, and simmer for 3 hours; skim the foam from the top of the pot every hour or so. Alternatively, you can place all of the ingredients in a 6-quart slow cooker set on high for 5 hours.

2. After cooking, pour the chicken stock through a mesh strainer. Let it cool, skim any fat off the top, and transfer the stock to a container to store in the fridge or freezer. You can shred the meat from the chicken pieces to use for a meal.

Vegetable Stock

4 carrots, cut into 2-inch pieces

3 stalks celery, cut into 2-inch pieces

2 leeks, cut into 2-inch pieces

5 cloves garlic, peeled

4 sprigs fresh thyme

4 sprigs fresh rosemary

2 bay leaves

10 cups water

1. Place the leek pieces in a bowl of water and leave them submerged for 5 minutes to loosen any dirt from between the leaves. Use a slotted spoon to remove the leeks from the water and transfer to a large pot.

2. Place all of the remaining ingredients in the pot over medium-high heat. Bring to a boil, then reduce the heat to low and simmer for 2 hours. Alternatively, you can use a 6-quart slow cooker set on high for 5 hours.

3. After cooking, pour the vegetable stock through a mesh strainer. Transfer to a container to store in the fridge or freezer.

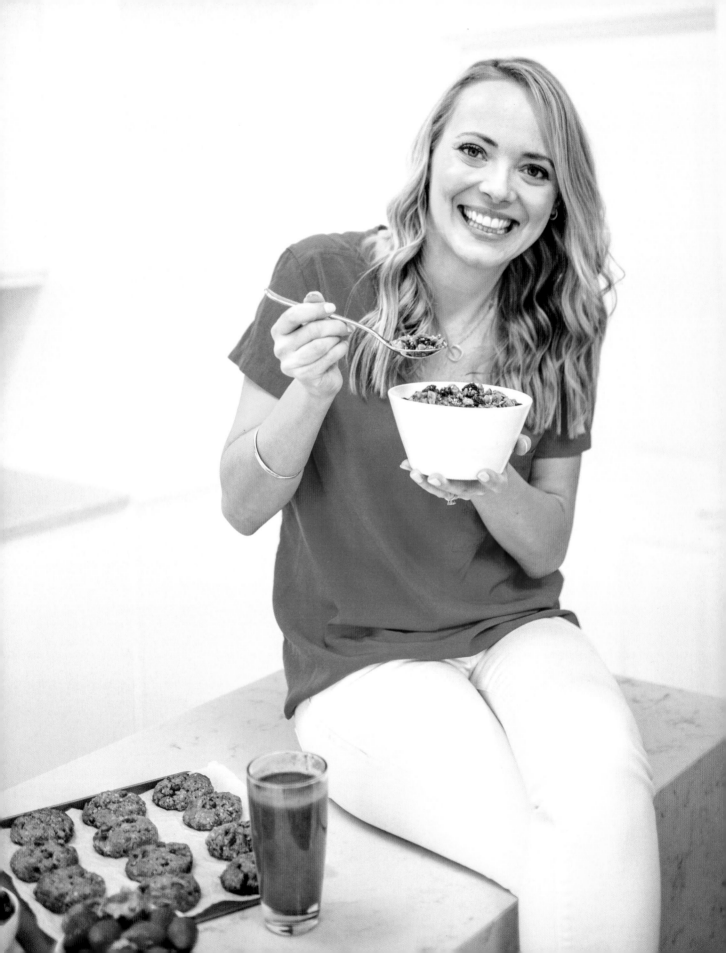

Breakfast

Butternut Squash Toast
FOUR WAYS

Make ahead · *<30 min*

Yield: 4 servings **Prep Time:** 10 minutes **Cook Time:** 7 minutes

You've probably heard of sweet potato toast, which was a big health food trend in 2017. Well, this is my SCD-legal spin on it. You can slice and grill the butternut squash all at once and then quickly reheat slices through the week for breakfast each morning. These are four of my favorite toppings, but the options are truly endless.

1 large butternut squash

2 tablespoons extra-virgin olive oil

½ teaspoon ground cumin

¼ teaspoon cayenne pepper

¼ teaspoon salt

SCD BASICS

Harissa (page 33)

Easy 3-Minute Mayonnaise (page 42)

Leftover Squash

Deseed and peel the base of the butternut squash, then shred it to use in Mexican Breakfast Casserole (page 60) or cut it into cubes for use in Chipotle Butternut Squash Salad (page 146).

1. Cut the long neck of the butternut squash from the round base. (Reserve the base for another use; see the tip.) Peel the neck, then cut it crosswise into eight ½-inch-thick slices.

2. In a bowl, whisk together the oil, cumin, cayenne pepper, and salt.

3. Heat a grill pan over medium-high heat (or you can use an electric panini press). Place the butternut squash slices on the grill and brush them with the seasoned oil. Allow to cook for 4 minutes, flip and brush with oil on the other side, and continue to cook for 3 minutes, or until tender.

4. Remove from the grill and top with one or more of the suggested topping combinations or with your favorite toppings.

STORAGE: *The grilled butternut squash will last in the fridge for up to 3 days. Reheat in a preheated 350°F oven for 6 to 8 minutes or in the microwave for 2 minutes.*

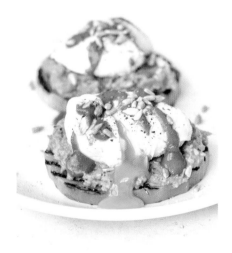

Avocado & Harissa Toast

1 avocado, mashed

2 medium eggs, poached

½ teaspoon harissa

1 teaspoon raw hulled sunflower seeds

Evenly spread 2 grilled butternut squash slices with the mashed avocado, then top each slice with a poached egg. Drizzle the harissa over the top and sprinkle with the sunflower seeds.

Salmon & Scrambled Eggs Toast

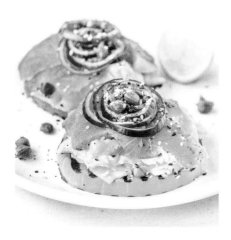

2 medium eggs, scrambled

4 slices Salmon Gravlax (page 120)

½ medium red onion, thinly sliced

1½ teaspoons capers

½ teaspoon sesame seeds

1 lemon wedge, for serving (optional)

Spoon the scrambled eggs onto 2 grilled butternut squash slices, then evenly top with the gravlax, red onion slices, capers, and sesame seeds. Serve with a lemon wedge, if desired.

BLT Toast

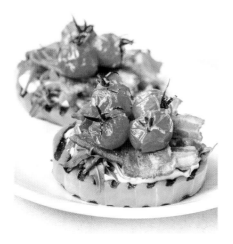

4 strips thick-cut bacon

8 cherry tomatoes

1 tablespoon mayonnaise

2 lettuce leaves, or ⅓ cup arugula

Preheat the oven to 375°F. Place the bacon and cherry tomatoes on a sheet pan and bake in the oven for 20 minutes, or until the bacon is crisp. To assemble, evenly spread 2 grilled butternut squash slices with the mayonnaise, then top with the lettuce or arugula, bacon strips, and tomatoes.

Spinach & Mushroom Toast

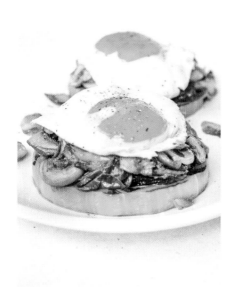

2 teaspoons extra-virgin olive oil, divided

1 cup spinach

1 cup mushrooms, thinly sliced

2 medium eggs

1. Heat ½ teaspoon of the oil in a medium-sized skillet over medium-high heat and add the spinach. Cook for 2 to 3 minutes, until wilted, then remove from the skillet.

2. Heat ½ teaspoon of the oil in the skillet and add the mushrooms. Cook for 5 minutes, or until tender, then remove from the skillet.

3. Heat the remaining 1 teaspoon of oil in the skillet and crack the eggs into the skillet. Fry the eggs until the whites are set and the yolks are cooked to your liking.

4. To assemble, top 2 grilled butternut squash slices with the cooked spinach and mushrooms, then top each with a fried egg.

KETO
LOW-FODMAP
PALEO
VEGETARIAN
DAIRY-FREE
NUT-FREE

Avocado, Bacon & Egg
BREAKFAST SANDWICHES

< 30 min

Yield: 2 servings **Prep Time:** 10 minutes **Cook Time:** 20 minutes

All it takes is a bit of creativity to turn your typical breakfast ingredients into a delicious sandwich that's fun to eat. When you make these sandwiches, grill extra portobello mushrooms to use for burger or sandwich buns.

4 large portobello mushrooms

1 tablespoon extra-virgin olive oil

Salt

4 strips thick-cut bacon, cut in half lengthwise

2 medium eggs

1 avocado, peeled and pitted

4 slices tomato (about ½ tomato)

2 pinches of red pepper flakes (optional)

Ground black pepper

1. Remove the stem from each of the portobello mushrooms and scoop out the gills using a spoon. Brush the mushrooms on both sides with the oil and sprinkle with the salt.

2. Heat a grill pan over medium heat and cook the mushrooms for 5 minutes per side or until tender. Place the cooked mushrooms on a plate and set aside. Note: If you don't have a grill pan, you can cook the mushrooms in a panini press or bake them in a preheated 400°F oven for 15 minutes.

3. Cook the bacon in a medium-sized skillet over medium heat for 6 minutes, or until crisp. Set the bacon on a paper towel-lined plate, leaving the grease in the skillet.

4. Reduce the heat to medium-low. Crack the eggs into the skillet and cook for 4 minutes, or until the whites are set but the yolks are still runny.

5. While the eggs are cooking, place the avocado in a bowl and smash it with a fork until it has a chunky consistency. Sprinkle with a pinch of salt.

6. To assemble: Evenly spread the smashed avocado on 2 of the portobello mushroom caps, then top each with 4 pieces of bacon, 2 slices of tomato, and a fried egg. Sprinkle each with a pinch of red pepper flakes, if desired, and season to taste with salt and pepper. Top with the other 2 portobello mushrooms and serve.

Ripe Avocado Test
Rather than squeeze (and bruise) an avocado to test ripeness, flick off the little nub at the top. If it doesn't come off easily, the avocado isn't ripe enough to eat. If you see brown under the nub, the avocado is likely overripe, and you will find brown spots inside. The perfect avocado will still be green under the nub.

SUBSTITUTIONS: *Use 2 slices of eggplant in place of the portobello mushrooms as buns and omit the avocado to make the sandwiches low-FODMAP. Skip the bacon to make these sandwiches vegetarian.*

STORAGE: *The cooked portobello mushrooms will last in the fridge for up to 4 days.*

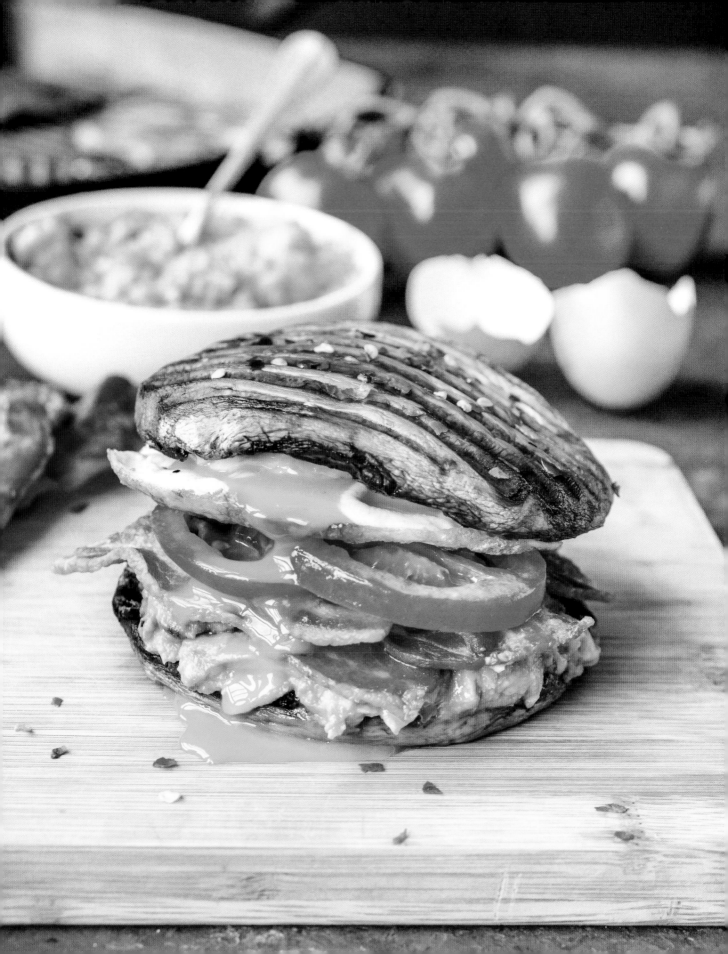

Mexican BREAKFAST CASSEROLE

Yield: 8 servings   **Prep Time:** 10 minutes   **Cook Time:** 50 minutes

Breakfast casseroles are a fantastic meal-prep dish. I like to make one on Sunday and then reheat portions throughout the week for a fast-and-easy breakfast. Everyone will love the bold Mexican flavors and kick of spice that make this dish so much more than the typical eggy breakfast casserole. For a change of pace, swap the pork for ground turkey, chicken, or beef.

1 tablespoon extra-virgin olive oil

1 medium yellow onion, finely diced

1 pound ground pork

1 tablespoon plus ½ teaspoon ground cumin, divided

1½ teaspoons paprika

½ teaspoon ground coriander

1 yellow or red bell pepper, diced

1 cup chopped tomatoes

2 cups shredded butternut squash

¼ teaspoon cayenne pepper

12 medium eggs

½ cup shredded cheddar cheese

⅓ cup unsweetened almond milk

½ teaspoon salt

½ teaspoon ground black pepper

For Garnish (Optional)

½ avocado, thinly sliced

2 tablespoons salsa, or 1 tablespoon finely diced tomatoes and 1 tablespoon sliced scallions

1 tablespoon chopped fresh cilantro

1. Preheat the oven to 350°F and grease an 8 by 11-inch casserole dish.

2. Heat the oil in a large skillet over medium heat. Add the onion and cook for 3 minutes, or until it begins to soften.

3. Add the ground pork. Season with 2 teaspoons of the cumin, the paprika, and coriander and cook for 5 minutes, or until the pork is no longer pink, using a wooden spoon to break the meat into a fine crumble as it cooks. Use a slotted spoon to transfer the seasoned pork to a bowl and set aside.

4. Add the bell pepper and tomatoes to the skillet and sauté for 5 minutes, or until the bell peppers have softened.

5. Add the butternut squash, the remaining 1½ teaspoons of the cumin, and the cayenne pepper to the skillet and cook for another 4 minutes, then return the ground pork to the skillet, stirring to ensure everything is well combined.

6. In a bowl, whisk together the eggs, cheese (if using), almond milk, salt, and pepper.

7. Spoon the ground pork and pepper mixture into the prepared casserole dish, then pour the egg mixture over the top.

8. Bake for 30 minutes, or until the eggs have set and the top of the casserole is firm to the touch. If desired, garnish with avocado, salsa, and/or cilantro before serving.

Make-Ahead Breakfast

Divide the casserole into single-serving portions and freeze separately. The night before, transfer a portion from the freezer to the fridge. In the morning, quickly reheat in the microwave for 3 minutes or bake in a preheated 350°F oven for 10 minutes.

SUBSTITUTIONS: *For keto, reduce the grated butternut squash to 1 cup. Use coconut milk in place of the almond milk to make this dish nut-free. For Paleo or dairy-free, omit the cheddar cheese.*

STORAGE: *Leftovers will last in the fridge for up to 5 days or in the freezer for up to a month.*

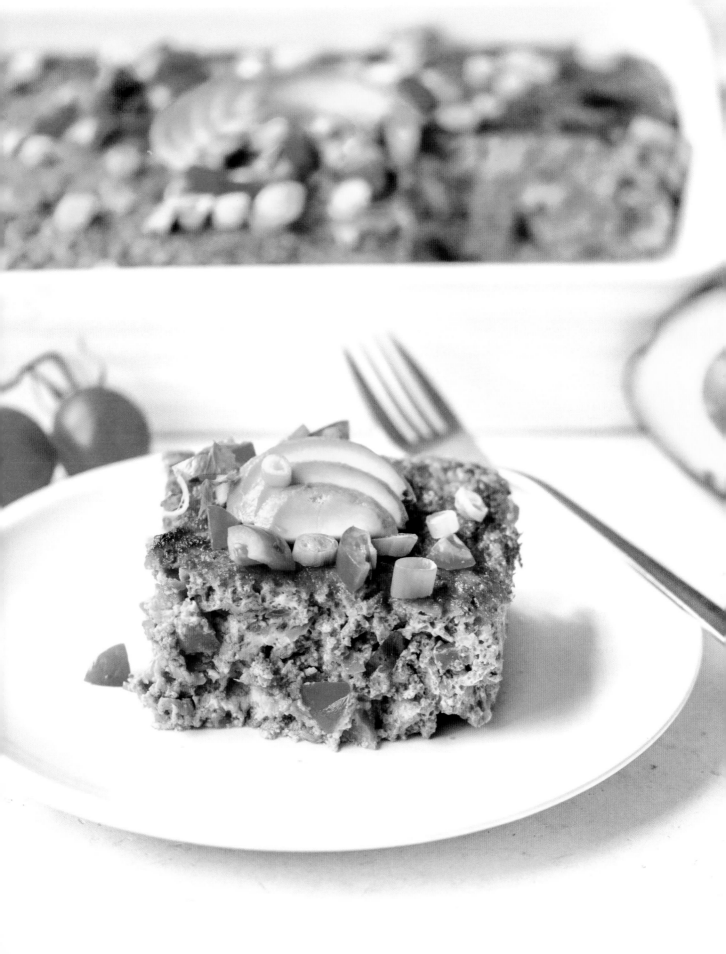

Salmon, Asparagus &
CAPER QUICHE

Make ahead

Yield: 8 servings   **Prep Time:** 20 minutes   **Cook Time:** 35 minutes

Quiche is a great brunch dish to serve when you want to impress guests. The flakes of salmon make it seem slightly fancy, while capers and herbs give it a fresh flavor. The crust is incredibly easy to make, even for those new to baking, but if you're short on time or ingredients, skip it and turn this into a crustless quiche (see below).

Crust

2½ cups blanched almond flour

1 medium egg

¼ teaspoon salt

3 tablespoons melted ghee, unsalted butter, or coconut oil

8 spears asparagus, woody stems removed

1 teaspoon extra-virgin olive oil

½ teaspoon ground black pepper

¼ teaspoon salt

10 ounces salmon fillets, skin on

5 medium eggs

2 tablespoons coconut cream

1 teaspoon dry mustard, or 1½ teaspoons Dijon mustard

2 tablespoons chopped red onions

2 tablespoons chopped fresh dill

1 tablespoon capers

SPECIAL EQUIPMENT: 9-inch tart pan with a removable bottom

MAKE AHEAD/STORAGE: *You can make this dish the day before and quickly reheat it in a 350°F preheated oven on the morning you're serving it. Alternatively, you can bake the crust and cook the salmon and asparagus up to two days in advance, leaving just the assembly and 15 minutes of baking to do before serving. Leftovers will last in the fridge for up to 4 days.*

1. Preheat the oven to 350°F and grease a 9-inch tart pan with a removable bottom.

2. To make the crust, place the almond flour, egg, and salt in a food processor and pulse for a few seconds until the mixture resembles crumbs. Slowly drizzle in the melted ghee while continuing to pulse until the mixture comes together to form a ball.

3. Remove the dough from the food processor and evenly press it into the bottom of and up the sides of the tart pan. Prick holes into the bottom using a fork and par-bake for 10 minutes, or until golden.

4. While the crust bakes, bring a medium-sized skillet filled with 2 inches of water to a gentle simmer over medium heat. Add the asparagus and cook for 5 minutes, or until fork-tender. Use tongs to remove the spears from the skillet; when the asparagus is cool enough to handle, cut the spears into 1-inch pieces. Pour the water out of the skillet.

5. Warm the oil in the skillet over medium heat. Season the salmon fillets with a pinch each of salt and pepper and cook them for 3 minutes per side. Once the salmon is cooked through (It will be opaque in the center), transfer it to a plate, remove the skin, and use a fork to break it into pieces.

6. In a bowl, whisk together the eggs, coconut cream, and mustard.

7. Evenly arrange the flaked salmon, pieces of asparagus, and chopped red onion in the quiche shell. Pour the egg mixture over the top and arrange the chopped dill and capers on top.

8. Bake for 15 minutes, or until the eggs have set. If the crust is browning too much, place a sheet of aluminum foil over the top of the quiche while it bakes.

SUBSTITUTIONS: *Skip the salmon to make it vegetarian. For nut-free, skip the crust and pour the filling into a greased baking dish.*

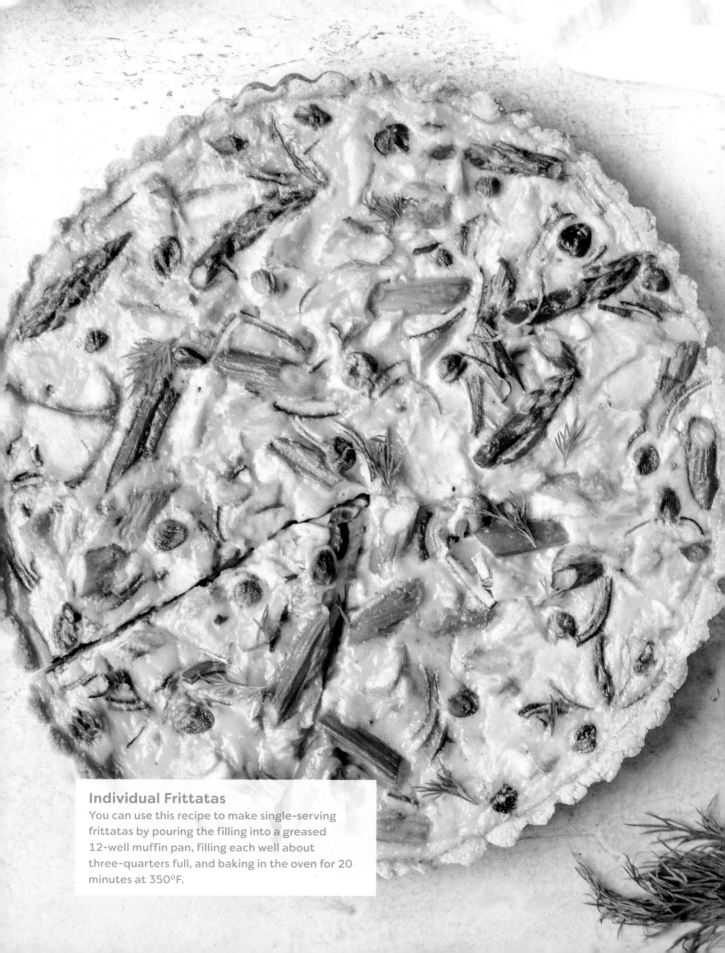

Individual Frittatas
You can use this recipe to make single-serving frittatas by pouring the filling into a greased 12-well muffin pan, filling each well about three-quarters full, and baking in the oven for 20 minutes at 350ºF.

Eggplant & Harissa
SHAKSHUKA

Yield: 4 servings **Prep Time:** 18 minutes **Cook Time:** 23 minutes

I always love the idea of serving a big breakfast when friends or family are staying over. But between waking up extra early and tiptoeing around my less-than-soundproof kitchen, I've come to realize that prepping the night before is the only way to achieve my hosting goals. You can completely prep the eggplant mixture for this recipe the day before; morning of, all you have to do is reheat the mixture, add the eggs, and cook—so easy!

2 medium eggplants, cubed (about 4 cups)

½ teaspoon salt

1 tablespoon extra-virgin olive oil

1 large yellow onion, finely diced

3 cloves garlic, minced

1½ cups roughly chopped Roma tomatoes

1½ teaspoons ground cumin

1½ teaspoons ground coriander

½ teaspoon paprika

1½ cups chunky tomato sauce or chopped canned tomatoes

1 tablespoon harissa

4 medium eggs

2 or 3 slices red chili pepper, such as Fresno, for garnish (optional)

2 tablespoons fresh cilantro leaves, for garnish (optional)

1. Place the cubed eggplant in a colander. Sprinkle with the salt and allow to rest for 10 minutes to draw out the moisture. Pat the eggplant with a paper towel to remove any excess moisture.

2. Heat the oil in a large skillet over medium heat. Add the onion and garlic and sauté for 3 minutes, or until the onion is translucent. Add the eggplant and cook for 6 to 7 minutes, until the eggplant begins to soften.

3. Add the tomatoes, cumin, coriander, and paprika and cook for 5 minutes, or until the tomatoes begin to release their liquid and soften.

4. Stir in the tomato sauce and harissa and bring the mixture to a gentle simmer over medium heat.

5. Using a spoon, form 4 hollows in the sauce and crack an egg into each one.

6. Cover the skillet with a lid and simmer for 5 to 6 minutes, or until the egg whites have set. If desired, garnish with sliced chili pepper and cilantro before serving.

MAKE AHEAD/STORAGE: *This is a great dish to meal-prep for the week. Complete Step 4 then equally divide the eggplant mixture into 4 microwave-safe serving bowls and store in the fridge. Each morning, microwave a single serving in a bowl for 3 minutes, or until warm, make a well in the sauce and crack an egg into it, cover with a damp paper towel, and then microwave for 1 minute 30 seconds or until the egg white is set.*

TIP: *Chopping garlic and onion manually can leave a lingering smell on your hands that doesn't wash off with soap. To rid your hands of the smell, rub them over anything made with stainless steel, such as the sink, the faucet, or a bowl.*

SCD BASICS
Harissa (page 33)
Tomato Sauce (page 36)

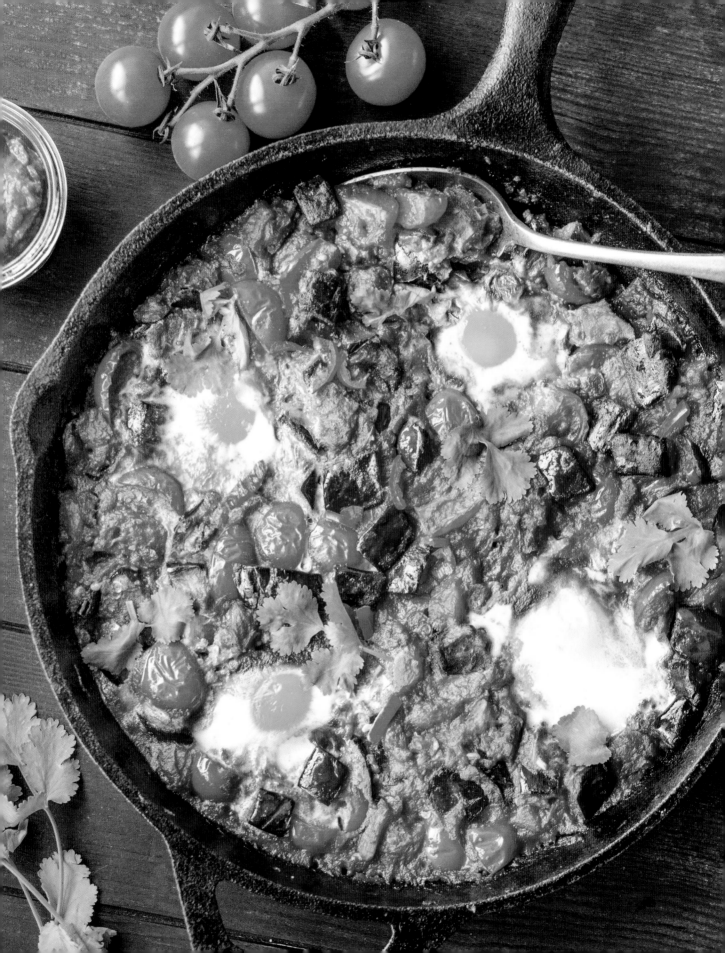

Portobello Baked Eggs
WITH CHIMICHURRI

Make ahead *< 30 min*

Yield: 4 servings **Prep Time:** 15 minutes **Cook Time:** 11 minutes

As someone who isn't a big fan of the texture of eggs, I'm always looking for new ways to hide them in breakfast dishes. Chimichurri, which in the past I have only served with steak, is a great condiment to brighten up the flavor of baked eggs.

Chimichurri

1 cup fresh Italian parsley leaves

⅓ cup extra-virgin olive oil

2 tablespoons finely diced red onions

2 tablespoons red wine vinegar

1 tablespoon chopped red chili pepper, such as Fresno

2 cloves garlic, peeled

¼ teaspoon salt

½ cup chopped spinach

½ cup chopped tomatoes

4 portobello mushrooms

4 medium eggs

1. Preheat the oven to 400°F.

2. Place all of the chimichurri ingredients in a food processor and pulse until minced. Transfer the chimichurri to a bowl.

3. In a separate medium-sized bowl, toss the spinach and tomatoes together with 1 tablespoon of the chimichurri.

4. Rub the outside of the portobello mushrooms with a damp paper towel to remove any dirt. Twist off the stem from each mushroom and use a spoon to gently scrape out the gills. Place the mushrooms on a sheet pan, and divide the tomato and spinach mixture among the 4 mushrooms.

5. Bake for 5 minutes, or until they begin to soften. Remove the mushrooms from the oven and tilt them to the side to drain excess moisture that may have been released during baking.

6. Crack an egg into each of the mushrooms and return them to the oven to bake for another 6 minutes, or until the egg whites have just set.

7. Spoon more of the chimichurri over each of the mushrooms before serving.

Chimichurri

Make extra chimichurri; it's great as a marinade for chicken or steak, a salad dressing, or a sauce served with grilled veggies.

MAKE AHEAD/STORAGE: *The chimichurri can be made up to 3 days in advance, and any leftover chimichurri will last in the fridge for up to 4 days. You can fill the mushrooms with the tomato and spinach mixture and parbake them a day in advance of serving; the day of, continue the recipe at Step 6.*

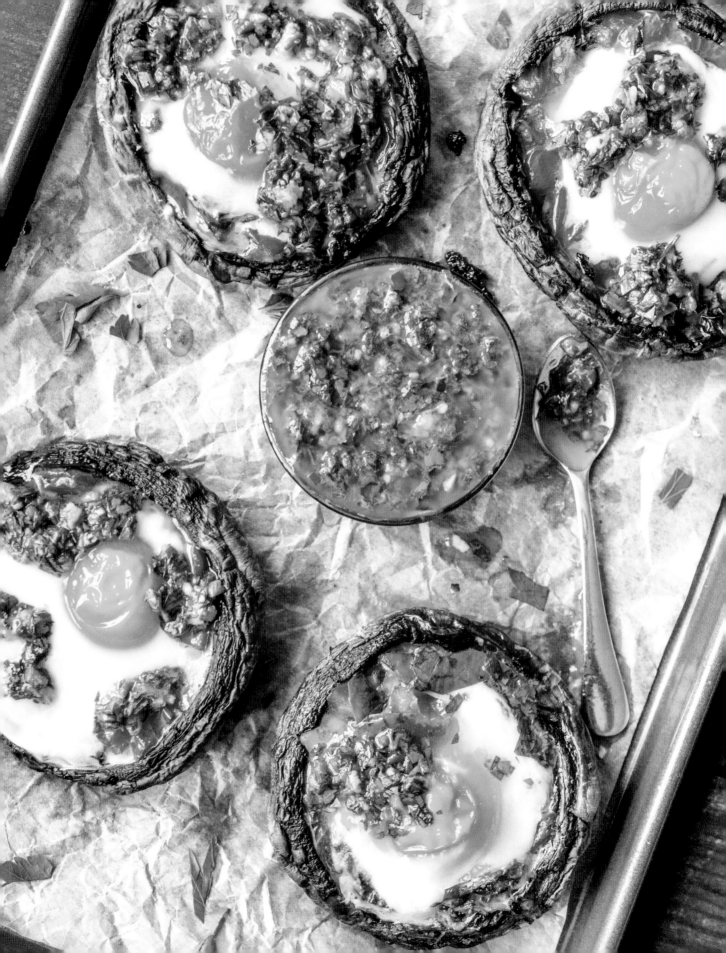

Asparagus
SOLDIERS & EGGS

Yield: 2 servings   **Prep Time:** 10 minutes   **Cook Time:** 18 minutes

When it comes to three-ingredient breakfasts, this one is hard to beat for both its simplicity and fanciness. I am a total sucker for an ooey gooey egg yolk, and it turns out that crispy bacon-wrapped asparagus is the perfect accompaniment for dipping in a runny yolk. I've tried many different methods for boiling eggs, and this is by far the most foolproof. Just be sure to set a timer because even an extra 20 seconds can make a massive difference. To make this dish more "brunchy," substitute prosciutto for the bacon and reduce the baking time by 5 minutes.

8 spears asparagus, woody stems removed

8 strips regular-cut bacon

4 medium eggs, directly from the refrigerator

1. Preheat the oven to 400°F and place a wire rack on top of a sheet pan. (This will help the bacon cook evenly.)

2. Starting at the bottom of an asparagus spear, wrap a strip of bacon around and up the spear, then place on the wire rack. Repeat with the remaining bacon and asparagus.

3. Bake for 16 to 18 minutes, until the bacon is crisp and the thicker end of the asparagus is tender.

4. While the bacon-wrapped asparagus spears are baking, prepare the eggs. Fill a small saucepan with 3 inches of water and bring to a boil over medium-high heat. Once the water is boiling, use a slotted spoon to slowly lower the eggs into the water. Set a timer for 4½ minutes and allow the eggs to cook in the boiling water. After 4½ minutes, transfer the eggs from the pan to a bowl and run under cold tap water for 10 seconds to cool slightly.

5. Place the eggs in egg cups or alternatively in cups that have been cut out of an egg carton. Gently tap a knife around the top of the egg to remove the cap. Serve with the asparagus spears on the side for dipping.

Boiling Eggs

Exactly 4½ minutes will give you a very runny yolk; increase the time to 5½ minutes for a less-runny but still liquid yolk, and to 6 to 7 minutes for a jammy yolk. If your eggs are room temperature, reduce the cooking time by 30 seconds.

SUBSTITUTIONS: *For low-FODMAP, swap the asparagus for bunches of 2 to 3 green beans wrapped in bacon.*

MAKE AHEAD: *You can wrap the asparagus in the bacon up to 12 hours in advance, but you shouldn't cook it until just before serving to ensure the asparagus doesn't become mushy.*

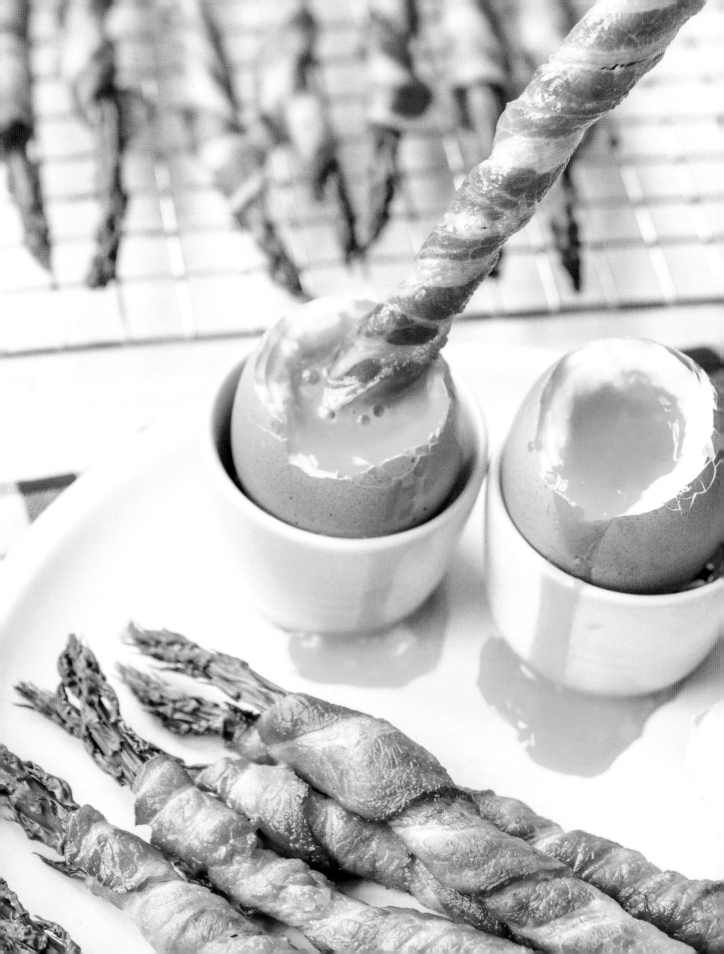

KETO
LOW-FODMAP
PALEO
VEGETARIAN
DAIRY-FREE
NUT-FREE

Roasted Vegetable
SHEET PAN FRITTATA

Yield: 10 servings   **Prep Time:** 15 minutes   **Cook Time:** 45 minutes

I originally made this frittata as a way to use leftover roasted vegetables, but it was such a hit I knew I had to create a recipe for it. Feel free to add any other vegetables you might have in your fridge; eggplant, broccoli, or asparagus are all great additions.

1 medium red onion, cut into eighths

1½ cups cubed butternut squash

1 yellow bell pepper, cut into thin strips

1 cup cherry tomatoes

1 medium zucchini, thinly sliced

1 tablespoon extra-virgin olive oil

6 medium eggs

½ cup unsweetened almond milk

1 teaspoon Dijon mustard

½ teaspoon salt

¼ teaspoon ground black pepper

½ cup chopped spinach

2 tablespoons chopped fresh Italian parsley

2 tablespoons chopped fresh basil

1. Preheat the oven to 350°F.

2. Place the onion, butternut squash, bell pepper, cherry tomatoes, and zucchini on a 9 by 13-inch sheet pan. Drizzle with the oil and roast for 20 minutes.

3. In a bowl, whisk together the eggs, almond milk, mustard, salt, and pepper. Stir in the spinach, parsley, and basil.

4. Remove the pan from the oven and pour the egg mixture over the roasted vegetables. Return the pan to the oven to bake for 25 minutes, or until the eggs have set. Allow to cool for 5 minutes before slicing and serving.

SUBSTITUTIONS: *Skip the red onion to make it low-FODMAP. Use coconut milk in place of almond milk to make this dish nut-free.*

STORAGE: *Leftovers will last in the fridge for up to 4 days.*

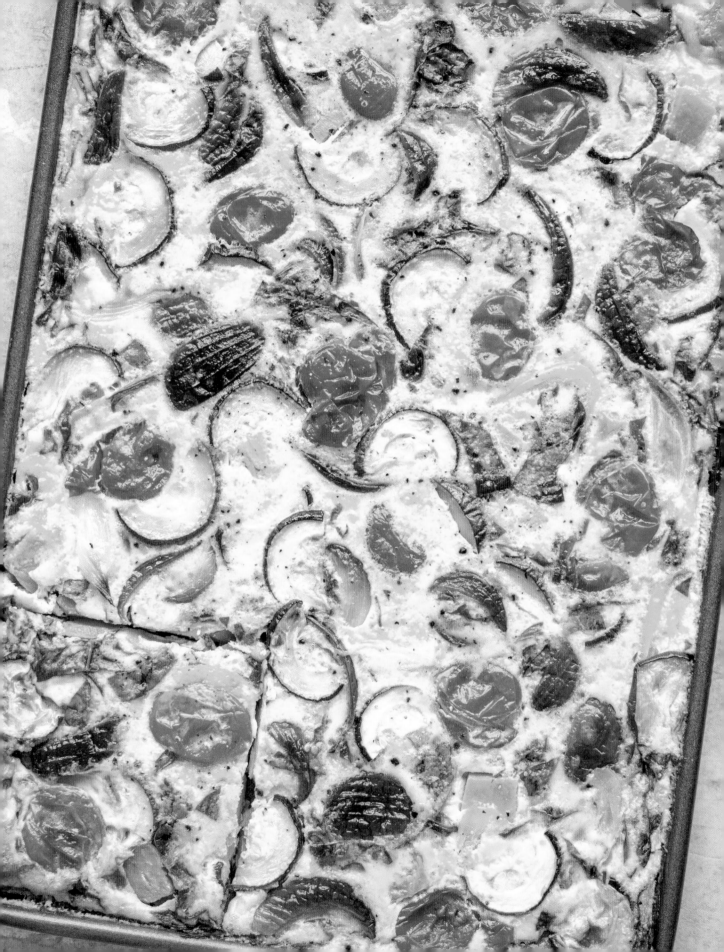

KETO
LOW-FODMAP
PALEO
VEGETARIAN
DAIRY-FREE
NUT-FREE

Mexican Eggs BENEDICT

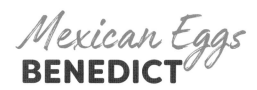

Yield: 2 servings **Prep Time:** 20 minutes **Cook Time:** 25 minutes

I don't like to play favorites, but for this recipe I'm willing to make an exception. This is my absolute favorite breakfast recipe, and readers of my blog seem to agree. One person even said they'd never go back to regular eggs Benedict! Butternut squash slices make a great base to top with smashed avocado, spicy chorizo, a perfectly poached runny egg, and creamy chipotle hollandaise. IT'S SO GOOD.

1 large butternut squash

1½ tablespoons extra-virgin olive oil, divided

6 ounces ground chorizo

1 teaspoon white vinegar

4 medium eggs

1 large avocado, mashed

Chipotle Hollandaise

2 medium egg yolks

1 tablespoon freshly squeezed lime juice

1 tablespoon chipotle paste, or 1 teaspoon chipotle chili powder

¼ teaspoon salt

¼ cup melted unsalted butter, ghee, or coconut oil

For Garnish

1 jalapeño pepper, thinly sliced

1 tablespoon chopped fresh cilantro

SPECIAL EQUIPMENT
Immersion blender

SCD BASICS
Chipotle Paste (page 34)
Chorizo (page 50)

1. Preheat the oven to 200°F.

2. Peel a butternut squash and cut the long neck from the round base. (See the tip on page 56 for using the leftover squash.) Then cut the neck into four ½-inch-thick slices.

3. Heat a grill to medium-high heat. Brush both sides of each butternut squash slice with 1 tablespoon of oil and grill the slices for 3 to 4 minutes per side, until grill marks appear and the squash is slightly tender. Transfer the slices to the oven to keep them warm while you prep the rest of the recipe.

4. To make the hollandaise, place the egg yolks, lime juice, chipotle paste, and salt in a wide-mouth 16-ounce mason jar or a 3-quart spouted mixing bowl. Insert an immersion blender into the container and blend for 30 seconds. Very slowly drizzle the melted butter into the container while blending. You also could use a small blender if you do not have an immersion blender. The mixture should begin to emulsify and thicken as you blend it. Dip a spoon into the hollandaise and run your finger over the back of the spoon; the sauce is done when you can create a clear line in the sauce on the back of the spoon.

5. Heat the remaining ½ tablespoon of oil in a medium-sized skillet over medium heat. Place the chorizo in the skillet and cook for 8 to 10 minutes, or until the chorizo is completely cooked through. While the chorizo cooks, use a wooden spoon to break up the meat into a crumbly texture.

6. Bring approximately 3 inches of water in a pot over medium-high heat to a boil and add the vinegar. Once the water is boiling, reduce the heat to medium-low and move a spoon quickly in a circular motion in the water to create a whirlpool and then crack an egg into the middle. Cook the egg for 4 minutes before removing from the water using a slotted spoon. Repeat with the remaining eggs.

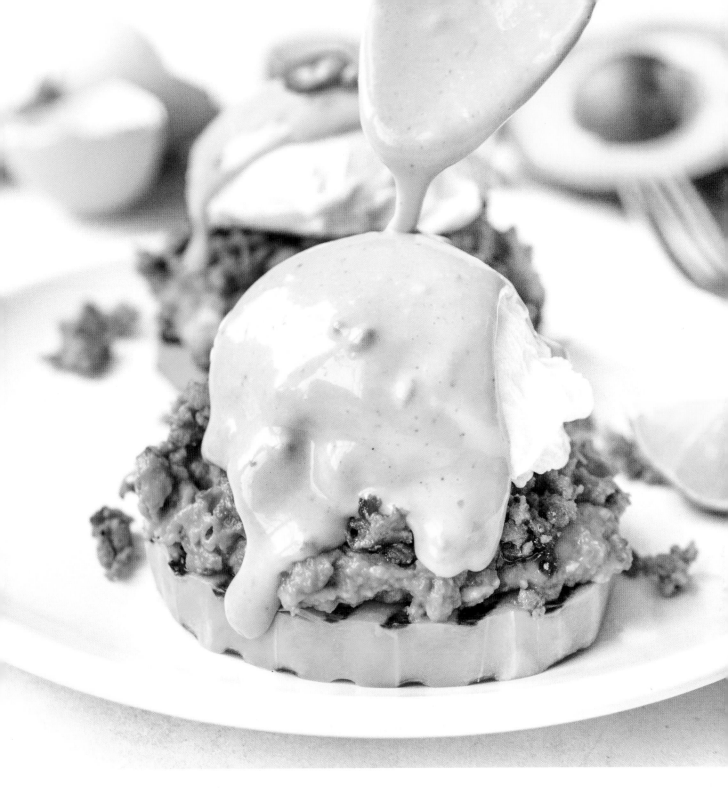

7. To assemble, place 2 butternut squash slices on a plate, top each with one-fourth of the smashed avocado, 2 large spoonfuls of the chorizo, and a poached egg. Then spoon one-quarter of the hollandaise over the top of each egg. Repeat with the remaining ingredients. Garnish with jalapeño slices and cilantro before serving.

SUBSTITUTIONS: *Skip the avocado to make it low-FODMAP. Skip the chorizo to make this vegetarian.*

KETO
LOW-FODMAP
PALEO
VEGETARIAN
DAIRY-FREE
NUT-FREE

Broccoli & Bacon
EGG MUFFINS

Yield: 12 muffins   **Prep Time:** 10 minutes   **Cook Time:** 34 minutes

These egg muffins are great for meal prepping on Sunday to eat throughout the week as a grab-and-go breakfast. Although they're primarily egg-based, the addition of coconut flour makes these muffins less eggy than they would be otherwise; for example, their texture is less eggy than a traditional frittata. (This is a huge bonus if, like me, you aren't a fan of the texture of eggs.)

2 cups broccoli florets

1½ teaspoons unsalted butter, ghee, or coconut oil

1 medium yellow onion, thinly sliced

¼ teaspoon salt

10 medium eggs

⅔ cup unsweetened almond milk

½ cup coconut flour

¼ cup shredded cheddar cheese, or 2 tablespoons nutritional yeast

¼ cup chopped fresh Italian parsley

1 teaspoon Dijon mustard

½ teaspoon cayenne pepper

½ teaspoon ground black pepper

5 strips bacon, cooked and roughly chopped

1. Preheat the oven to 400°F and grease a 12-well muffin pan or line it with muffin liners.

2. Bring ¼ inch of water in a medium-sized skillet over medium heat to a boil and add the broccoli florets. Cover with a lid and steam for 4 minutes, or until the florets are tender but not soft. Remove from the water and allow to cool before cutting the florets into small pieces, about ½ inch.

3. Pour out any water remaining in the skillet before melting the butter over medium heat. Add the onion and salt, cover with a lid and cook for 5 minutes until the onion is soft.

4. In a bowl, whisk together the eggs, almond milk, coconut flour, cheddar cheese, parsley, mustard, cayenne pepper, and pepper. Stir in the broccoli florets and the bacon.

5. Spoon the mixture into the prepared muffin pan, filling each well to the top. Bake for 25 minutes, or until golden and the tops are completely dry to the touch. Allow the muffins to cool for 10 minutes before removing from the muffin pan and transferring to a cooling rack. If the muffins appear to be stuck in the pan, run a knife around the outside of each to loosen them.

SUBSTITUTIONS: *Skip the onion for low-FODMAP. Swap the bacon for sautéed mushrooms to make them vegetarian. Use coconut milk in place of almond milk to make these nut-free.*

STORAGE: *The muffins will last in the fridge for up to 5 days or in the freezer for up to 2 months. Reheat in a preheated 350°F oven for 10 minutes. Reheating in the microwave may cause them to become slightly mushy.*

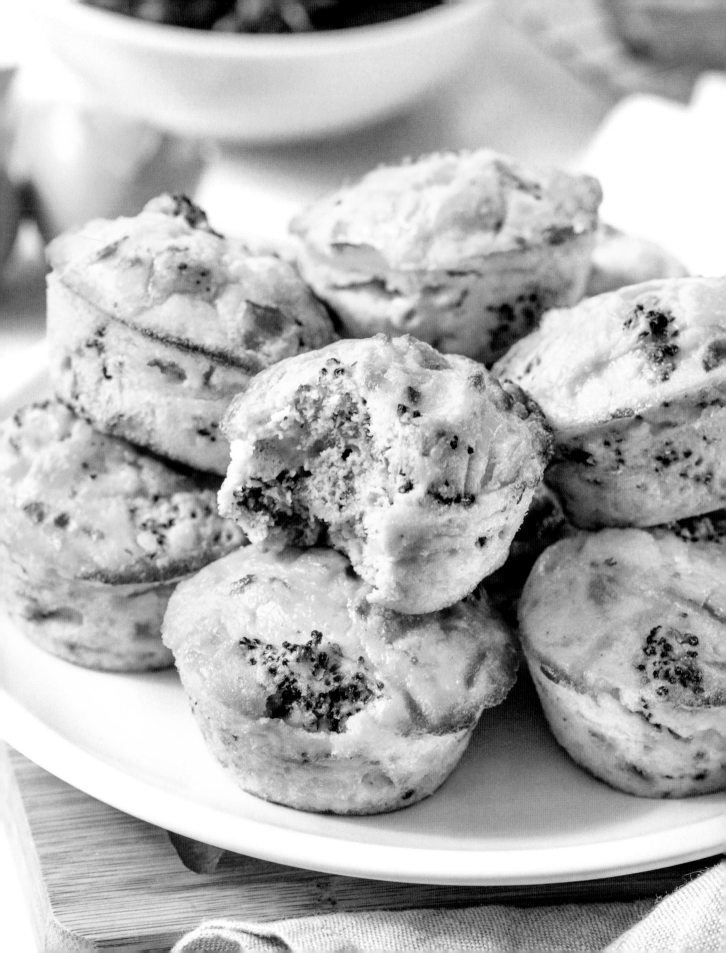

Chunky Banana &
PECAN MUFFINS

Yield: 10 muffins **Prep Time:** 15 minutes **Cook Time:** 30 minutes

Through a lot of trial and error, I've learned a few secrets to making the perfect grain-free banana muffins. First, you have to be patient (and be okay with the odd fruit fly) because the bananas need to be compost-on-your-countertop ripe for the best flavor. Second, saving one banana to add to the batter in Step 3 results in moist little clumps of banana goodness in each bite. And third, there is no point in trying to resist a batch of these when they're fresh out of the oven—just give in. They'll be a bit crumbly when hot, but they're soooo good.

4 very ripe bananas, divided

2 medium eggs

3 tablespoons melted coconut oil

2 tablespoons honey

1 teaspoon vanilla extract

½ teaspoon apple cider vinegar

2½ cups blanched almond flour

⅓ cup roughly chopped raw pecans

2 tablespoons unsweetened shredded coconut

1 tablespoon coconut flour

1 teaspoon ground cinnamon

½ teaspoon baking soda

¼ teaspoon salt

STORAGE: *The muffins will last in the fridge for up to a week or in the freezer for up to 2 months.*

1. Preheat the oven to 350°F and line 10 wells of a 12-well muffin pan.

2. Put 3 of the bananas, the eggs, coconut oil, honey, vanilla extract, and vinegar in a large mixing bowl. Using an electric mixer, beat until thoroughly combined. Next, add the almond flour, pecans, shredded coconut, coconut flour, cinnamon, baking soda, and salt and mix into a thick batter.

3. Cut 10 thin slices off the remaining banana and set them aside. Break the rest of the banana into chunks and use a wooden spoon to stir it into the batter.

4. Divide the batter among the lined wells of the muffin pan, filling each cup to the top. Add a slice of banana to the top of each muffin.

5. Bake for 25 to 30 minutes, until a toothpick inserted in the center comes out clean. If the top of the muffins are browning too quickly, cover with a sheet of aluminum foil.

6. Remove the muffin pan from the oven and allow to cool for 10 minutes before attempting to remove the muffins from the pan.

Ripening Bananas

Bananas release a gas called ethylene, which causes other fruit around them to ripen more quickly. To prevent apples, melon, and so on from going bad too soon, store your bananas separately. However, if you have a hard avocado, you can place it in a paper bag with a banana to make it ripen faster.

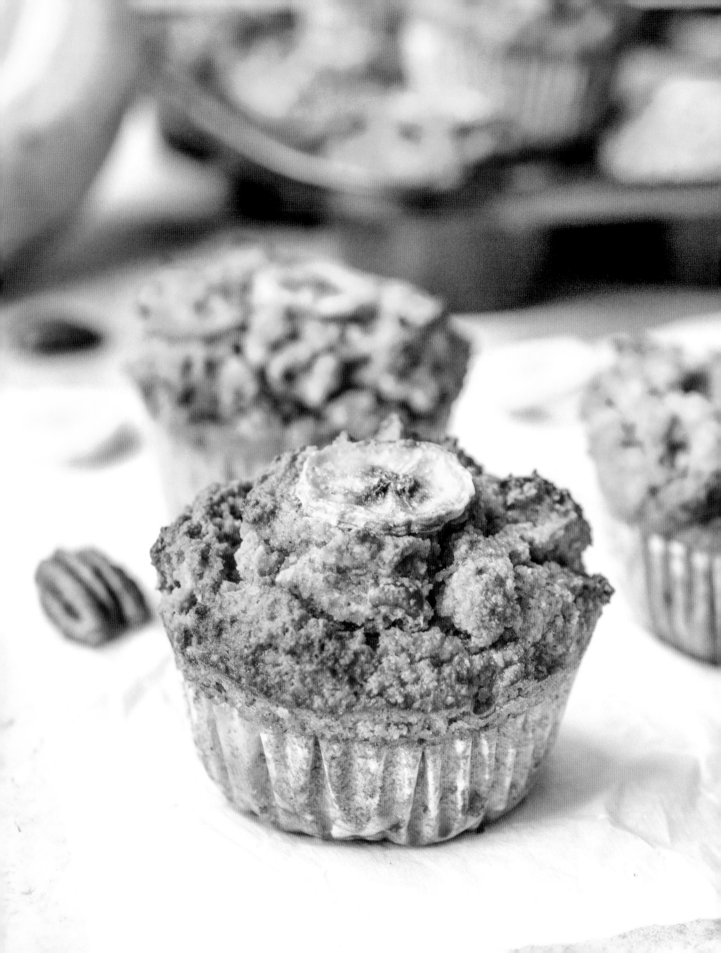

Apple Cinnamon
BREAKFAST COOKIES

Yield: 15 cookies **Prep Time:** 12 minutes **Cook Time:** 15 minutes

I call these cookies, but they're really just like a muffin top (which, let's be honest, is the best part of a muffin anyway). An entire batch only contains 1 tablespoon of honey, which you can omit completely if you use a very ripe banana. I try to always have a batch of these breakfast cookies in my freezer because they are a perfect grab-and-go breakfast for busy mornings when I'm rushing out the door.

2 medium eggs

1 ripe banana

⅓ cup melted coconut oil

1 tablespoon honey

1 teaspoon vanilla extract

1½ cups blanched almond flour

1½ cups shredded apple (about 2 medium-sized apples)

½ cup unsweetened shredded coconut

½ cup chopped raw walnuts

½ cup raisins

1 tablespoon coconut flour

2 teaspoons ground cinnamon

½ teaspoon ground nutmeg

½ teaspoon ginger powder

½ teaspoon baking soda

¼ teaspoon salt

1. Preheat the oven to 350°F and line a sheet pan with parchment paper.

2. Place the eggs, banana, melted coconut oil, honey, and vanilla extract in a large bowl and use an electric mixer to beat the mixture together until well combined and the banana is completely mashed into the batter.

3. Add the almond flour, apple, shredded coconut, walnuts, raisins, coconut flour, cinnamon, nutmeg, ginger, baking soda, and salt to the liquid mixture and beat on low speed until the batter is well combined.

4. Drop large spoonfuls (about 2 tablespoons each) of the batter onto the prepared sheet pan and gently press down on the cookies to flatten them. Bake for 15 minutes, until evenly golden.

5. Let the cookies cool on the sheet pan for 5 minutes before transferring them to a cooling rack to cool completely.

STORAGE: *These cookies will keep in an airtight container in the fridge for up to 5 days or in the freezer for up to 3 months. (They are delicious frozen, too!)*

TIP: *You can substitute shredded pear or even zucchini for the shredded apple. Feel free to swap the raisins and chopped walnuts for any other dried fruit and nuts.*

Measuring Honey

Before measuring honey, pour a bit of melted coconut oil into the measuring spoon or cup; this will help the honey easily slide out.

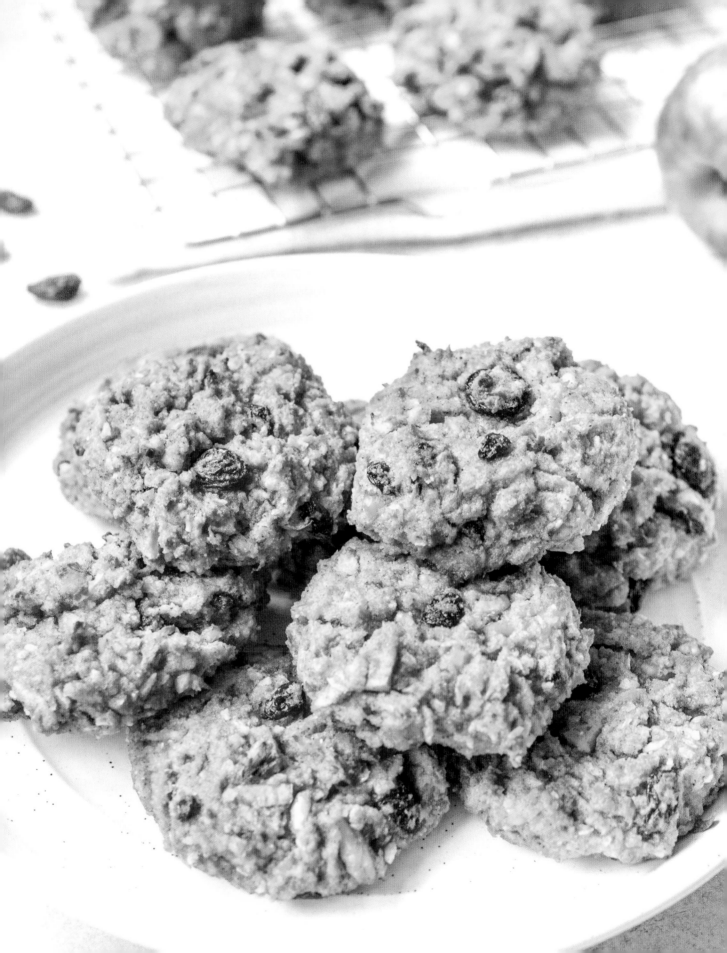

Raspberry Orange
MUFFINS

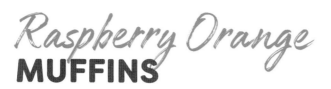

Yield: 9 muffins   **Prep Time:** 10 minutes   **Cook Time:** 25 minutes

Pulling a fresh batch of muffins out of the oven always makes me feel a little bit like Martha Stewart. The house can be a disaster, but with the smell of fresh-baked muffins in the air, I really feel like a domestic goddess, even if it's just for a moment or two. These muffins couldn't be easier to make; all you need is a bowl and a few minutes to stir everything together, then you can just sit back and relax while they bake. I love the combination of orange with little bits of juicy raspberry in each bite. If you're a newbie to grain-free baking, this is a great recipe to start with.

4 medium eggs

⅓ cup melted coconut oil or unsalted butter

2 tablespoons orange zest

¼ cup freshly squeezed orange juice

3 tablespoons honey

1 teaspoon vanilla extract

2 cups blanched almond flour

¼ cup coconut flour

½ teaspoon baking soda

¼ teaspoon salt

¼ teaspoon apple cider vinegar

1 cup raspberries

1. Preheat the oven to 350°F and line 9 wells of a 12-well muffin pan with liners.

2. Using an electric mixer, beat the eggs, melted coconut oil, orange zest, orange juice, honey, and vanilla extract until well mixed.

3. Add the almond flour, coconut flour, baking soda, salt, and vinegar and mix until just combined; don't overmix.

4. Add the raspberries and stir with a spoon to incorporate them throughout the batter. You can break them into smaller pieces with the spoon, but don't overmix them into a puree.

5. Fill each lined well of the muffin pan to the top with the batter and bake for 25 minutes, or until a toothpick inserted in the center comes out clean. If the muffins brown on the top too quickly, cover the pan with aluminum foil. Allow the muffins to cool for 5 minutes before removing them from the pan.

STORAGE: *These muffins are best stored in the fridge rather than at room temperature and will last in the fridge for up to 5 days. They will last in the freezer for up to 2 months.*

Grain-Free Baking

Keep in mind when doing any grain-free baking that most things don't rise or change shape as they bake, which is unlike regular baked items. Always fill the wells of the muffin pan right to the top and smooth over the surface of breads, cakes, and so on. The shape of the item as it goes into the oven is similar to how it'll look when it comes out.

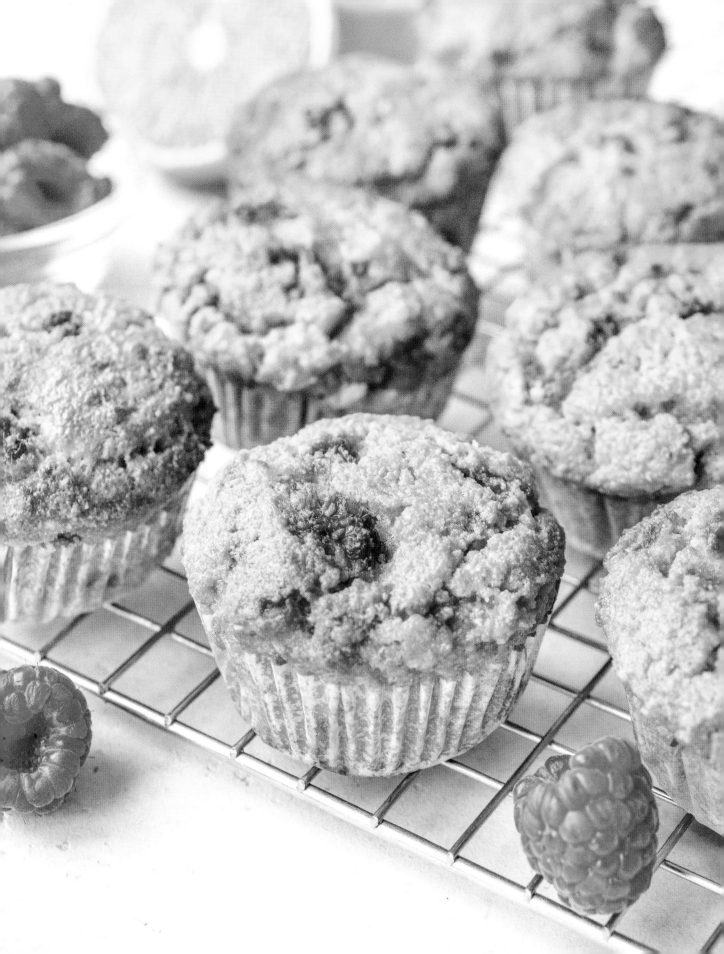

Pancakes with
BERRY COMPOTE

Yield: 8 to 10 small pancakes (2 servings)   **Prep Time:** 8 minutes   **Cook Time:** 20 minutes

These easy-to-make almond flour pancakes are light and fluffy and a family favorite on Sunday mornings. Berry compote is a delicious SCD-legal alternative to maple syrup that you can make using any frozen berries you have stashed in your freezer.

Quick Berry Compote

2 cups frozen berries (blueberries, blackberries, raspberries, or a mixture)

2 tablespoons water

1 teaspoon vanilla extract

1 teaspoon freshly squeezed lemon juice

Pancakes

2 cups blanched almond flour

½ cup unsweetened almond milk or water

4 medium eggs

¼ cup honey, plus more for serving if desired

1 teaspoon vanilla extract

1 teaspoon ground cinnamon

½ teaspoon salt

½ teaspoon baking soda

1 tablespoon coconut oil, divided, for the pan

1. To make the compote, place the berries, water, vanilla extract, and lemon juice in a small saucepan over medium heat. Simmer for 15 minutes, or until the berries have broken down into a syrup consistency, adding more water if needed to ensure the mixture doesn't burn.

2. While the compote is simmering, make the pancakes: In a bowl, whisk together the almond flour, almond milk, eggs, honey, vanilla extract, cinnamon, salt, and baking soda until smooth.

3. Heat 1 teaspoon of the oil in a large nonstick skillet over medium heat. Once hot, pour in about 3 tablespoons of the batter per pancake. (You should be able to cook 3 pancakes per batch.) Cook for 3 minutes, or until the edges begin to turn golden and bubbles appear, then flip and cook for another 2 minutes. Repeat with the remaining batter.

4. Serve the pancakes with the compote spooned over the top and a drizzle of honey, if desired.

MAKE AHEAD/STORAGE: *The berry compote can be made a day or two in advance and freezes well. The pancakes will keep in the fridge for up to 2 days or in the freezer for up to 1 month.*

Compote

The berry compote is incredibly versatile and can be modified depending on what fruit you have on hand. You could use pitted cherries, diced strawberries, or diced peaches in place of the berries. Serve any leftover compote on vanilla ice cream (like the one on page 334).

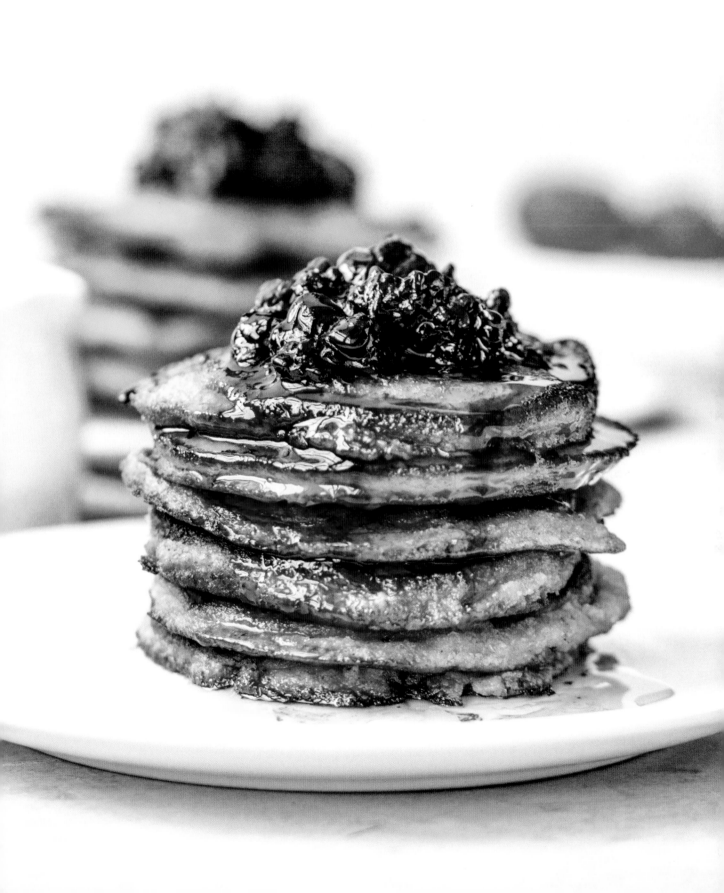

Tahini Cherry GRANOLA

Make ahead

Yield: 4 cups   **Prep Time:** 15 minutes   **Cook Time:** 35 minutes

Granola is my go-to for a quick-and-easy breakfast when I need something that will keep me full well into the afternoon. The tahini helps to bind the nuts together and reduces the amount of oil and honey required as well as creating a delicious creaminess that is a nice contrast to the tart chewy cherries (but feel free to swap in pistachios, pecans, hazelnuts, or any other nuts you have on hand). I like to keep a bag of this in the bottom of my purse to grab a handful of when I'm out and in need of a quick snack.

½ cup raw Brazil nuts

½ cup raw almonds

1 cup raw walnuts

1 cup unsweetened coconut flakes

½ cup unsweetened shredded coconut

⅓ cup sesame seeds

½ cup tahini

2 tablespoons honey

2 tablespoons melted coconut oil

2 teaspoons vanilla extract

1 teaspoon ground cinnamon

¾ teaspoon salt

1 cup unsweetened dried cherries

⅓ cup raisins

1. Preheat oven to 300°F.

2. Place the Brazil nuts and almonds in a food processor and pulse for a few seconds, until they break down into small pieces.

3. Add the walnuts and pulse for a few more seconds. Transfer the nuts to a large bowl and stir in the coconut flakes, shredded coconut, and sesame seeds.

4. In a small bowl, whisk together the tahini, honey, coconut oil, vanilla extract, cinnamon, and salt. Pour the liquid mixture over the nut mixture and stir until everything is well coated. Transfer the granola onto a sheet pan and spread it out evenly.

5. Bake for 30 to 35 minutes, stirring every 10 minutes, until golden. Watch the granola closely to ensure nothing burns.

6. Remove from the oven and stir in the dried cherries and raisins. Allow the granola to cool before storing.

Homemade Tahini

If you'd like to make your own tahini, see page 17 for a recipe.

SUBSTITUTIONS: *Swap the honey for maple syrup to make it vegan.*

STORAGE: *This granola is best stored in an airtight container in the pantry for up to 4 weeks.*

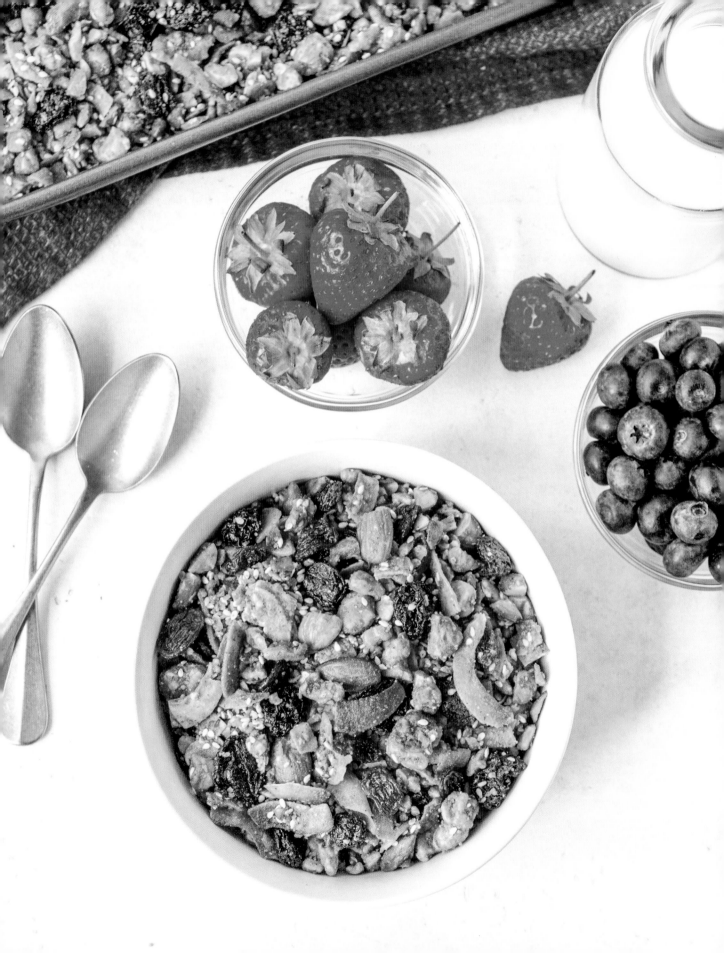

PALEO
VEGAN
VEGETARIAN
DAIRY-FREE
EGG-FREE
NUT-FREE

< 30 min

Pear & Chai
SPICED PORRIDGE

Yield: 2 servings   **Prep Time:** 5 minutes   **Cook Time:** 15 minutes

This truly has the same consistency as traditional porridge but is made with a rather unexpected ingredient—cauliflower! Cooking cauliflower rice with almond milk and a mashed banana makes it soft, thick, and creamy, and the mix of chai spices masks any hint of cauliflower flavor. Add more almond milk near the end of cooking, if you prefer your porridge milky.

1 very ripe banana

2 cups fresh or frozen cauliflower rice

1¼ cups unsweetened almond milk, plus more if desired

1½ teaspoons ground cinnamon, plus more for garnish

½ teaspoon ginger powder

½ teaspoon allspice

¼ teaspoon ground nutmeg

¼ teaspoon ground cloves

½ teaspoon vanilla extract

1 pear, plus 6 or 8 slices for garnish

2 tablespoons chopped raw pecans, for garnish

2 tablespoons raisins, for garnish (optional)

1. Peel the banana, place it in a bowl, and mash it with a fork into a smooth consistency.

2. Place the cauliflower rice and almond milk in a medium-sized saucepan over medium heat. Stir in the mashed banana, cinnamon, ginger, allspice, nutmeg, cloves, and vanilla extract and simmer, uncovered, for 8 to 10 minutes.

3. Use a box grater to shred the pear, then add to the saucepan. Continue to cook the mixture for another 4 to 5 minutes, until the cauliflower rice is tender, and all of the liquid has been absorbed. Add a splash more almond milk if needed until the porridge reaches your desired consistency.

4. Top each serving with half of the chopped pecans, raisins (if using), and pear slices, then sprinkle with cinnamon.

SUBSTITUTIONS: *For nut-free, substitute coconut milk for the almond milk and skip the pecans. You can replace the banana with 1 tablespoon of honey (or maple syrup to make it vegan).*

STORAGE: *Leftovers will last in the fridge for up to 2 days, after which time the smell of cauliflower may become more apparent.*

Softening Bananas

If you have bananas that are yellow but still quite firm and not soft enough to be used in this porridge or in batter for baking, bake the unpeeled bananas in a preheated 300°F oven for 30 minutes. The heat will soften them and make them easy to mash with a fork.

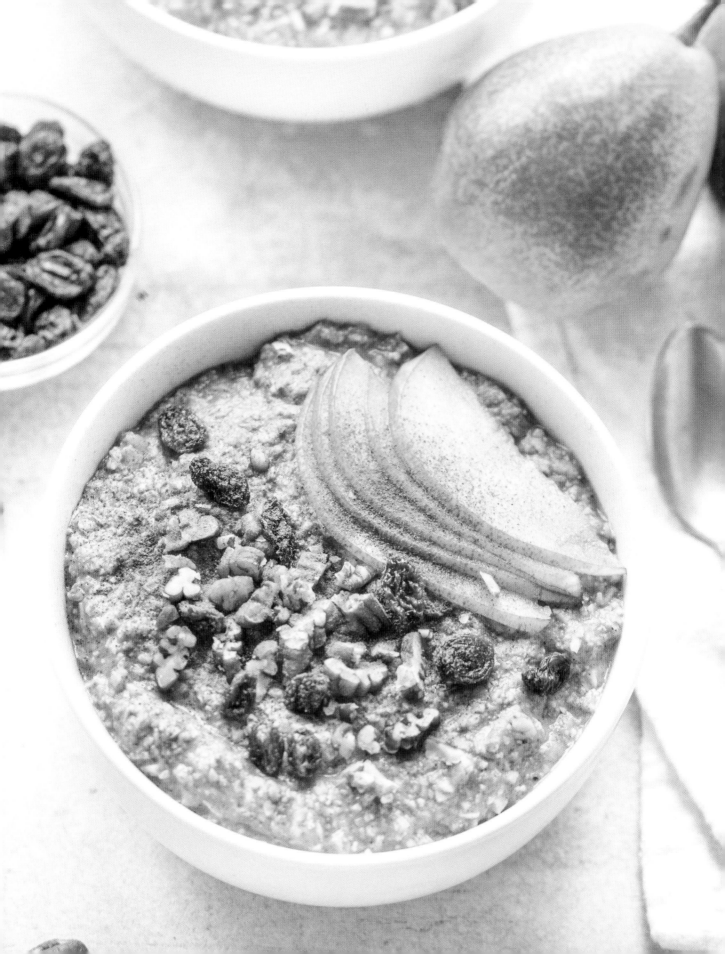

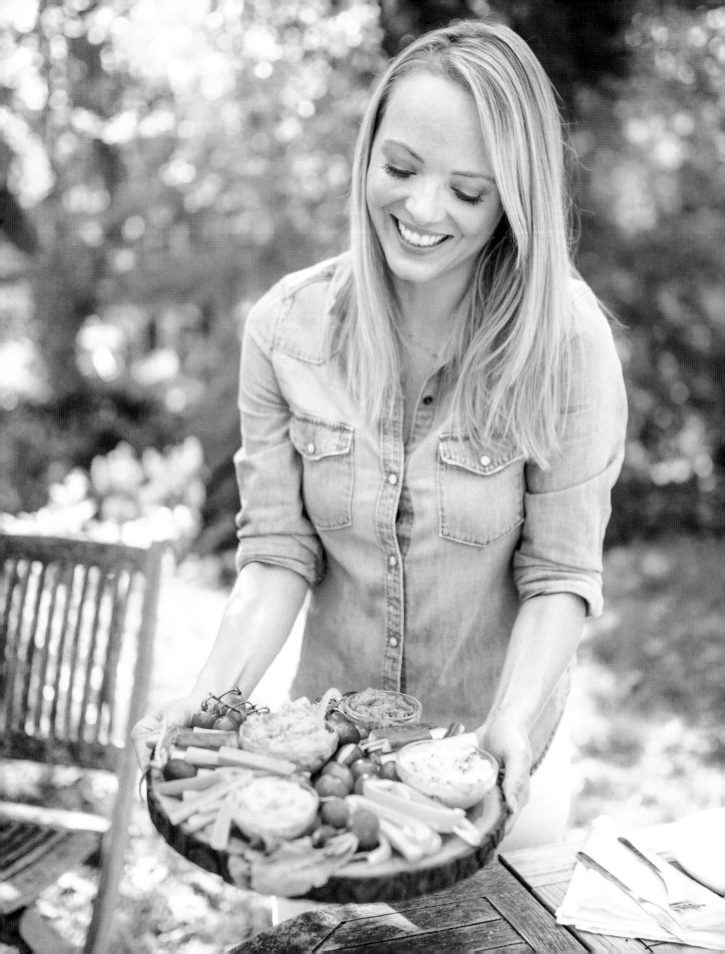

Appetizers

KETO
LOW-FODMAP
PALEO
VEGAN
VEGETARIAN
DAIRY-FREE
EGG-FREE

MUHAMMARA

Yield: 4 servings **Prep Time:** 12 minutes **Cook Time:** 30 minutes

Muhammara is a spicy roasted red pepper and walnut dip that is originally from Syria. It's a great alternative to hummus and is delicious served with veggies or crackers (page 292). I find that the flavors only get better after a day in the fridge, so I like to make a batch of this dip on Sunday so I can snack on it throughout the week.

3 red bell peppers

2 tablespoons extra-virgin olive oil, divided

¾ cup raw walnuts, plus 1½ teaspoons chopped for garnish

1 Medjool date, pitted and soaked in boiling water for 10 minutes to soften, or 1½ teaspoons honey

2 cloves garlic, peeled

1 tablespoon freshly squeezed lemon juice

1 teaspoon ground cumin

½ teaspoon salt

2 tablespoons blanched almond flour

¾ teaspoon crushed Aleppo chili flakes, or ½ teaspoon red pepper flakes, plus extra for garnish

1. Preheat the oven to 400°F and place the bell peppers in a baking dish. Drizzle with 1 tablespoon of the oil and arrange the walnuts around the peppers. Bake in the oven for 12 minutes until the walnuts are golden; then remove the walnuts from the baking dish, flip the peppers, and return the dish to the oven for another 18 minutes, until the peppers are charred.

2. While the peppers continue baking, pulse the toasted walnuts in a food processor for 5 seconds until they have broken into a crumbly texture; be sure not to over pulse into a powder. Transfer the walnut crumble to a bowl and set aside.

3. Place the charred bell peppers on a cutting board and invert a bowl over them; let rest for 10 minutes. (The trapped steam will make the peppers much easier to peel.) Remove the bowl and peel the skin from the peppers, then remove the stem and seeds.

4. Drain the date and place in the food processor. Add the bell peppers, garlic, lemon juice, cumin, salt, and the remaining 1 tablespoon of oil and pulse for 5 seconds or until the peppers have broken down into a smooth consistency. Add the walnut crumble and almond flour and pulse quickly—2 to 3 seconds—just to combine. The dip should be slightly chunky rather than completely smooth.

5. Transfer to a bowl and garnish with additional chopped walnuts and extra chili flakes, if desired, before serving.

Storing Nuts

Store shelled nuts in the freezer in a sealed container to extend their shelf life to up to a year.

SUBSTITUTIONS: *For keto, skip the dates. Omit the garlic and dates for low-FODMAP.*

STORAGE: *Leftovers will last in the fridge for up to 5 days.*

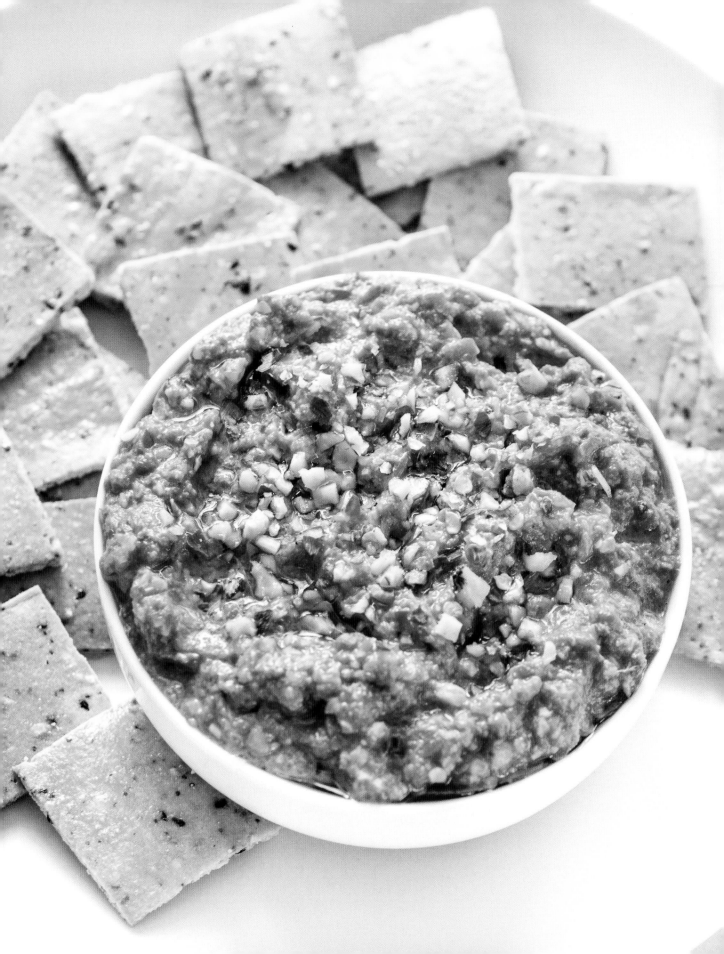

KETO
PALEO
VEGAN
VEGETARIAN
DAIRY-FREE
EGG-FREE

Jalapeño CASHEW DIP

Yield: 4 servings **Prep Time:** 12 minutes **Cook Time:** —

I must warn you that this dip is highly addicting. I have been known to polish off an entire batch in minutes. It has a real garlic-and-jalapeño kick to it, so if you're spice averse, I recommend starting with one jalapeño and then adding more as needed. I love eating this as a dip with veggies or grain-free crackers (page 292), but it's also great as a sauce served with grilled chicken or shrimp.

1 cup raw cashews, soaked in boiling water for 10 minutes

½ cup water

¼ cup fresh cilantro leaves

2 jalapeño peppers, seeds removed for a milder spice level

3 tablespoons freshly squeezed lime juice, plus more if needed

1½ tablespoons coconut aminos

2 cloves garlic, peeled

½ teaspoon salt, plus more if needed

SPECIAL EQUIPMENT
High-powered blender

1. Drain the cashews and place in a high-powered blender. Add the remaining ingredients and blend until completely smooth.

2. Taste and adjust the flavors, adding more salt, lime juice, or jalapeño as needed.

SUBSTITUTIONS: *Use macadamia nuts in place of cashews to reduce the net carbs for keto.*

STORAGE: *Leftovers will last in the fridge for up to 5 days.*

SCD BASICS
Coco-not Aminos (page 47)

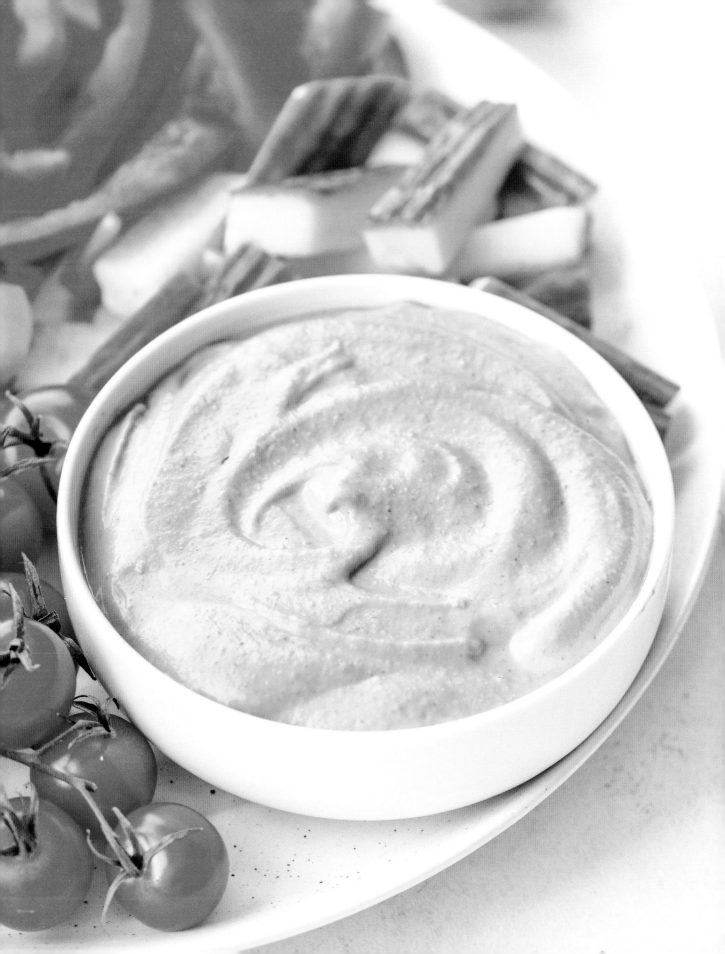

KETO
PALEO
VEGAN
VEGETARIAN
DAIRY-FREE
EGG-FREE
NUT-FREE

Roasted Cauliflower
HUMMUS

Yield: 4 servings   **Prep Time:** 12 minutes   **Cook Time:** 20 minutes

When you're trying to eat healthy or stick to a restrictive diet such as SCD, snacking can be a struggle. I remember feeling ravenous when I came home from work most evenings, which meant I was easily tempted by the packaged cookies and chips in my cupboard. Stocking my fridge with a batch of hummus and some precut veggies, such as carrots, cucumber, peppers, and celery, gave me a snack that was readily available. I've included some flavor variations to keep things interesting.

3 cups cauliflower florets (1 small head)

1 bulb garlic

3 tablespoons extra-virgin olive oil, divided, plus more for drizzling

¼ cup tahini

2 tablespoons freshly squeezed lemon juice

½ teaspoon salt

¼ teaspoon paprika

1 to 2 tablespoons water

STORAGE: *This hummus will last in the fridge for up to 5 days or in the freezer for up to 4 months. I recommend storing it in a freezer bag; to thaw, place the sealed bag in a large dish of warm water.*

1. Preheat the oven to 350°F.

2. Place the cauliflower florets on a sheet pan. Remove the outer papery skin of the garlic bulb and cut off the top one-third to expose the top of the cloves; place on the sheet pan with the florets. Drizzle the cauliflower and exposed garlic cloves with 1 tablespoon of the oil and bake for 20 minutes, or until the cauliflower is tender and golden and the garlic cloves are soft.

3. Squeeze the cloves of garlic out of the roasted bulb into a food processor. Add the roasted cauliflower, tahini, lemon juice, salt, paprika, and the remaining 2 tablespoons of oil and blend.

4. Add 1 tablespoon of water to the mixture and continue to blend until smooth. If the mixture is still not smooth enough, add 1 tablespoon more water until it reaches your desired consistency. To serve, transfer the hummus to a bowl and drizzle with olive oil, if desired.

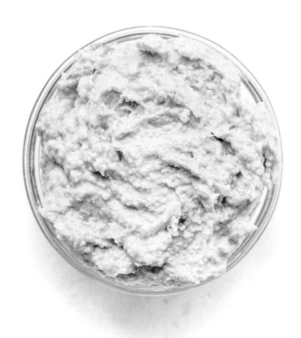

Harissa Hummus

3 cups cauliflower florets (1 small head)

2 tablespoons extra-virgin olive oil, divided, plus more for drizzling

¼ cup tahini

2 tablespoons freshly squeezed lemon juice

1½ tablespoons harissa

1 tablespoon tomato paste

2 cloves garlic, peeled

½ teaspoon salt

¼ teaspoon paprika

1 to 2 tablespoons water

SCD BASICS
Harissa (page 33)
Tomato Paste (page 35)

1. Preheat the oven to 350°F.

2. Place the cauliflower florets on a sheet pan, drizzle with 1 tablespoon of the oil and bake for 20 minutes, or until the cauliflower is tender and golden.

3. Place the roasted cauliflower in a food processor and add the tahini, lemon juice, harissa, tomato paste, garlic, salt, paprika, and the remaining 1 tablespoon of oil and blend.

4. Add 1 tablespoon of water to the mixture and continue to blend until completely smooth. If the mixture is still not smooth enough, add more water until it reaches your desired consistency. To serve, transfer the hummus to a bowl and drizzle with oil, if desired.

Jalapeño Cilantro Hummus

3 cups cauliflower florets (1 small head)

2½ tablespoons extra-virgin olive oil, divided, plus more for drizzling

¼ cup tahini

¼ cup fresh cilantro leaves

1 tablespoon freshly squeezed lemon juice

1 tablespoon freshly squeezed lime juice

1 jalapeño pepper

2 cloves garlic, peeled

½ teaspoon salt

1. Preheat the oven to 350°F.

2. Place the cauliflower florets on a sheet pan, drizzle with 1 tablespoon of the oil and bake for 20 minutes, or until the cauliflower is tender and golden.

3. Place the roasted cauliflower in a food processor and add the tahini, cilantro, lemon juice, lime juice, jalapeño, garlic, salt, and the remaining 1½ tablespoons of oil and pulse until smooth. To serve, transfer the hummus to a bowl and drizzle with oil, if desired.

Roasted Pepper Hummus

3 cups cauliflower florets (1 small head)

1 red bell pepper

2½ tablespoons extra-virgin olive oil

¼ cup tahini

1½ tablespoons freshly squeezed lemon juice

2 cloves garlic, peeled

1 teaspoon smoked paprika

½ teaspoon salt

1. Preheat the oven to 350°F.

2. Place the cauliflower florets on a sheet pan. Cut the bell pepper in half and remove the stem and seeds, then place the halves cut side down on the sheet pan with the florets. Drizzle the vegetables with 1 tablespoon of oil and bake for 20 minutes, or until the cauliflower is tender and golden and the bell pepper is soft and charred.

3. Remove the sheet pan from the oven. Invert a bowl over the charred bell pepper and steam for 10 minutes. (This will make the bell pepper much easier to peel.) Then peel the skin off the pepper using your fingers.

4. Place the peeled bell pepper in a food processor and add the roasted cauliflower, tahini, lemon juice, garlic, smoked paprika, salt, and the remaining 1½ tablespoons of oil and pulse until smooth. To serve, transfer the hummus to a bowl and drizzle with olive oil, if desired.

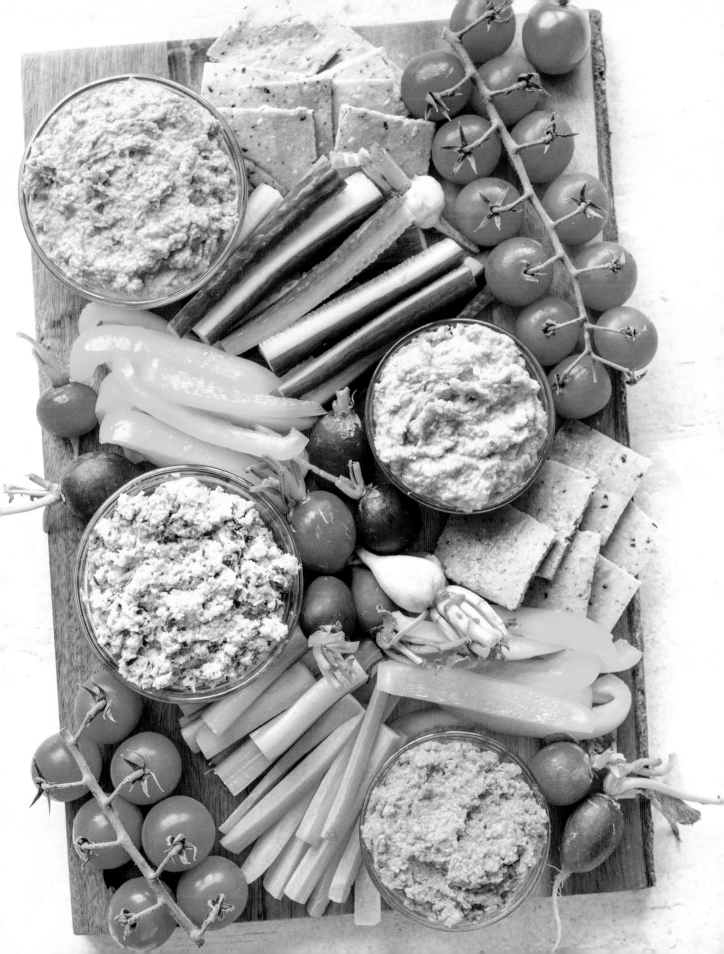

KETO

PALEO

VEGAN

VEGETARIAN

DAIRY-FREE

EGG-FREE

TZATZIKI

Yield: 2 cups   **Prep Time:** 15 minutes   **Cook Time:** —

This tzatziki is a great multipurpose dip that comes together in less than 15 minutes. You can serve it with veggies and crackers (page 292) for dipping as a quick appetizer, or you can use it as a sauce to jazz up simple grilled chicken, fish, or veggies.

1 large seedless cucumber

½ teaspoon salt, plus more if needed

¾ cup raw cashews, soaked in boiling water for 10 minutes and drained

½ cup water

2 tablespoons freshly squeezed lemon juice, plus more if needed

2 cloves garlic, peeled

1 tablespoon chopped fresh dill, plus more if needed, or 1 teaspoon dried dill weed

SPECIAL EQUIPMENT
High-powered blender or food processor

1. Cut both ends off the cucumber. Use a grater to shred the cucumber, then place the shredded cucumber in a sieve placed over a bowl, sprinkle with the salt, and allow to drain for about 10 minutes.

2. Place the cashews in a high-powered blender or food processor. Add the water, lemon juice, and garlic and blend until completely smooth. This might take a few minutes; I like using a NutriBullet to get the smoothest consistency.

3. Pour the blended cashew mixture into a medium-sized bowl and add the dill. Squeeze the shredded cucumber with your hands to get as much of the water out as possible, then add it to the cashew mixture. Stir everything together to ensure it is well mixed, then taste and add more salt, dill, or lemon juice as desired.

SUBSTITUTIONS: *Using macadamia nuts in place of cashews will reduce the carbs for keto.*

STORAGE: *Leftovers will last in the fridge for up to 4 days. Because cucumber has such a high water content, the dip may become slightly watery after a few days in the fridge; just give it a good stir before you serve it.*

Cleaning Your Blender

After emptying the blender, fill it one-third full with warm water and a splash of soap, secure the lid, and turn it on for 20 seconds. This will help loosen any bits of food that have stuck to the blade and sides, making it much easier to clean.

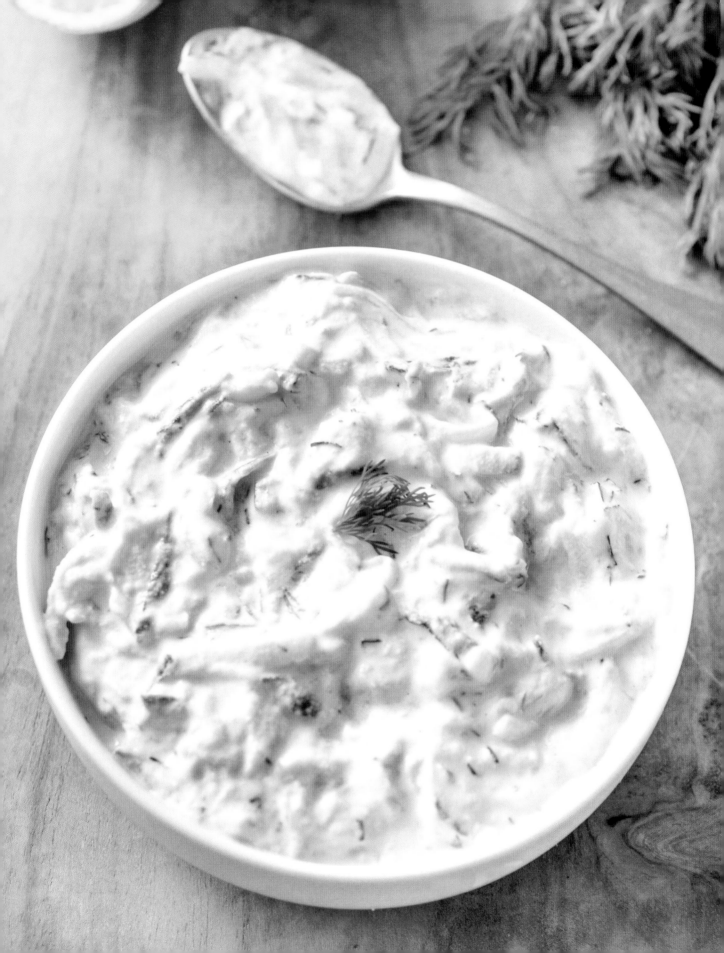

KETO
LOW-FODMAP
PALEO
VEGAN
VEGETARIAN
DAIRY-FREE
EGG-FREE

"Goat Cheese," Sun-Dried
TOMATO & PESTO TOWER

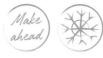

Yield: 6 servings **Prep Time:** 20 minutes, plus 4 hours for chilling

The inspiration for this recipe came from a rather unexpected place: a gas station outside of Cape Town where I spotted a small container filled with layers of goat cheese, sun-dried tomatoes, and pesto. The flavor combination stuck in my head, and I knew that I needed to try to re-create it in a dairy-free way. This recipe has quickly become my go-to appetizer for guests, and it's a reader favorite on my blog. Not only does it look pretty, but it has a deliciously creamy texture that everyone will assume is goat cheese. It's a great make-ahead dish that you can quickly flip onto a plate with some crackers (page 292) as guests arrive. This spread is also good with sliced vegetables.

"Goat Cheese" Layer

1 cup raw cashews, soaked in boiling water for 10 minutes and drained

1 tablespoon freshly squeezed lemon juice

1 tablespoon apple cider vinegar

1 tablespoon melted coconut oil

1 clove garlic, peeled

¼ teaspoon salt

¼ teaspoon ground black pepper

2 to 3 tablespoons water, divided

Pesto Layer

1 cup packed fresh basil leaves

2 tablespoons extra-virgin olive oil

2 tablespoons pine nuts

1 clove garlic, minced

¼ teaspoon salt

Sun-Dried Tomato Layer

⅓ cup oil-packed sun-dried tomatoes, roughly chopped

1 tablespoon pine nuts, toasted, for garnish

SCD BASICS
Sun-Dried Tomatoes (page 38)

1. To make the "goat cheese," place the cashews in a food processor along with the lemon juice, vinegar, coconut oil, garlic, salt, pepper, and 1 tablespoon of the water. Blend, adding 1 tablespoon more water as needed until the mixture is smooth and creamy. Remove the cashew cheese from the food processor and set aside. Wipe out the food processor bowl.

2. To make the pesto, place the basil, pine nuts, oil, garlic, and salt in the food processor and blend.

3. Line a 1-cup bowl with plastic wrap so that the wrap overhangs the edges of the bowl.

4. Spoon enough of the cheese mixture into the bowl to form a 1-inch-thick layer. Next, spoon in an even layer of the pesto. (You will likely use only about half of the pesto; see the tip, opposite, for leftover suggestions.) Top with the remaining cheese mixture and spread evenly, then add a layer of the sun-dried tomatoes. Cover with the loose ends of the plastic wrap.

5. Put the bowl in the fridge for 3 to 4 hours to become firm.

6. When ready to serve, place a serving plate upside down on top of the bowl and then flip the plate and bowl over. Lift the bowl; the tower should remain on the plate. Gently peel off the plastic wrap. Place the pine nuts on top of the tower and serve with crackers or sliced vegetables.

SUBSTITUTIONS: *Skip the garlic and use macadamia nuts in place of the cashews to make this tower low-FODMAP.*

MAKE AHEAD/STORAGE: *This tower can be made in advance and placed in the fridge for up to 4 days or in the freezer for up to 2 months. Store the tower in the bowl and only flip it onto a plate right before serving. To allow to thaw completely, take the tower out of the freezer 2 to 3 hours before serving and let it rest at room temperature.*

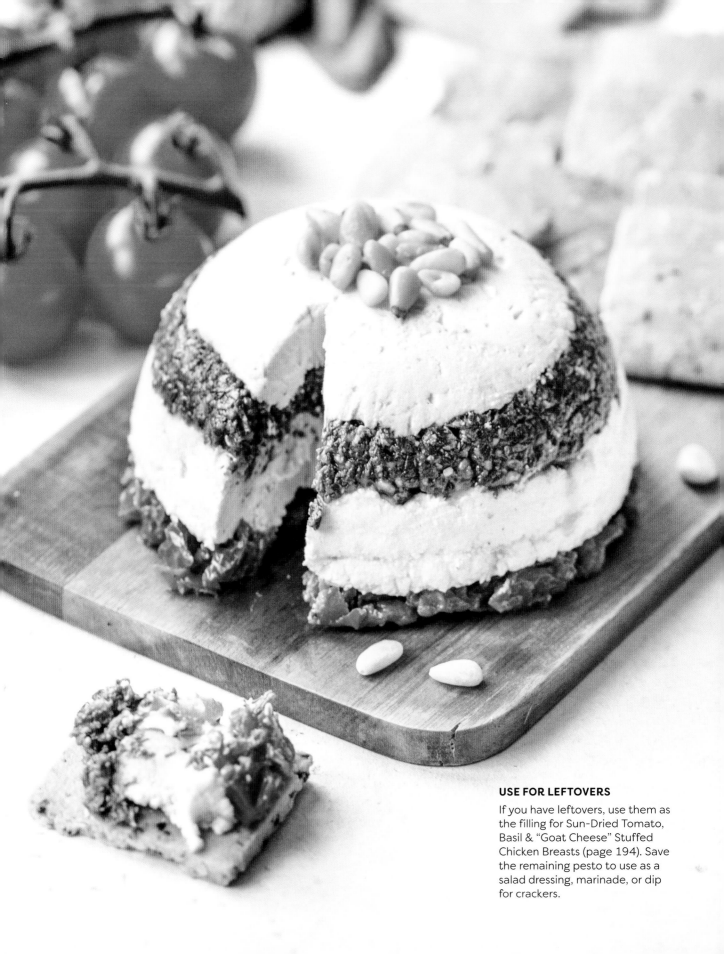

USE FOR LEFTOVERS

If you have leftovers, use them as the filling for Sun-Dried Tomato, Basil & "Goat Cheese" Stuffed Chicken Breasts (page 194). Save the remaining pesto to use as a salad dressing, marinade, or dip for crackers.

Grilled Prosciutto-Wrapped Peaches with
HONEY THYME "CHEESE"

Yield: 4 servings   **Prep Time:** 20 minutes, plus 20 minutes to chill   **Cook Time:** 5 minutes

This is a great appetizer to serve during the summer when peaches are in season. They require only a few simple steps to prepare but can really steal the show at a cookout and are great for those times when you want to impress. If you don't have a barbecue grill, you can use a panini press or bake the peaches in a preheated 375°F oven for 20 minutes for equally delicious results. Serve as an appetizer or on top of a simple salad.

⅔ cup cashews, soaked in boiling water for 10 minutes and drained

1 tablespoon coconut oil

1½ teaspoons honey

1½ tablespoons freshly squeezed lemon juice

1 tablespoon water, plus more if needed

1 teaspoon ground black pepper

½ teaspoon salt

1 teaspoon grated lemon zest

2 teaspoons roughly chopped fresh thyme, plus more for garnish

4 ripe peaches, halved and pitted

8 slices prosciutto

1 tablespoon honey

Flaked sea salt

SPECIAL EQUIPMENT
High-powered blender

1. Place the cashews in a high-powered blender. Add the coconut oil, honey, lemon juice, water, pepper, and salt and blend until smooth. If the mixture isn't becoming smooth, add a splash more water. Once the mixture is completely smooth and creamy, stir in the lemon zest and thyme and then place the cashew mixture in the fridge for a minimum of 20 minutes.

2. Heat a grill or panini press to medium-high heat.

3. Use a spoon to scoop out some of the center of each of the peach halves to slightly enlarge the hole where the pit was. Fill each of the holes with a spoonful of the cashew "cheese," then wrap each peach half with a slice of prosciutto.

4. Place the peach halves onto the grill and cook for 3 minutes, or until grill marks form, then flip and cook on the other side for another 2 minutes. Remove the cooked peaches from the grill and drizzle with a touch of honey. Sprinkle with sea salt and garnish with thyme before serving immediately.

SUBSTITUTIONS: *If you can't find nitrate-free prosciutto, use bacon instead.*

MAKE AHEAD/STORAGE: *The peaches can be filled and wrapped with prosciutto a day in advance and then grilled right before serving. These do not reheat well because the texture of the prosciutto changes.*

Crystallized Honey
Honey has a long shelf life; however, after a few months in the cupboard, it may begin to crystallize. Don't throw it out! Instead, place the jar in a bowl of warm water. The honey should return to its liquid state within 10 minutes.

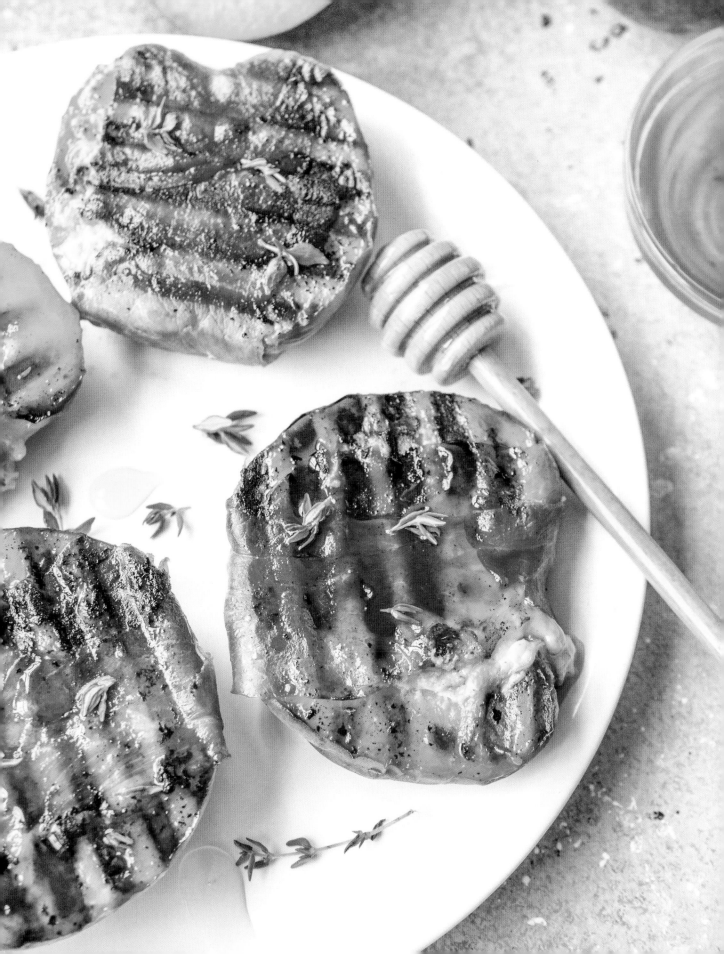

KETO
LOW-FODMAP
PALEO
VEGAN
VEGETARIAN
DAIRY-FREE
EGG-FREE

Zucchini Roll-Ups with Sun-Dried Tomatoes & BLACK PEPPER "CHEESE"

Make ahead *<30 min*

Yield: 12 rolls   **Prep Time:** 30 minutes   **Cook Time:** —

This recipe is a great choice when your group includes a few vegans or vegetarians. The rolls are light and flavorful and a great one-bite appetizer that you can easily pop in your mouth. Due to the amount of liquid in zucchini, these rolls can become quite soggy if you make them too far in advance; however, you can still prepare the cashew "cheese" up to four days ahead and then assemble the rolls right before serving.

Black Pepper "Cheese"

⅔ cup raw cashews, soaked in boiling water for 10 minutes and drained

1½ tablespoons water, plus more if needed

1 tablespoon melted coconut oil

1½ teaspoons freshly squeezed lemon juice

1 clove garlic, peeled

¾ teaspoon ground black pepper

¼ teaspoon salt

1 medium zucchini (about 5 ounces)

⅓ cup oil-packed sun-dried tomatoes, chopped

⅔ cup arugula

SPECIAL EQUIPMENT
High-powered blender

1. To make the black pepper "cheese," place the cashews in a high-powered blender. Add the water, melted coconut oil, lemon juice, garlic, pepper, and salt and blend until completely smooth and creamy. You may need to add another splash of water if the mixture isn't blending properly. Transfer to a bowl and place in the fridge to firm up for a few minutes while you prepare the zucchini.

2. Lay a ribbon of zucchini on the cutting board and spread it with a thin layer (about 1 teaspoon) of the cashew cheese. Scatter 4 to 5 pieces of the sun-dried tomatoes on the filling, then top with a few leaves of arugula.

3. Starting at one of the shorter ends of a zucchini strip, roll tightly. Place a small amount of the cashew cheese at the very end of the roll to help keep it firmly closed. Repeat Steps 2 and 3 with the remaining zucchini strips.

SUBSTITUTIONS: *Use macadamia nuts in place of cashews for keto. Omit the garlic to make these roll-ups low-FODMAP.*

MAKE AHEAD/STORAGE: *The cashew filling can be made and refrigerated up to 4 days in advance. You also can store the cashew filling in the freezer for up to 1 month. I recommend eating these rolls within a few hours of assembly to prevent them from becoming soggy.*

SCD BASICS
Sun-Dried Tomatoes (page 38)

Switch It Up
Swap the sun-dried tomatoes for chopped olives or pesto.

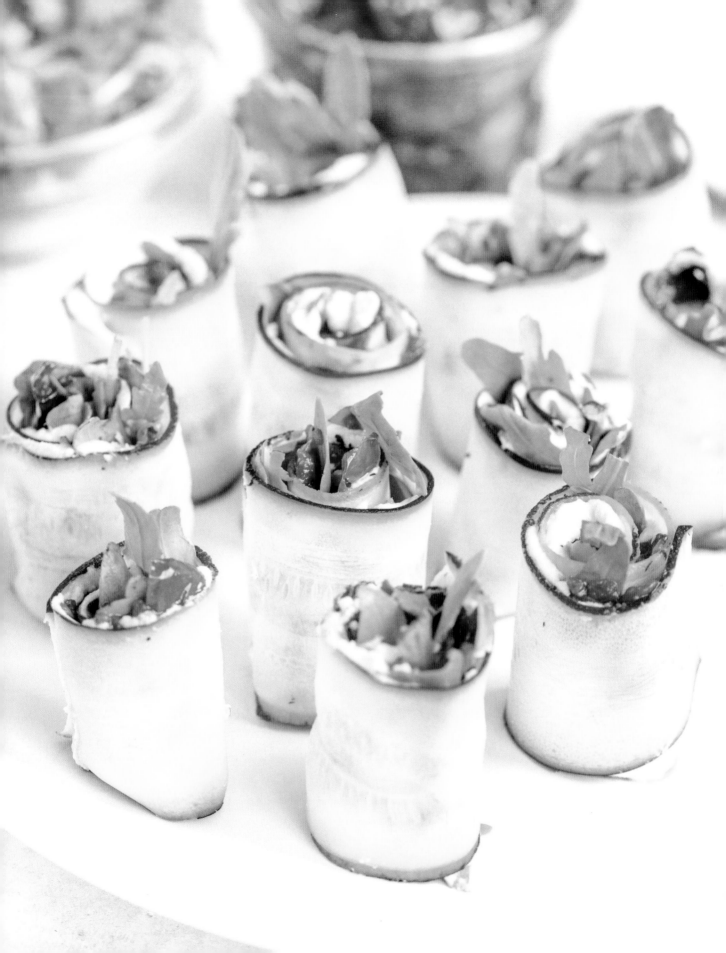

Bacon & Scallion
SPAGHETTI SQUASH FRITTERS

Yield: 12 fritters   **Prep Time:** 20 minutes   **Cook Time:** 18 minutes

Although I originally created this recipe as a fun appetizer, I ended up using the leftovers as a base for a poached egg for breakfast, which was fantastic.

Spicy Dip

½ cup mayonnaise

1 teaspoon paprika

1 teaspoon freshly squeezed lemon juice

½ teaspoon cayenne pepper

Fritters

3 cups cooked spaghetti squash (see sidebar)

2 medium eggs

⅔ cup blanched almond flour

1½ teaspoons Dijon mustard

½ teaspoon cayenne pepper

½ teaspoon ground black pepper

¼ teaspoon salt

⅓ cup chopped cooked bacon, plus 2 tablespoons for garnish, if desired

¼ cup sliced scallions, plus 1 tablespoon for garnish

1½ tablespoons chopped jalapeño peppers

2½ tablespoons extra-virgin olive oil, for frying

1. In a small bowl, whisk together the ingredients for the spicy dip. Set aside.

2. To make the fritters, place the cooked spaghetti squash in a kitchen towel and wring out as much liquid as possible. Set aside.

3. In a bowl, stir the eggs, almond flour, mustard, cayenne pepper, black pepper, and salt until well combined. Next, add the bacon, scallions, and jalapeño. Finally, add the spaghetti squash, stirring gently to ensure you don't break up the strands of "spaghetti."

4. Heat 1 tablespoon of the oil in a medium-sized skillet over medium-high heat. Scoop about 2 tablespoons of batter into the skillet and flatten with a spatula; repeat until you've made 4 fritters. Cook the fritters for 3 minutes per side or until golden brown. Repeat with the remaining batter, adding more oil to the skillet as needed.

5. Garnish with the extra scallions and bacon, if desired, and serve with the spicy dip on the side.

SUBSTITUTIONS: *In place of bacon, use an additional 2 tablespoons of diced bell pepper to make these vegetarian.*

STORAGE: *The fritters will last in the fridge for up to 3 days. Reheat with a splash of olive oil in a skillet for 3 to 4 minutes to crisp them up.*

How to Cook Spaghetti Squash

Preheat the oven to 400°F. Microwave the uncut spaghetti squash for 3 minutes to soften slightly, and then cut the squash in half lengthwise. Scoop out the seeds and stringy pulp, then place the two squash halves on a sheet pan with the cut sides facing up. Drizzle with 1½ teaspoons of extra-virgin olive oil and bake for 40 minutes. Once cooked, remove from the oven and allow to cool slightly before using a fork to scrape out the long strings of "spaghetti." As a general rule, a 4-pound squash will make approximately 5 cups of "spaghetti."

SCD BASICS
Easy 3-Minute Mayonnaise
(page 42)

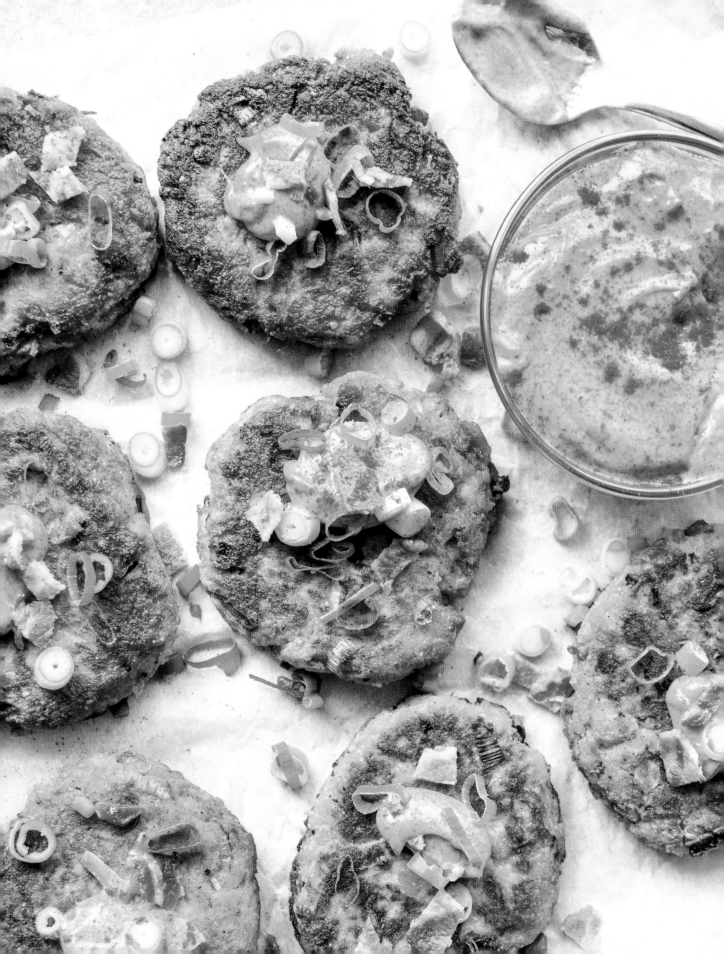

KETO
PALEO
VEGAN
VEGETARIAN
DAIRY-FREE
EGG-FREE
NUT-FREE

Vietnamese
SUMMER ROLLS

Yield: 12 rolls   **Prep Time:** 30 minutes   **Cook Time:** —

These grain-free summer rolls are packed with fresh herbs, crunchy cucumber, carrots, and juicy shrimp, just like the traditional rolls. The only thing that makes them different is the rice-paper wrapper, which I've replaced with thinly sliced daikon radish that gives the rolls a refreshing crunchy texture. These rolls hold up well in the fridge for a couple of days, so make extra to enjoy as an easy snack or packed lunch. Just don't skip the dipping sauce; it's want-to-drink-it-through-a-straw good and really elevates the flavor of these rolls.

Dipping Sauce

3 tablespoons unsweetened, unsalted peanut butter

1 tablespoon toasted sesame oil

1½ teaspoons coconut aminos

1 red chili pepper, such as Fresno

1 (1-inch) piece ginger, peeled

1 teaspoon freshly squeezed lime juice

1 clove garlic, peeled

2 tablespoons water

Summer Rolls

1 long and thin daikon radish

1 large carrot

½ cucumber

12 large cooked shrimp, cut in half lengthwise

6 iceberg or butter lettuce leaves, torn into large pieces

1 large handful fresh Thai basil leaves

1 large handful fresh cilantro leaves

1 large handful fresh mint leaves

3 tablespoons chopped roasted peanuts or cashews, for garnish

SCD BASICS
Coco-not Aminos (page 47)

1. To make the dipping sauce, place all of the sauce ingredients in a blender and pulse until smooth. If the sauce is too thick, add a little more water and blend again. Transfer to a bowl and refrigerate until ready to serve.

2. To make the rolls, wash the daikon radish and use a vegetable peeler to remove the outer skin. Using a cheese slicer (or mandoline), cut thin, wide ribbons running the length of the radish. After a few slices, flip the radish over and continue slicing on the other side until you have a total of 10 to 12 long ribbons. The ribbons should be about 7 inches in length, so trim longer ribbons accordingly.

3. Wash the carrot and cucumber and use a julienne peeler to cut the vegetables into long matchstick-thin pieces about 2 inches long. If you don't have a julienne peeler, you can cut the carrot and cucumber into thin slices, then cut those slices into matchstick-sized strips.

4. To assemble the rolls, lay two ribbons of daikon radish down on a cutting board side by side, allowing them to just slightly overlap lengthwise. Place two shrimp halves at one end of the ribbons, then add 3 carrot strips, 3 cucumber strips, a piece of lettuce, and 2 to 3 leaves each of Thai basil, cilantro, and mint. Lift the end of the daikon ribbons over the filling and press firmly down while tightly rolling up the summer rolls. Place the rolls on a plate with the seam side down and trim any excessively long filling that hangs out either side of the roll. Repeat with the remaining daikon slices and filling ingredients.

5. Sprinkle the rolls and dipping sauce with the chopped peanuts and serve with the dipping sauce on the side.

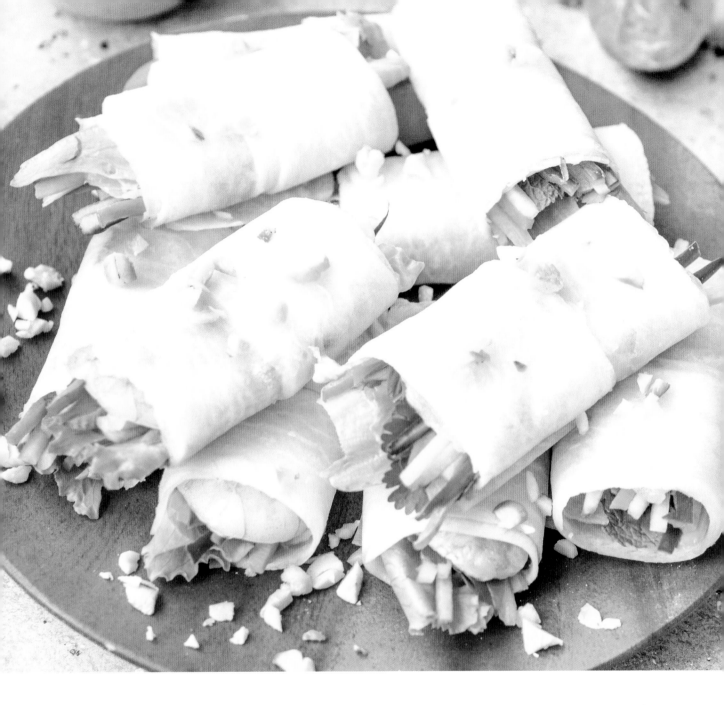

What's Daikon Radish?

Daikon radish is a winter radish that is most commonly used in Asian cooking. You might recognize it as a garnish with sushi. It resembles a massive white carrot, and you can usually find it at most farmers markets or Asian grocery stores.

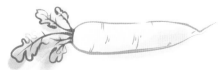

SUBSTITUTIONS: *To make these rolls Paleo, use almond butter for the sauce and cashews as the garnish. To make the rolls vegan or vegetarian, swap the shrimp for thin slices of bell pepper or avocado. To make them nut-free, use sunflower butter in place of nut butter and skip the nut garnish.*

MAKE AHEAD/STORAGE: *The rolls will last in the fridge for up to 2 days. I don't recommend storing the rolls any longer because of the shrimp. The sauce can be made and stored in the fridge up to 4 days in advance and can be stored in the freezer for up to 1 month.*

Crab & Shrimp-Stuffed MUSHROOMS

Make ahead

Yield: 15 mushrooms **Prep Time:** 10 minutes **Cook Time:** 24 minutes

These stuffed mushrooms are a great dish to serve to guests as either an appetizer or side dish. The small pieces of shrimp give the filling some texture, and the crab makes them seem a bit fancy. Use double the amount of shrimp and skip the crab meat for a more economic option.

15 button or cremini mushrooms

4 ounces medium-sized shrimp, peeled and deveined

1½ teaspoons unsalted butter or ghee

1 small shallot, finely diced (about 2 tablespoons)

2 cloves garlic, minced

2 tablespoons mayonnaise

1½ tablespoons thinly sliced scallions, plus extra for garnish

1½ tablespoons chopped fresh Italian parsley, divided

1 teaspoon freshly squeezed lemon juice

½ teaspoon dry mustard

¼ teaspoon salt

¼ teaspoon ground black pepper

Pinch of cayenne pepper

4 ounces fresh crab meat

1. Preheat the oven to 350°F.

2. Remove the stems from the mushrooms and use a spoon to scoop out the gills. Place the mushroom caps on a sheet pan. Chop the shrimp into small pieces.

3. In a medium-sized skillet over medium heat, melt the butter. Add the shallot, garlic, and chopped shrimp and cook for 4 minutes, or until the shrimp is pink and the shallot has softened. Remove the skillet from the heat.

4. In a bowl, stir together the mayonnaise, scallions, 1 tablespoon of the parsley, lemon juice, dry mustard, salt, pepper, and cayenne pepper. Once well mixed, stir in the crab meat and the shrimp mixture.

5. Fill each mushroom cap with a large spoonful of the mixture and bake for 20 minutes, or until the mushrooms have softened. Garnish the stuffed mushrooms with the remaining ½ tablespoon of parsley before serving.

SUBSTITUTIONS: *Use olive oil in place of the butter to make these mushrooms dairy-free.*

MAKE AHEAD/STORAGE: *The filling can be made a day in advance, and you can stuff the mushrooms up to 6 hours before baking. Once baked, they will last in the fridge for up to 3 days and can be quickly reheated in the microwave or oven.*

Avoid Soggy Mushrooms

Whether you're baking mushrooms in the oven or sautéing them in a skillet, for best results, don't crowd the mushrooms! Mushrooms have a high water content, so the moisture they release needs space to evaporate; otherwise, you'll be left with steamed and soggy mushrooms. When in doubt, cook them in small batches.

SCD BASICS
Easy 3-Minute Mayonnaise
(page 42)

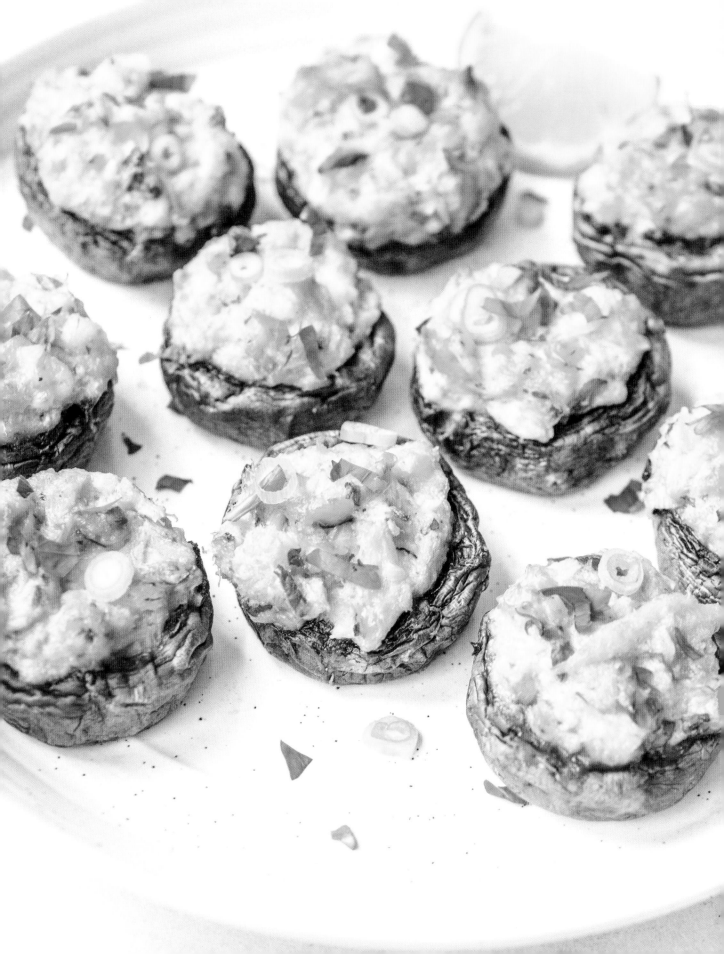

Chicken-Stuffed
JALAPEÑO POPPERS

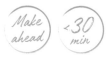

Yield: 20 poppers **Prep Time:** 10 minutes **Cook Time:** 18 minutes

This is a healthy spin on my all-time favorite game day dish. Spicy, creamy, and highly addicting, these poppers are guaranteed to be a big hit with junk food eaters, too!

10 jalapeño peppers

1 tablespoon extra-virgin olive oil

½ cup mayonnaise

¼ cup chopped tomatoes

2 tablespoons thinly sliced scallions, divided

1 tablespoon finely diced red onions

1 teaspoon ground cumin

½ teaspoon paprika

¼ teaspoon salt

¼ teaspoon ground black pepper

1 (4-ounce) boneless, skinless chicken breast, cooked and cut into ¼-inch pieces

1 strip bacon, cooked crisp and minced, for garnish

1. Preheat the oven to 400°F and line a sheet pan with parchment paper.

2. Cut the jalapeños in half lengthwise and remove the seeds. Place the jalapeño halves on the prepared sheet pan and toss them with the oil.

3. Place the mayonnaise, tomatoes, 1 tablespoon of the scallions, red onion, cumin, paprika, salt, and pepper in a medium-sized bowl and stir until well mixed. Add the chicken and stir until well coated. Evenly divide the filling among the jalapeño halves.

4. Bake for 18 minutes, or until the jalapeños have softened and the filling is hot and bubbly. Garnish with the bacon and the remaining 1 tablespoon of scallions before serving.

SUBSTITUTIONS: *Omit the red onion and scallions to make these poppers low-FODMAP.*

MAKE AHEAD/STORAGE: *The filling can be made a day in advance and then spooned into the jalapeño halves and baked for 20 minutes before serving. Leftover poppers will last in the fridge for up to 3 days and can be reheated in the oven or microwave; although the flavors will still be great, the jalapeños may soften slightly.*

SCD BASICS
Easy 3-Minute Mayonnaise
(page 42)

Try This
The chicken filling can also be served cold in lettuce wraps, stuffed in avocado halves, or even baked in the oven and served warm as a dip.

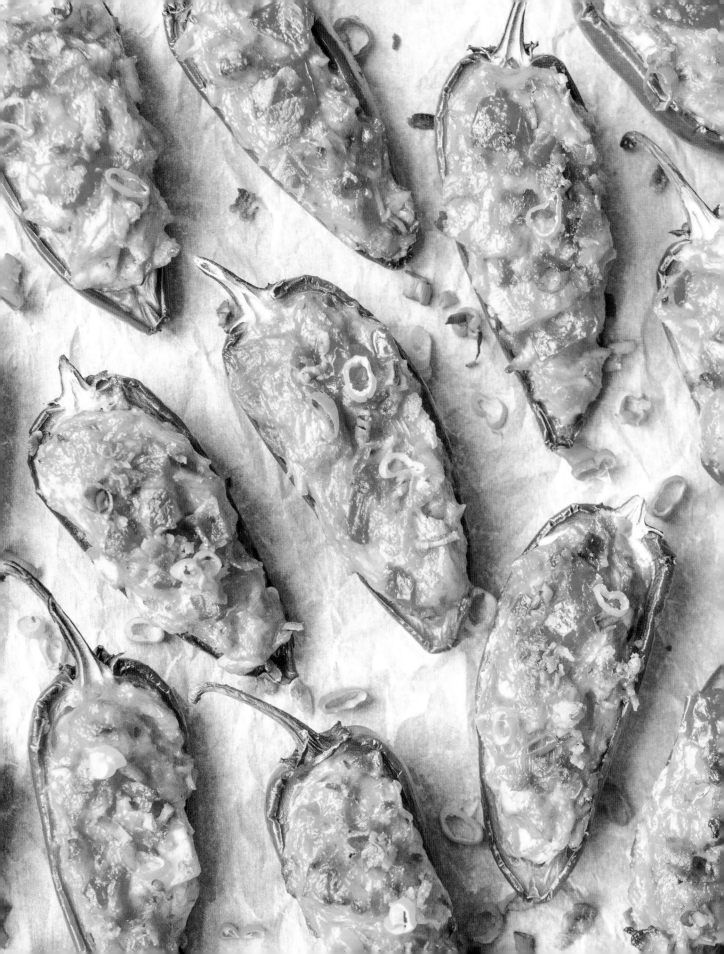

Make ahead

Spicy Orange CHICKEN WINGS

Yield: 4 servings **Prep Time:** 10 minutes **Cook Time:** 25 minutes

Let's be honest: When it comes to chicken wings, it's all about the sauce. These wings are coated in a spicy orange sauce that's sticky and slightly sweet, and it's guaranteed to have you licking your fingers between bites.

1 pound chicken wings

1 tablespoon extra-virgin olive oil

½ teaspoon ground black pepper

¼ teaspoon salt

Spicy Orange Sauce

1½ cups freshly squeezed orange juice, or no-sugar-added store-bought orange juice

⅓ cup honey

2 tablespoons coconut aminos

2 cloves garlic, peeled

1 red chili pepper, such as Fresno

1 (1-inch) piece ginger, peeled

2 tablespoons chopped scallions or cilantro, for garnish

½ teaspoon white sesame seeds (optional), for garnish

1. Preheat the oven to 410°F. Set a wire rack inside a sheet pan.

2. Place the chicken wings in a bowl and toss with the oil, pepper, and salt. Lay the wings evenly on the wire rack. Bake for 20 to 25 minutes, flipping halfway through cooking to ensure they are evenly crispy and golden.

3. While the wings are baking, place all of the spicy orange sauce ingredients in a blender and blend until smooth. Pour the mixture into a small saucepan and simmer for 15 minutes, or until the liquid has reduced by three-fourths to a thick sticky sauce.

4. Place the baked wings in a large bowl and pour the sauce over the top. Toss until the wings are well coated. Serve garnished with scallions or cilantro and sesame seeds and serve.

SUBSTITUTIONS: *Omit the red chili and ground black pepper to make these wings AIP.*

MAKE AHEAD/STORAGE: *If making the wings in advance, store the wings and sauce separately. Baked wings will last in the fridge for up to 4 days. To reheat and re-crisp, toss the wings in the sauce and then bake them on a sheet pan topped with a wire rack in a preheated 350°F oven for 5 to 6 minutes.*

SCD BASICS
Coco-not Aminos
(page 47)

Crisp and Delicious

Using a wire rack is one of my favorite tricks when I'm trying to make something crispy in the oven. It increases airflow around the food, preventing the bottom from becoming mushy and allowing the surface to crisp on all sides. It's a great way to cook bacon, chicken, or sliced veggies that you want to be crispy.

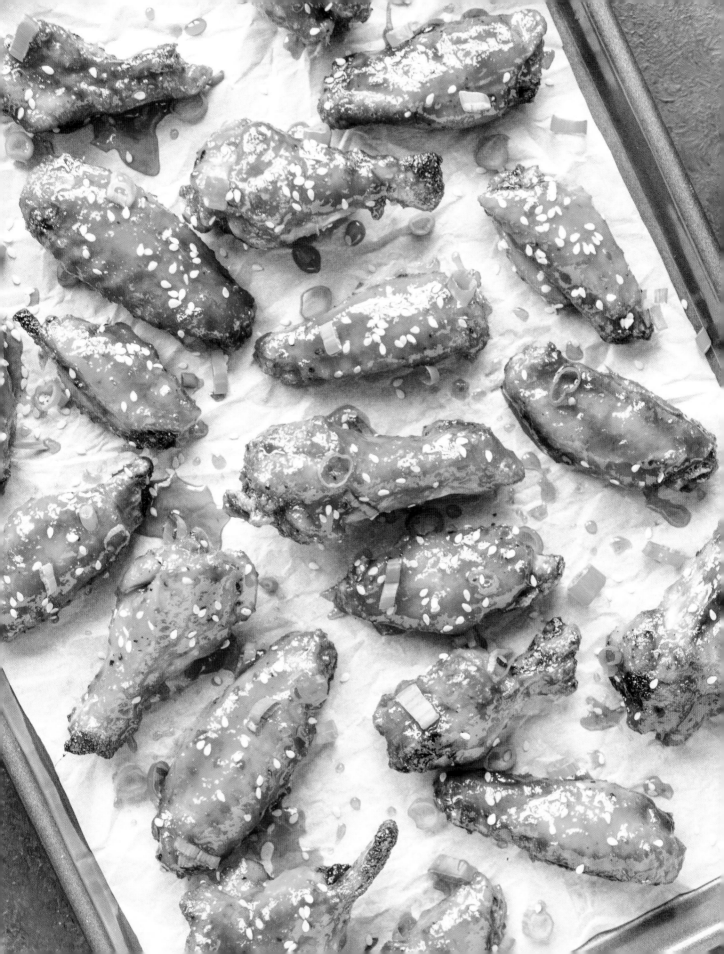

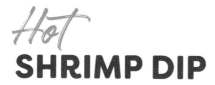

SHRIMP DIP

Yield: 6 servings **Prep Time:** 10 minutes **Cook Time:** 27 minutes

In my view, nothing brings a crowd together faster than a bubbly hot dip. I regularly get requests to bring this shrimp dip to parties, and it's always the first plate to be wiped clean. Although the Parmesan adds a nice cheesy flavor, the Paleo version of this dip—made with nutritional yeast—is just as creamy and delicious, so don't feel like you're missing out. I like serving this with grain-free crackers (page 292) and slices of cucumber, but don't be surprised if you catch people eating it with a spoon, too.

1 cup mayonnaise

½ cup grated Parmesan cheese

¼ cup chopped scallions, plus more for garnish

1½ tablespoons freshly squeezed lemon juice

¼ teaspoon cayenne pepper

1 tablespoon olive oil or avocado oil

½ medium yellow onion, finely diced

½ red bell pepper, finely diced

½ cup chopped tomatoes

1 pound medium-sized shrimp, peeled, deveined, and cut into ¼-inch pieces

3 cloves garlic, minced

1. Preheat the oven to 350°F.

2. In a large bowl, stir together the mayonnaise, Parmesan cheese (or nutritional yeast), scallions, lemon juice, and cayenne pepper.

3. Heat the oil in a medium-sized skillet over medium heat. Add the onion, bell pepper, and tomatoes and cook for about 8 minutes, until soft. Using a slotted spoon, transfer the cooked vegetables into the bowl with the mayonnaise mixture, leaving any excess liquid from the tomatoes in the skillet.

4. Add the shrimp and garlic to the skillet and cook for 3 to 4 minutes, until the shrimp is pink and the garlic is fragrant. Transfer the shrimp and garlic to the bowl and stir until the mixture is well combined.

5. Pour the mixture into a 1-quart ovenproof dish or a 6-inch cast-iron skillet and bake for 15 minutes, until golden and bubbling. Garnish with chopped scallions before serving.

SUBSTITUTIONS: *For low-FODMAP, skip the garlic and onion and use 1 tablespoon garlic-infused oil in place of the olive oil. For Paleo or dairy-free, replace the Parmesan cheese with 2 tablespoons of nutritional yeast.*

MAKE AHEAD/STORAGE: *You can make this dip a day in advance and bake it before serving. Leftovers will last in the fridge for up to 2 days.*

SCD BASICS
Easy 3-Minute Mayonnaise
(page 42)

Seafood Stock
Save the shrimp shells and store them in a zip-top bag in the freezer. Later, you can use them to make a fantastic seafood stock.

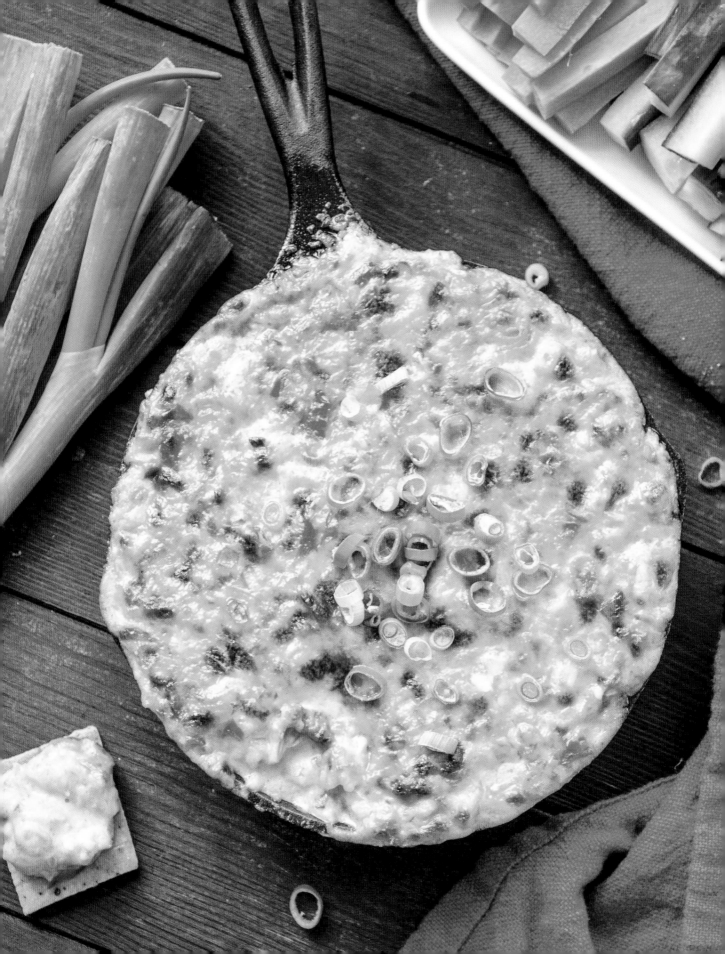

KETO
PALEO
VEGAN
VEGETARIAN
DAIRY-FREE
EGG-FREE

Queso DIP

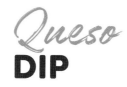

Yield: 6 servings **Prep Time:** 10 minutes **Cook Time:** 20 minutes

This ooey gooey queso is a great party dip to serve to a crowd. It's thick and creamy and great for dipping with veggies or crackers. For a Paleo dairy-free version, you can replace the cheddar cheese with nutritional yeast. This cheesy sauce can also be served over roasted cauliflower or broccoli, on top of tacos or enchiladas, or drizzled over a Mexican salad.

2 cups cauliflower florets

½ cup diced carrots

1 tablespoon extra-virgin olive oil

½ medium yellow onion, finely diced

½ cup diced tomatoes

3 cloves garlic, minced

1 jalapeño pepper, finely chopped

½ cup raw cashews, soaked in boiling water for 10 minutes and drained

⅔ cup unsweetened almond milk

1 tablespoon apple cider vinegar

2 teaspoons chipotle paste

1½ teaspoons ground cumin

1 teaspoon salt

⅓ cup shredded cheddar cheese

For Garnish (Optional)

2 tablespoons finely chopped tomatoes

1 jalapeño pepper, sliced

2 tablespoons fresh cilantro leaves

1 tablespoon sliced scallions

1. Place the cauliflower florets and carrots in a medium-sized saucepan with ½ inch of water, cover with a lid, and steam for 8 to 10 minutes (alternatively, you can use a steamer basket), until they are fork-tender. While the cauliflower and carrots are steaming, prepare the rest of the vegetables.

2. Warm the oil in a medium-sized skillet over medium heat. Add the onion, tomatoes, garlic, and jalapeño and sauté for 8 to 10 minutes, until the onion is translucent and the tomatoes are tender.

3. Drain the steamed cauliflower and carrots and place in a blender; transfer the sautéed vegetables to the blender.

4. Add the cashews to the blender along with the almond milk, vinegar, chipotle paste, cumin, and salt and blend until smooth.

5. Pour the mixture into the skillet, add the cheese, and heat over medium heat until the cheese has melted. If desired, garnish with the chopped tomatoes, jalapeño slices, cilantro, and scallions.

SUBSTITUTIONS: *Omit the carrots to make this dip keto. For Paleo, vegan, or dairy-free, replace the cheese with 3 tablespoons of nutritional yeast.*

MAKE AHEAD/STORAGE: *You can make the dip up to 2 days in advance. Leftovers will last in the fridge for up to 4 days. The queso can be reheated for 2 minutes in the microwave or in the oven for 10 minutes at 350°F until heated through.*

SCD BASICS
Chipotle Paste (page 34)

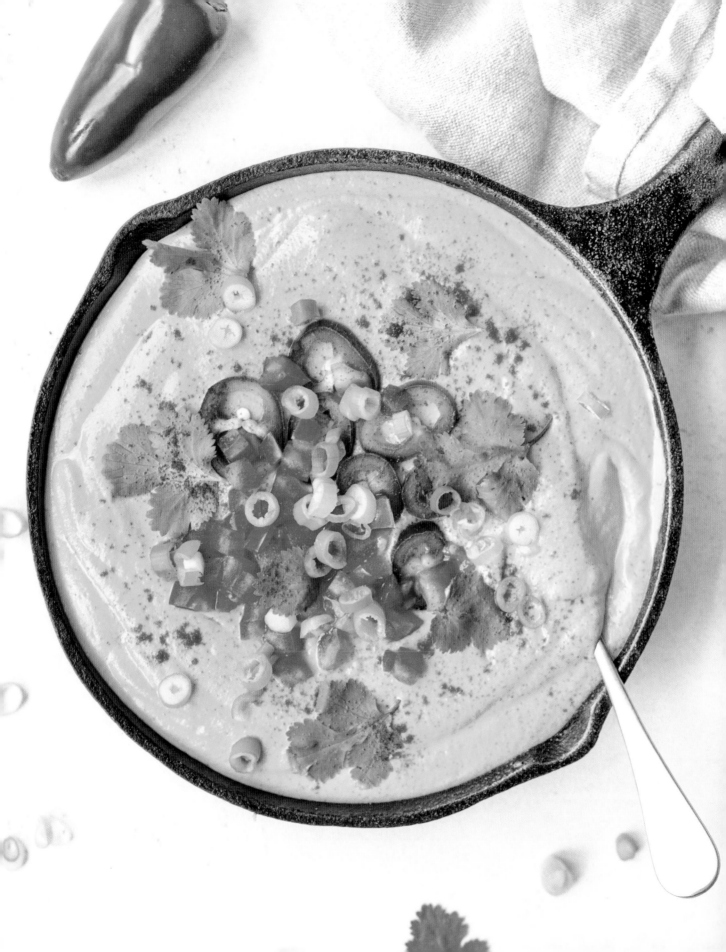

Make ahead

Salmon Gravlax & "CREAM CHEESE" PLATTER

Yield: 8 servings   **Prep Time:** 25 minutes, plus 2 days to cure   **Cook Time:** —

I love salmon gravlax, but it can be a struggle to find any that is sugar- and nitrate-free. Curing salmon at home is incredibly easy: just a few minutes of hands-on work and two days of resting to allow the salt to draw the moisture out of the fish. You can serve the gravlax with scrambled egg on Butternut Squash Toast (page 56), on Celery Root Latkes (page 122) for a fun appetizer, or as part of this impressive platter.

Salmon Gravlax

2 tablespoons grated lemon zest

1 tablespoon black peppercorns

1 tablespoon coriander seeds

¾ cup rock salt

⅔ cup chopped fresh dill, divided

1 pound salmon fillets, skin removed

Cashew "Cream Cheese"

½ cup raw cashews, soaked in boiling water for 10 minutes and drained

2 tablespoons freshly squeezed lemon juice

1 tablespoon apple cider vinegar

¾ teaspoon coconut cream

½ teaspoon salt

For the Platter

½ cucumber, thinly sliced

6 radishes, thinly sliced

1 lemon, cut into wedges

½ medium red onion, thinly sliced

2 tablespoons capers

Seeded Crackers (page 292)

1 tablespoon chopped fresh chives, for garnish

1½ teaspoons black or pink peppercorns

SPECIAL EQUIPMENT
High-powered blender

1. To make the gravlax, place the lemon zest, peppercorns, and coriander seeds in a spice grinder or mortar and pestle and grind into a fine texture. Transfer it to a small bowl, add the rock salt, and stir until well mixed.

2. Lay a large piece of plastic wrap on the counter and spread about half of the salt mixture into a shape about the size of the salmon. Top with a layer of half of the dill and place the salmon on top. Spread the remaining dill over the salmon, then top with the remaining salt mixture.

3. Pull the plastic wrap up and over the salmon to seal it as tightly as possible in a small parcel. Place the wrapped salmon in a dish in which it fits snugly, then put a heavy object (such as a wine bottle or pot) on top. Allow to cure in the fridge for 48 hours. Flip the parcel over every 12 hours.

4. After 2 days, the salmon should feel very firm to the touch. Unwrap the parcel and use a damp paper towel to brush off the salt cure. Then thinly slice the salmon, transfer to a serving platter, and garnish with the chives.

5. An hour before serving, make the "cream cheese": Place the cashews, lemon juice, vinegar, coconut cream, and salt in a high-powered blender and blend until completely smooth. Transfer to the fridge to firm up for a minimum of 1 hour.

6. Serve the gravlax with the sliced vegetables, lemon, capers, cream cheese, and crackers arranged around it on the platter. Sprinkle with the peppercorns.

SUBSTITUTIONS: *For keto and low-FODMAP, swap the cashews for blanched almonds or macadamia nuts. For low-FODMAP, omit the red onion from the platter.*

STORAGE: *Once cured, the gravlax will last in the fridge for up to 5 days or in the freezer for up to 2 months. The "cream cheese" also freezes well; just blend it for a few seconds in a blender after it's thawed to lighten the texture.*

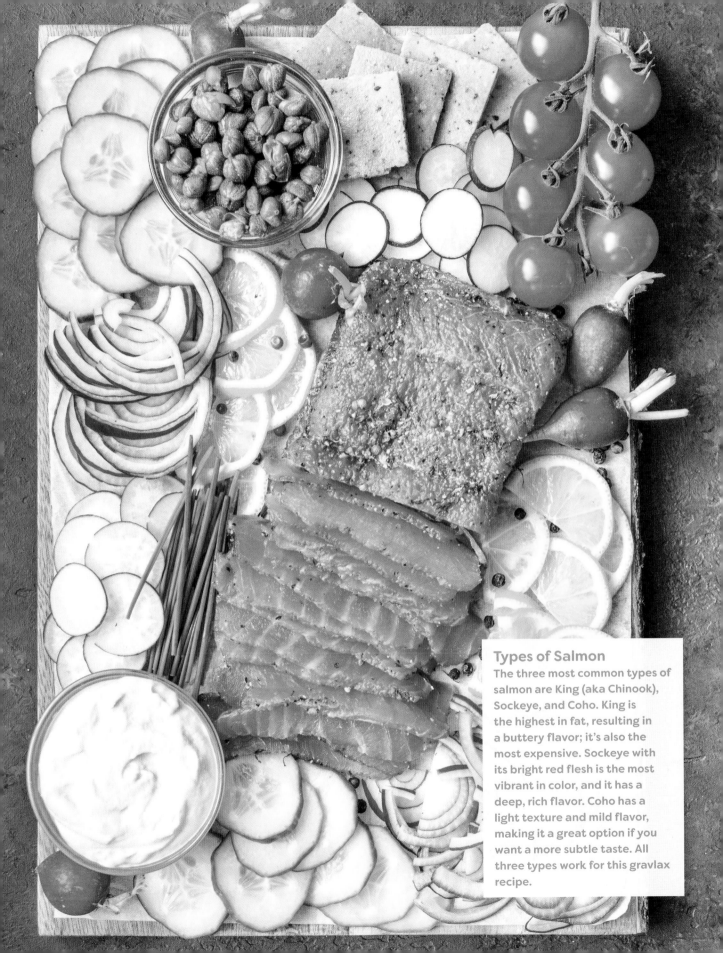

Types of Salmon

The three most common types of salmon are King (aka Chinook), Sockeye, and Coho. King is the highest in fat, resulting in a buttery flavor; it's also the most expensive. Sockeye with its bright red flesh is the most vibrant in color, and it has a deep, rich flavor. Coho has a light texture and mild flavor, making it a great option if you want a more subtle taste. All three types work for this gravlax recipe.

Celery Root Latkes
WITH GRAVLAX

Yield: 6 servings   **Prep Time:** 15 minutes   **Cook Time:** 16 minutes

Latkes become a thing of the past when you're on a potato-free diet—or so I thought. After creating the Salmon Gravlax & "Cream Cheese" recipe (page 120) for this book, I knew that I had to find a way to make latkes because cream cheese and gravlax-topped latkes is a combination not to be missed. Celery root is a fantastic replacement for potatoes because it binds together when shredded and has a mild flavor. These latkes reheat well, so you can warm the leftovers in the oven before serving; try them as hash browns topped with an egg for breakfast.

1 small celery root (1½ to 2 pounds)

1 medium yellow onion

2 medium eggs

½ cup blanched almond flour

½ teaspoon paprika

½ teaspoon ground black pepper

¼ cup light olive oil or avocado oil

1 teaspoon flaked sea salt

For Serving

½ batch Cashew "Cream Cheese" (page 120)

½ batch Salmon Gravlax (page 120)

¼ red onion, thinly sliced

1 tablespoon capers

1 teaspoon chopped fresh chives

1. Peel the celery root and use the largest holes on a box grater to shred it until you have 4 cups; reserve any remaining celery root for another use. (You may find it easier to handle the celery root if it's cut in halves or quarters before grating.) Place the shredded celery root in a large bowl.

2. Using the largest holes on the box grater, grate the onion and add it to the bowl with the celery root. Add the eggs, almond flour, paprika, and pepper and stir until well mixed.

3. Heat the oil in a large nonstick skillet over medium-high heat. Form the shredded celery root mixture into small patties, about 2 inches in size, gently squeezing out any liquid with your hands as you flatten them. Making the patties small helps to ensure that they hold together when cooking and flipping.

4. Place half of the flattened patties in the skillet and cook for 4 minutes, or until golden; then gently flip and cook for another 4 minutes. Transfer the cooked latkes to a paper towel and season with ½ teaspoon of the flaked sea salt. Repeat with the remaining latkes and flaked sea salt.

5. To serve the latkes, top them with a small spoonful of cream cheese, a piece of gravlax, sliced red onion, capers, and chives.

STORAGE: *These latkes will last in the fridge for up to 2 days.*

Flaked Sea Salt

Flaked sea salt is a fantastic finishing salt that elevates the flavors of both sweet and savory dishes. The salt flakes are crunchy and have a clean taste. You can substitute fleur de sel, but it has a slightly stronger taste. My preferred brand of flaked sea salt is Maldon.

Fried Capers

After you have finished frying the latkes, while the oil in the skillet is still hot, add the capers and cook them for 2 to 3 minutes before transferring to a paper towel to cool. The capers become light and crispy and are highly addicting. Serve them on the latkes, or you can use them as a flavorful garnish for fish.

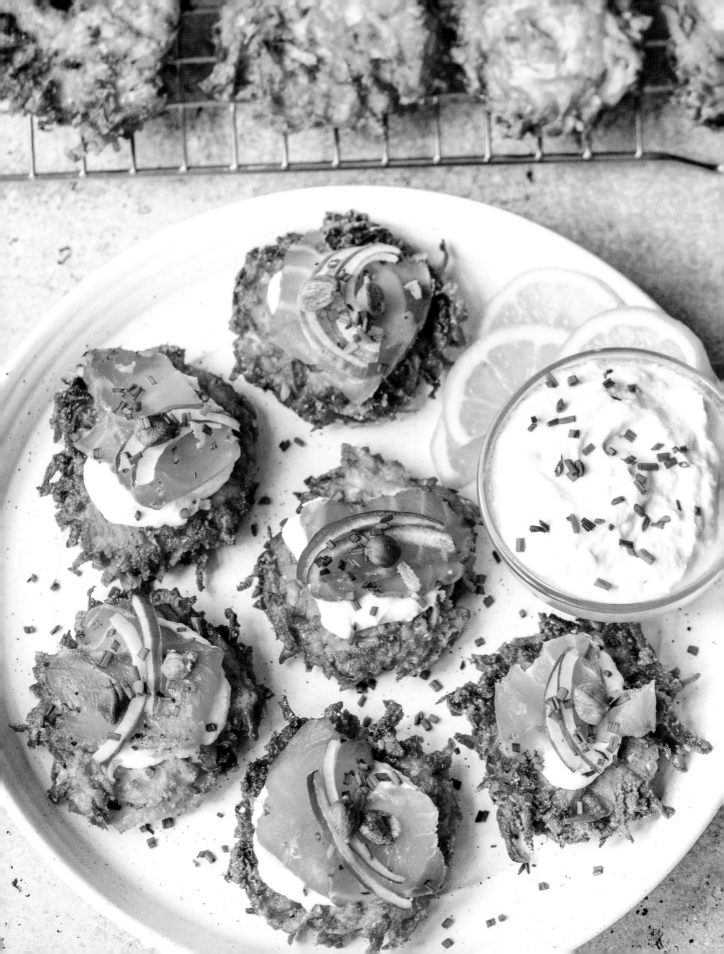

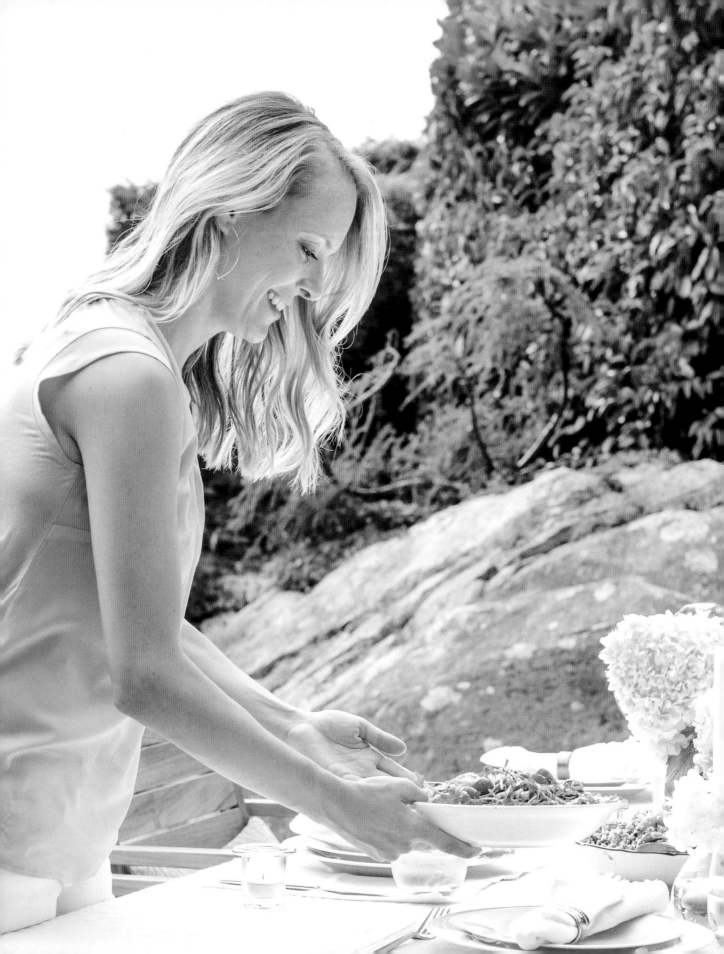

Salads

PALEO
VEGAN
VEGETARIAN
DAIRY-FREE
EGG-FREE
NUT-FREE

Charred Snap Pea & Bacon Salad with
CREAMY HERB DRESSING

Yield: 4 servings   **Prep Time:** 10 minutes   **Cook Time:** 5 minutes

My mom had a massive vegetable garden that produced an abundance of snap peas each summer. I remember the frustration in her voice after she picked yet another basket of crunchy peas: "What the heck am I supposed to do with even more of these?" She got creative in some good (and not-so-good) ways, but her charred pea salad was always a favorite. The trick is to leave some of the snap peas raw, giving you a wonderful contrast in texture and flavor. This summer salad, made with radishes, peas, shallot, and a variety of herbs, is a great way to showcase fresh produce from your garden (or the farmers market).

Creamy Herb Dressing

¼ cup mayonnaise

2 tablespoons extra-virgin olive oil

2 tablespoons apple cider vinegar

1 teaspoon Dijon mustard

2 tablespoons chopped fresh tarragon

1 tablespoon chopped fresh mint

1 tablespoon chopped fresh dill

½ teaspoon ground black pepper

¼ teaspoon salt

1 pound sugar snap peas, divided

1½ teaspoons extra-virgin olive oil

1 cup thinly sliced radishes (about 5 ounces whole radishes)

5 strips bacon, cooked and chopped

1 shallot, finely diced

1 tablespoon chopped fresh dill, for garnish

1. To make the dressing, whisk together the mayonnaise, oil, vinegar, and mustard in a small bowl. Add the chopped herbs and stir until well combined. Season with the pepper and salt, then set the dressing aside.

2. Heat a grill pan or medium-sized skillet over high heat until very hot. In a bowl, toss half of the sugar snap peas with the oil until well coated. Place the peas on the grill pan or skillet and cook for 2 minutes, until grill marks form, then flip and cook on the other side for another minute.

3. Transfer the cooked peas to a salad bowl and add the remaining raw peas, radishes, bacon, and shallot. When ready to serve, toss the salad in the herb dressing and garnish with the chopped dill.

SUBSTITUTIONS: *Omit the bacon and use Egg-Free Mayonnaise (page 40) to make this salad vegan.*

MAKE AHEAD/STORAGE: *If making them ahead, store the dressing and salad separately and toss right before serving. Once tossed with the dressing, the salad will last in the fridge for up to 2 days.*

SCD BASICS
Easy 3-Minute Mayonnaise
(page 42)

Storing Herbs
To extend the life of fresh leafy herbs like mint, dill, parsley, and cilantro, store them in the fridge in a glass or jar with the stems in an inch of water.

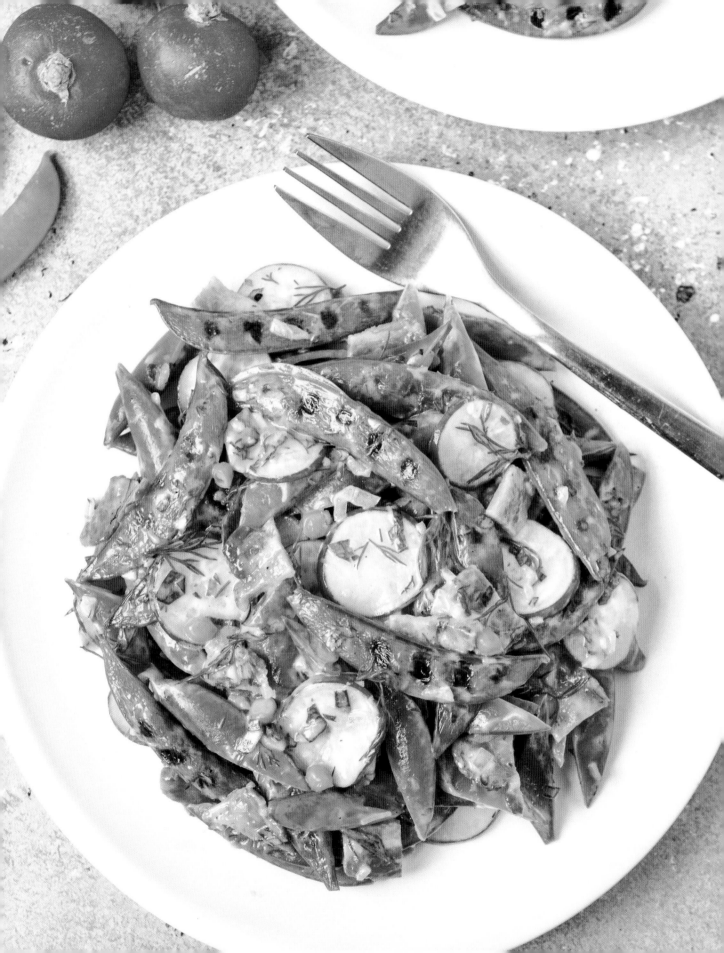

KETO
PALEO
VEGAN
VEGETARIAN
DAIRY-FREE
EGG-FREE
NUT-FREE

Make ahead   < 30 min

Roasted Broccoli, Butternut Squash & Kale
SALAD WITH CREAMY ROASTED GARLIC DRESSING

Yield: 4 servings   **Prep Time:** 10 minutes   **Cook Time:** 20 minutes

This is my favorite warm winter salad. The veggies are roasted until tender and slightly caramelized and then added to the salad and coated with a creamy roasted garlic dressing. I love kale-based salads because they don't go mushy like a lettuce base, so you can enjoy leftovers for a day or two.

1 head broccoli, cut into small florets

3 cups cubed butternut squash

1 red onion, cut into thick slices

1 bulb garlic

1½ tablespoons extra-virgin olive oil

½ teaspoon plus 1 pinch salt, divided

1 bunch Tuscan ("dino") kale, destemmed and chopped into bite-size pieces

⅓ cup raw almonds, roughly chopped

Creamy Roasted Garlic Dressing

Cloves from 1 bulb roasted garlic (from above)

⅓ cup extra-virgin olive oil

2 tablespoons aged balsamic vinegar, or 1 tablespoon red wine vinegar

½ teaspoon ground black pepper

1 medium egg yolk (optional)

1. Preheat the oven to 425°F.

2. Place the broccoli florets, butternut squash, and red onion on a sheet pan. Cut the top one-third off of the garlic bulb to expose the top of the cloves and place on the sheet pan. Drizzle the vegetables and exposed garlic cloves with the oil and season with the salt. Bake for 20 minutes, or until the squash is tender and the garlic has softened.

3. Place the kale in a salad bowl and sprinkle the leaves with a pinch of salt. Massage the kale leaves by scrunching them between your hands for about 1 minute. The kale will become softer and darker. Set aside.

4. To make the dressing, squeeze the cloves out of the roasted head of garlic and place them in a blender. Add the oil, vinegar, pepper, and egg yolk (if using). Blend until smooth and creamy.

5. To assemble the salad, top the kale with the roasted butternut squash, broccoli, and red onion. Then top with the chopped almonds and toss with the roasted garlic dressing.

SUBSTITUTIONS: *For keto, reduce the butternut squash to 1 cup. Omit the egg yolk to make the salad vegan. Swap the almonds for pepitas to make it nut-free.*

MAKE AHEAD/STORAGE: *If making it ahead, store the dressing and salad separately and toss right before serving. Once tossed with the dressing, the salad will last in the fridge for up to 2 days.*

Massaging Kale
Massaging kale might seem like an unnecessary step, but it makes a massive difference in the texture of the leaves. By scrunching the kale between your hands for about a minute, the leaves become soft, tender, and less bitter.

SCD BASICS
SCD Balsamic Vinegar (page 46)

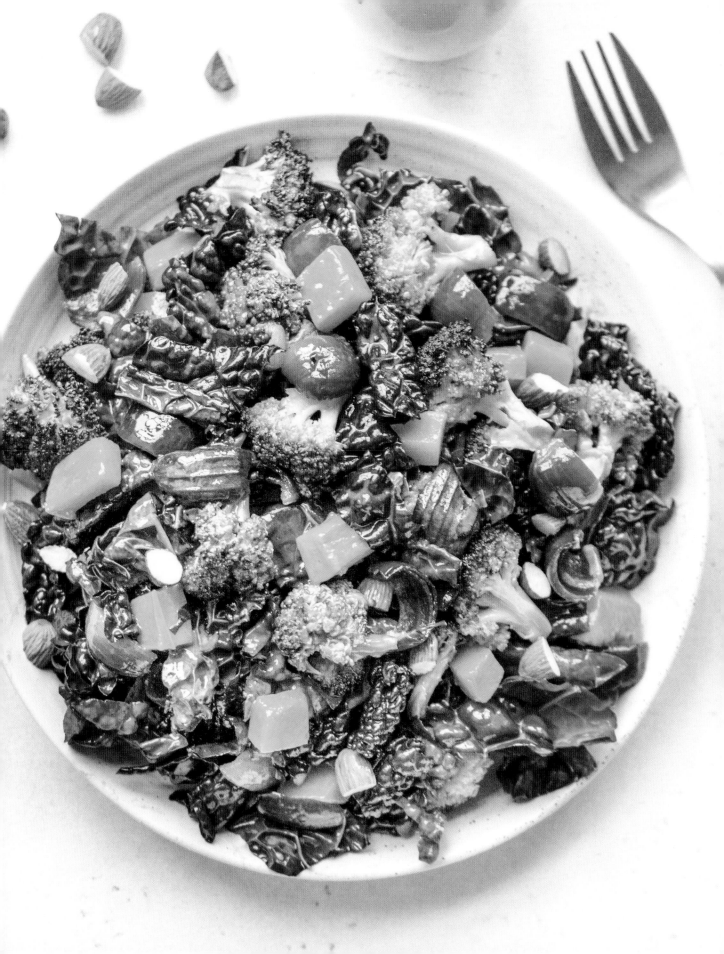

KETO
LOW-FODMAP
PALEO
VEGAN
VEGETARIAN
DAIRY-FREE
EGG-FREE
NUT-FREE

Cajun Shrimp
CAESAR SALAD

Yield: 4 servings   **Prep Time:** 15 minutes   **Cook Time:** 20 minutes

I love Caesar salad but wanted to come up with a recipe for one with a unique spin. I switched up the base by using finely shredded kale, Brussels sprouts, and romaine lettuce; this combination gives the salad a lot more texture (and more places for the dressing to coat!). The dressing, which is made with tahini, has a deliciously creamy consistency, and it's lighter and less oily then traditional egg- or mayonnaise-based Caesar dressings. Finally, the salad is topped with spicy Cajun-spiced shrimp and crunchy hazelnut "croutons" that really pack a punch.

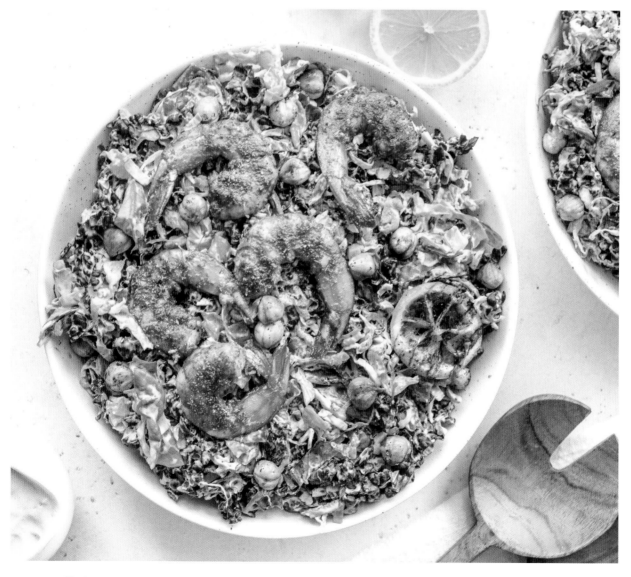

Cajun Shrimp and Croutons

1 teaspoon ground dried oregano

1 teaspoon paprika

¾ teaspoon ground black pepper

½ teaspoon salt

½ teaspoon ground dried thyme

¼ teaspoon cayenne pepper

⅓ cup blanched hazelnuts

2 tablespoons extra-virgin olive oil, divided

12 large shrimp, peeled and deveined

½ lemon

Salad Base

6 leaves Tuscan ("dino") kale

Pinch of salt

10 to 12 Brussels sprouts, or 2 cups packaged shredded Brussels sprouts

1 medium head romaine lettuce, or 2 cups packaged shredded romaine lettuce

Caesar Dressing

⅓ cup tahini

¼ cup water, plus more if needed

1 tablespoon Dijon mustard

2 cloves garlic, peeled

2 tablespoons freshly squeezed lemon juice

1½ teaspoons red wine vinegar, or 2 tablespoons aged balsamic vinegar

2 teaspoons capers

½ teaspoon ground black pepper

Grilled Lemon

Grilled lemon halves make a great garnish for salads or for serving alongside grilled fish or meat. Simply cut a lemon in half and grill it on a BBQ or grill pan on medium-high heat for 8 to 10 minutes until grill marks form.

SCD BASICS
SCD Balsamic Vinegar (page 46)

1. Preheat the oven to 350°F.

2. In a small bowl, mix together the oregano, paprika, pepper, salt, thyme, and cayenne pepper.

3. To make the "croutons," place the hazelnuts on a sheet pan, drizzle with 1 tablespoon of the oil and 1 teaspoon of the spice mixture, and toss until the nuts are well coated. Bake for 20 minutes, stirring halfway through baking to ensure they brown evenly.

4. While the hazelnuts are baking, place the shrimp in a medium-sized bowl, drizzle with the remaining 1 tablespoon of oil, and sprinkle with the remaining spice mixture. Toss to coat, then set aside to marinate while you prep the rest of the salad.

5. To prepare the base of the salad, remove the stems of the kale and finely shred the leaves. You will have about 2 cups. Place the shredded kale in a salad bowl, sprinkle with a pinch of salt, and massage the leaves for about a minute by scrunching them between your hands until the leaves become softer and darker.

6. To shred the Brussels sprouts, you can use the shredding disc on a food processor or cut them by hand. To cut them by hand, halve the Brussels sprouts and then use a box grater to shred each half. (You should have about 2 cups.) Place the shredded Brussels sprouts in the salad bowl with the kale. To shred the romaine lettuce, cut the head in half lengthwise and then thinly slice each half. When you have about 2 cups, add it to the salad bowl.

7. To make the dressing, put all of the dressing ingredients in a blender and blend until smooth. If the dressing is too thick, add a little more water and blend again.

8. Heat a medium-sized skillet over medium-high heat. Place the shrimp in the skillet and cook for 2 minutes, or until the shrimp turn pink, then flip and cook for another minute. Squeeze the juice from the lemon over the shrimp, then remove the pan from the heat.

9. To serve, toss the salad greens with the dressing, then top with the toasted hazelnuts and sautéed shrimp.

SUBSTITUTIONS: *Omit the garlic and Brussels sprouts and increase the kale and romaine to 3 cups each to make it low-FODMAP. Skip the shrimp and add some avocado to make this dish vegan and vegetarian. For nut-free, use pepitas in place of hazelnuts.*

Spicy Shrimp, Avocado & PEACH SALAD

Yield: 2 servings   **Prep Time:** 10 minutes   **Cook Time:** 3 minutes

This salad is summer in a bowl. It's packed with sweet sliced peaches, avocado, spicy jalapeño pepper, and shrimp that are quickly marinated in a sweet and spicy–chipotle chili sauce and then sautéed until pink. This is one of those salads that I could eat again and again without ever becoming bored because it's so flavorful.

2 tablespoons freshly squeezed lime juice

2 tablespoons extra-virgin olive oil

1 tablespoon honey

1 teaspoon chipotle chili powder

1 teaspoon ground cumin

½ teaspoon ground black pepper

¼ teaspoon salt

12 large shrimp or 8 prawns, peeled and deveined

2 peaches

1 avocado

1 small red onion

1 jalapeño pepper

6 cups torn butter, Bibb, or romaine lettuce leaves

1. In a bowl, whisk together the lime juice, oil, honey, chipotle chili powder, cumin, pepper, and salt. Add the shrimp to the bowl, toss gently until well coated, and set aside to marinate for 10 minutes.

2. While the shrimp are marinating, prepare the rest of the salad. Cut the peaches and avocado into wedges and thinly slice the red onion and jalapeño. Arrange all of the fruit and vegetables in a salad bowl with the lettuce.

3. Heat a medium-sized skillet over medium-high heat. Spoon the marinated shrimp with the marinade into the skillet and cook for 1 to 2 minutes, until the shrimp turn pink. Then flip the shrimp and cook for another minute.

4. Top the salad with the shrimp and pour the sauce from the pan over the salad as a dressing. This salad is best served immediately.

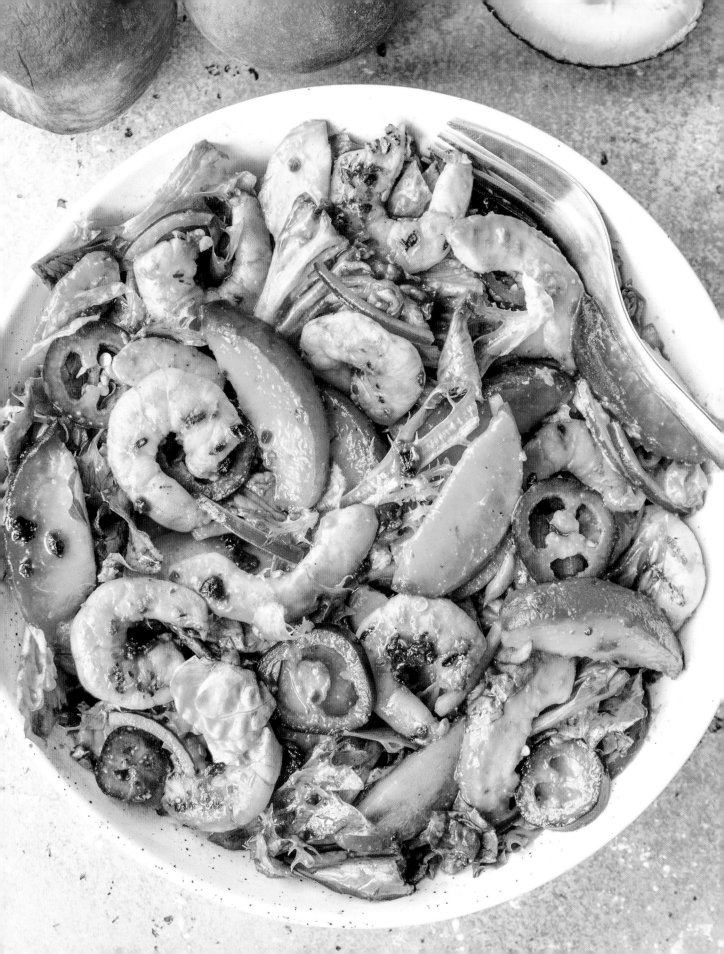

Sun-Dried Tomato, Chicken & Cauliflower Salad
WITH CREAMY BALSAMIC DRESSING

Make ahead   **<30 min**

Yield: 4 servings   **Prep Time:** 10 minutes   **Cook Time:** 20 minutes

This recipe has quickly become my go-to summer salad to bring to cookouts. Roasted cauliflower makes the perfect blank canvas base for a salad; and in this recipe, it's mixed with sun-dried tomatoes, chicken, and spinach and coated in a creamy balsamic and roasted garlic dressing.

1 large or 2 small heads cauliflower

1 bulb garlic

1 tablespoon extra-virgin olive oil

1¼ cups spinach, roughly chopped

1 (4-ounce) boneless, skinless chicken breast, cooked and cut into bite-sized pieces

½ small red onion, thinly sliced

½ cup oil-packed sun-dried tomatoes, roughly chopped

⅓ cup pine nuts, toasted, plus more for garnish

Creamy Balsamic Dressing

⅓ cup mayonnaise

2 tablespoons aged balsamic vinegar

¼ teaspoon salt

¼ teaspoon ground black pepper

Cloves from 1 bulb roasted garlic (from above)

1. Preheat the oven to 350°F.

2. Cut the cauliflower into bite-sized florets and place them on a sheet pan. Cut the top one-third off of the garlic bulb to expose the cloves. Place the bulb on the sheet pan and drizzle it and the cauliflower with the oil. Bake for 20 minutes, or until the cauliflower is tender and golden and the garlic cloves are soft. Set the cauliflower and garlic aside to cool slightly.

3. To make the dressing, put the mayonnaise, vinegar, salt, and pepper in a blender. Squeeze the cloves out of the roasted bulb of garlic into the blender and blend until completely smooth.

4. Transfer the roasted cauliflower to a salad bowl. Add the spinach, chicken, onion, sun-dried tomatoes, and pine nuts. Pour the dressing over the salad and toss until well coated. Garnish with pine nuts before serving.

SUBSTITUTIONS: *o make it vegan, skip the chicken, use Egg-Free Mayonnaise (page 40), and omit the roasted garlic because the mayonnaise already has a strong garlic flavor. Skip the chicken to make this salad vegetarian. T*

MAKE AHEAD/STORAGE: *If you make them ahead, store the dressing and salad separately, for up to 5 days, and toss right before serving. Once tossed in the dressing, the salad will last in the fridge for up to 3 days.*

SCD BASICS
Easy 3-Minute Mayonnaise (page 42)

SCD Balsamic Vinegar (page 46)

Sun-Dried Tomatoes (page 38)

Roasting Garlic

When roasted in the oven, the strong flavor of garlic mellows, and it becomes deliciously caramelized and sweet. Roast a few extra bulbs of garlic, squeeze the cloves out of the skins, and store them in extra-virgin olive oil in the fridge for up to 2 weeks. You can add the garlic to salad dressings, sauces, or dips or use it to flavor mayonnaise.

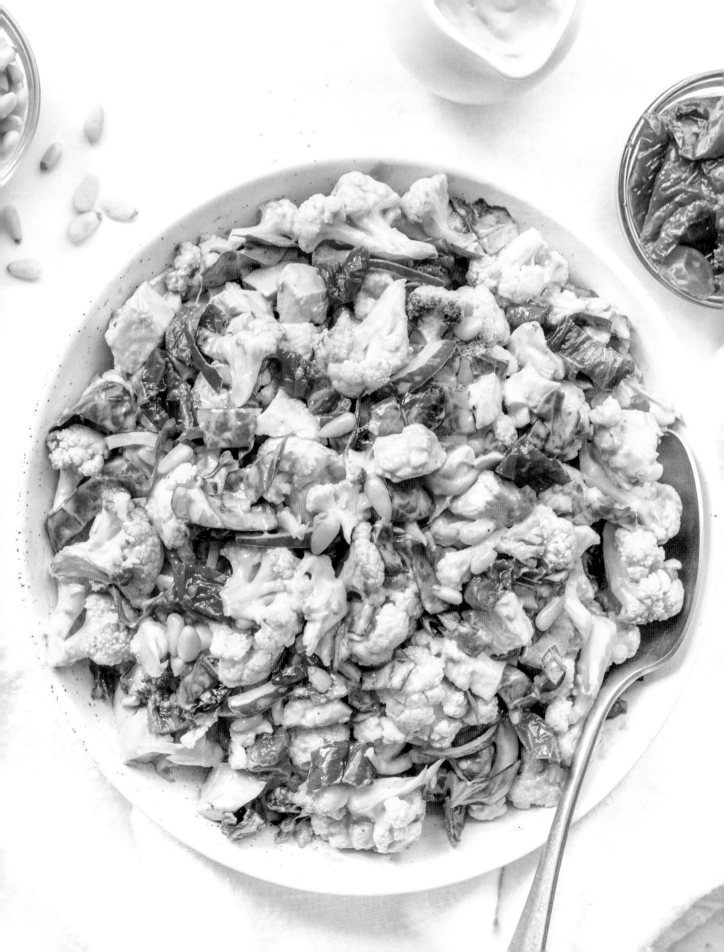

KETO
LOW-FODMAP
PALEO
DAIRY-FREE
EGG-FREE
NUT-FREE

Chicken, Avocado & Bacon Salad with
RANCH DRESSING

Yield: 2 servings   **Prep Time:** 15 minutes   **Cook Time:** 14 minutes

This is a great recipe for anyone who says salads can't be a meal. It's packed with all the good stuff—crispy bacon, flavorful marinated chicken, avocado, and a deliciously creamy ranch dressing that is egg- and dairy-free. The dressing will last for up to 5 days in the fridge and is great for amping up a simple salad or for serving as dip with veggies.

2 tablespoons extra-virgin olive oil

2 tablespoons apple cider vinegar

2 cloves garlic, minced

½ teaspoon paprika

½ teaspoon ground black pepper

¼ teaspoon salt

4 boneless, skinless chicken thighs

6 to 8 cups roughly chopped romaine or Bibb lettuce

1 cup cherry tomatoes, halved

½ small red onion, thinly sliced

½ cup thinly sliced cucumbers

1 avocado, halved and thinly sliced

6 strips bacon, cooked and chopped

Ranch Dressing

¼ cup tahini

2 tablespoons freshly squeezed lemon juice

1 teaspoon Dijon mustard

1 clove garlic, peeled

¼ cup water

2 tablespoons chopped fresh dill

1 tablespoon chopped fresh chives

1 tablespoon chopped fresh Italian parsley

1. In a large bowl, whisk together the oil, vinegar, garlic, paprika, pepper, and salt. Add the chicken thighs and allow to marinate for 10 minutes.

2. Meanwhile, make the dressing: Place the tahini, lemon juice, mustard, garlic, and water in a blender and blend until smooth. If the dressing seems too thick, add more water to thin it out. Transfer the dressing to a bowl, then stir in the chopped herbs. Set aside.

3. Heat a large skillet over medium-high heat. Add the marinated chicken thighs plus any excess marinade to the skillet and cook for 6 to 7 minutes per side, until the chicken is golden and cooked through.

4. While the chicken is cooking, assemble the rest of the salad ingredients: Place the lettuce in a salad bowl, then top with the tomatoes, red onion, cucumbers, avocado, and bacon.

5. Once the chicken is cooked, slice the thighs into strips and add them to the salad.

6. Wait until right before serving to toss the salad in the dressing because this salad is best served immediately.

SUBSTITUTIONS: *Omit the red onion and garlic to make this salad low-FODMAP.*

MAKE AHEAD/STORAGE: *The dressing will last in the fridge for up to 5 days. If you make the components ahead, store the dressing and salad separately in the fridge for up to 5 days and toss right before serving.*

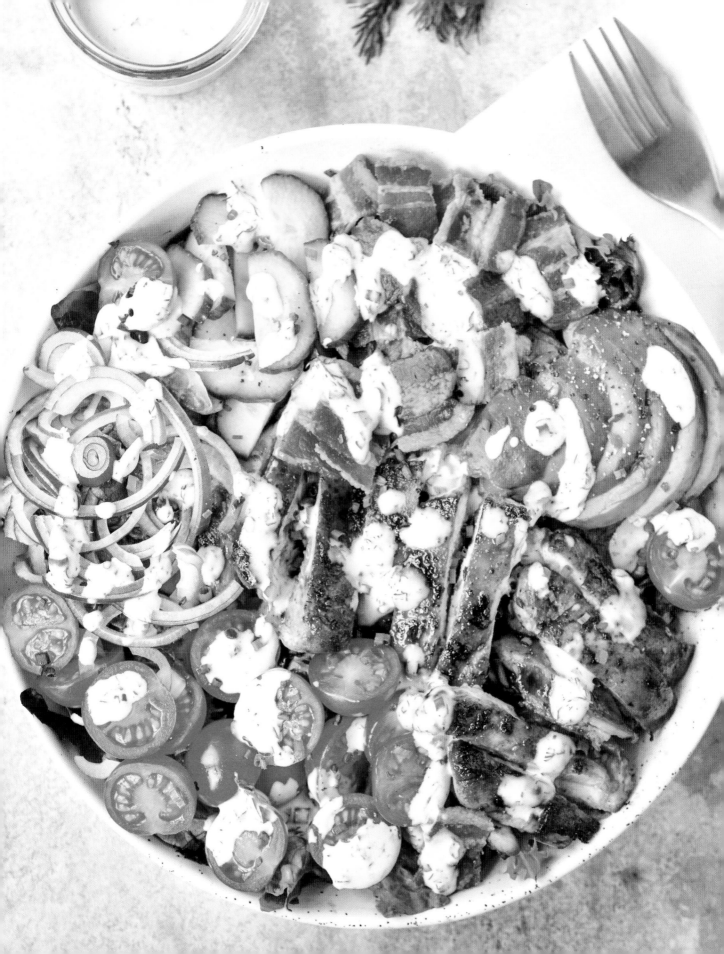

AIP
KETO
PALEO
DAIRY-FREE
EGG-FREE
NUT-FREE

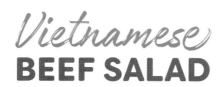

Vietnamese
BEEF SALAD

Make ahead

Yield: 2 servings **Prep Time:** 25 minutes, plus 30 minutes to marinate **Cook Time:** 3 minutes

I love the combination of fresh herbs and spicy flavors in this Vietnamese salad. It's a great make-ahead dish; just prep all the components, including cooking the beef, and then assemble individual salads throughout the week. Julienned daikon radish adds a refreshing crunch, but don't stress if you can't find any; thinly sliced radishes also work.

Marinade/Dressing

¼ cup apple cider vinegar

2 tablespoons honey

1 lemon grass stalk, tougher outer leaves and top removed

1 (1-inch) piece ginger, peeled

1 tablespoon toasted sesame oil

1 tablespoon fish sauce

2 cloves garlic, peeled

12 ounces beef steak (sirloin, rump, or filet), cut into ¼-inch-thick slices

1 large carrot

1 small cucumber

½ daikon radish (about 1 pound)

4 cups shredded romaine or butter lettuce

1 shallot, thinly sliced

¼ cup shredded fresh mint leaves, plus more leaves for garnish if desired

1½ teaspoons avocado oil

For Garnish

1 lime, cut into wedges

1 red chili pepper, such as Fresno, thinly sliced

¼ cup chopped toasted cashews

1 tablespoon chopped fresh cilantro (optional)

1 tablespoon chopped Thai basil

1. Put all of the ingredients for the marinade in a blender and blend until smooth. Place the beef in a container or zip-top bag, pour half of the marinade over the top, and allow to marinate for at least 30 minutes or up to 4 hours. Store the remaining marinade in the fridge to use as a salad dressing.

2. Prepare the vegetables for the salad: Use a julienne peeler to cut the carrot, cucumber, and daikon radish into long thin strips. Divide the lettuce, carrot, cucumber, radish, shallot, and mint between 2 serving bowls.

3. Heat the avocado oil in a large skillet over high heat. Once hot, add the marinated beef and cook for 2 to 3 minutes, until the beef is lightly browned on the edges and still pink in the center. Work in batches to cook the beef if you don't have a large enough pan; overcrowding will prevent the meat from browning.

4. Once the beef is cooked, divide between the serving bowls. Drizzle the reserved dressing over the top and garnish with the lime, red chili pepper, cashews, cilantro, and additional mint (if using). Serve immediately.

SUBSTITUTIONS: *Use olive oil in place of the sesame oil and skip the chili pepper and cashew garnishes for AIP. For keto, omit the honey and carrot. For nut-free, skip the cashew garnish. If you aren't a fan of fish sauce, I suggest adding ½ teaspoon salt to the marinade for a similar salty flavor.*

MAKE AHEAD/STORAGE: *This salad can be made up to 2 days in advance, but you should store the meat and vegetables/herbs separately. Once tossed, the salad should be eaten immediately.*

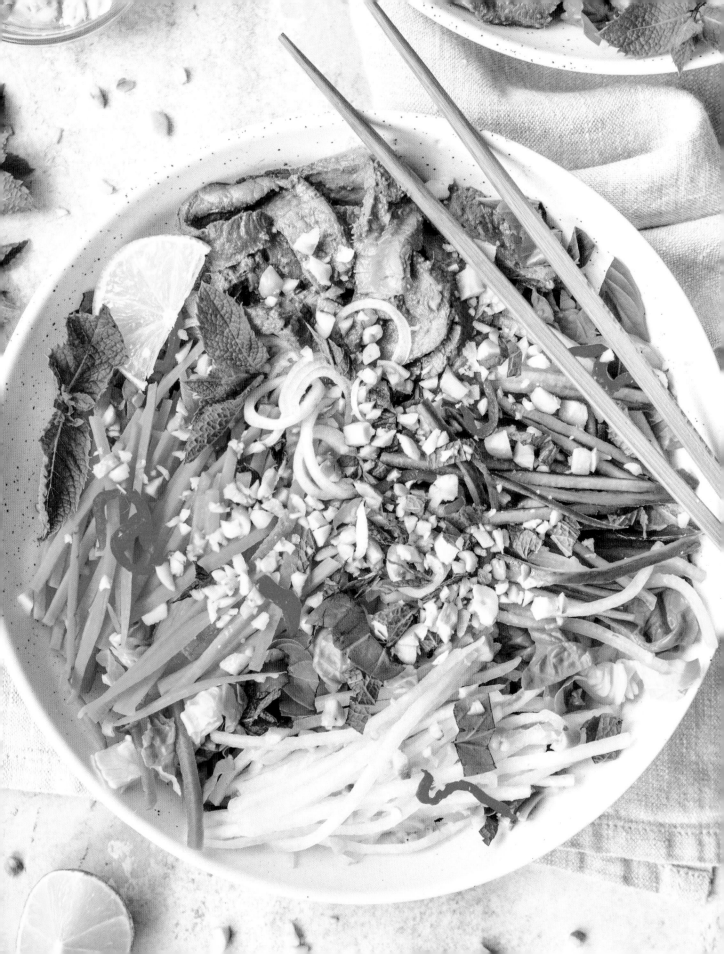

Moroccan "COUSCOUS" SALAD

Make ahead

Yield: 4 servings **Prep Time:** 15 minutes, plus 10 minutes to rest **Cook Time:** 17 minutes

This salad is made of finely riced raw cauliflower, which has a similar texture and consistency to couscous. On multiple occasions, I've served this salad to groups of friends who devoured it and thought it was couscous until I admitted otherwise. I recommend tossing the cauliflower "couscous" with the dressing 10 minutes before serving to give the raw cauliflower time to soften.

2 medium zucchini

2 bell peppers (preferably 1 red and 1 orange or yellow)

1 tablespoon extra-virgin olive oil

1 small head cauliflower

½ red onion, finely diced

½ cup sliced almonds, toasted

⅓ cup chopped fresh Italian parsley, plus more for garnish

¼ cup dried apricots, cut into small pieces

Dressing

⅓ cup extra-virgin olive oil

¼ cup aged balsamic vinegar, or 1½ tablespoons red wine vinegar

½ teaspoon ground black pepper

¼ teaspoon salt

1. Preheat the oven to 350°F.

2. Cut the zucchini and bell peppers into ½-inch-wide strips. Place on a sheet pan, drizzle with the oil, and bake for 15 to 17 minutes, until the vegetables begin to soften. (Alternatively, you can cook them on a barbecue grill.)

3. While the veggies are baking, make the "couscous": Cut the cauliflower into large chunks and put in a food processor. Pulse for about 10 seconds, until it is all broken down to a uniform size and resembles couscous. (See the tip; you should have 3 to 3½ cups.) Transfer the couscous to a salad bowl.

4. Once the zucchini and bell pepper strips are cooked, allow to cool before cutting them crosswise into ½-inch pieces; add to the salad bowl with the couscous. Add the red onion, toasted almonds, parsley, and apricots.

5. To prepare the dressing, whisk the oil, vinegar, pepper, and salt in a bowl, then drizzle over the salad. Toss to combine and garnish with more parsley before serving.

SUBSTITUTIONS: *For AIP, skip the almonds and replace the bell peppers with more red onion. For keto, omit the dried apricots. Skip the almonds to make the salad nut-free.*

MAKE AHEAD/STORAGE: *You can make this salad and toss with the dressing up to a day in advance, but store the toasted sliced almonds separately and add right before serving so that they remain crunchy. Leftovers will last in the fridge for up to 3 days.*

Cauliflower "Couscous"

Cauliflower couscous has a very fine texture, which is much easier to digest when raw than cauliflower rice. If you are using premade cauliflower rice, place it in a food processor and pulse for 5 seconds to break it into finer "couscous." Whenever you're serving cauliflower in raw form, I recommend using cauliflower "couscous" rather than cauliflower rice.

SCD BASICS
SCD Balsamic Vinegar (page 46)

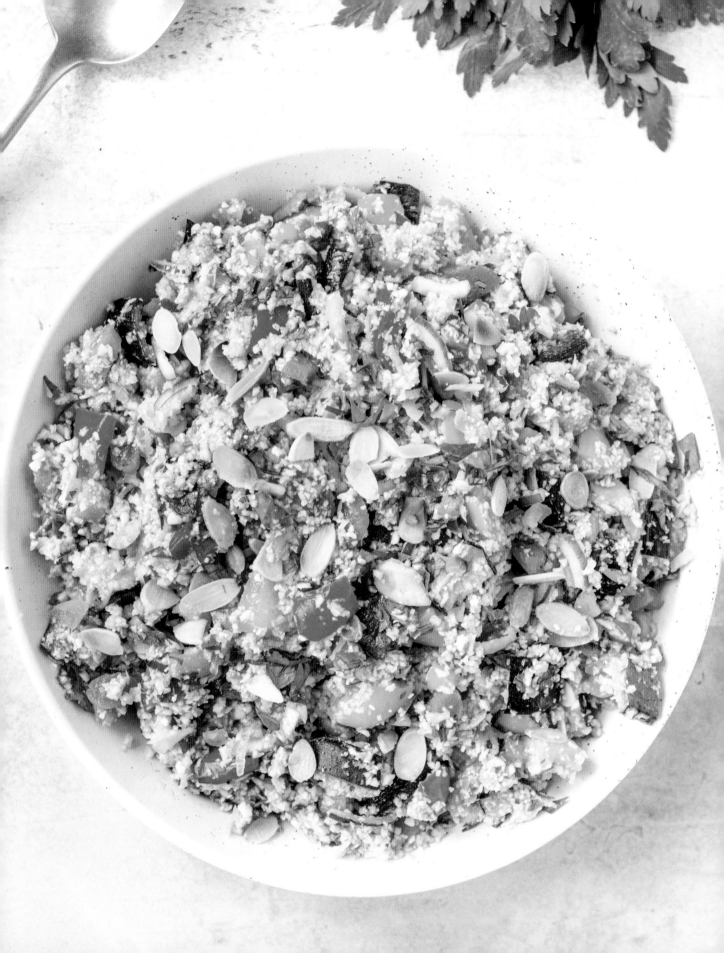

KETO
PALEO
VEGAN
VEGETARIAN
DAIRY-FREE
EGG-FREE
NUT-FREE

Roasted Cauliflower, Date, Red Onion &
PARSLEY SALAD

Yield: 4 servings   **Prep Time:** 10 minutes   **Cook Time:** 20 minutes

The ingredients in this salad might seem like a weird combination (cauliflower and dates?), but when tossed in a tart lemon and tahini dressing, the flavors combine amazingly well. As one of my blog readers said, the dates add the perfect sweetness. You can serve this warm as a side dish or at room temperature as a salad—it works well either way—and if you don't have any dates, you can use ⅓ cup of raisins instead.

1 medium head cauliflower, cut into florets

1 tablespoon extra-virgin olive oil

1 teaspoon dried oregano leaves

½ teaspoon paprika

¼ teaspoon salt

½ cup chopped fresh Italian parsley

⅓ cup chopped dates

¼ cup thinly sliced red onions

¼ cup pine nuts, toasted

Lemon Tahini Dressing

2 tablespoons extra-virgin olive oil

1 tablespoon tahini

½ teaspoon grated lemon zest

1 teaspoon freshly squeezed lemon juice

1 teaspoon apple cider vinegar

¼ teaspoon salt

¼ teaspoon ground black pepper

1. Preheat the oven to 400°F.

2. In a bowl, toss the cauliflower florets in the oil, then sprinkle with the oregano, paprika, and salt. Use your hands to toss the florets to make sure they are evenly coated with the seasoning. Place the cauliflower on a sheet pan and roast for 20 minutes, or until the cauliflower is tender and golden.

3. Meanwhile, make the dressing: In a bowl, whisk together the oil, tahini, lemon zest, lemon juice, vinegar, salt, and pepper. Set aside.

4. Transfer the cooked cauliflower to a salad bowl and add the parsley, dates, red onion, and pine nuts. Pour the vinaigrette over the top and toss until coated. Serve warm or at room temperature.

SUBSTITUTIONS: *For keto, omit the dates.*

MAKE AHEAD/STORAGE: *If making ahead, I recommend keeping the parsley on the side and adding it just before serving to prevent it from wilting. Leftovers will last in the fridge for up to 3 days.*

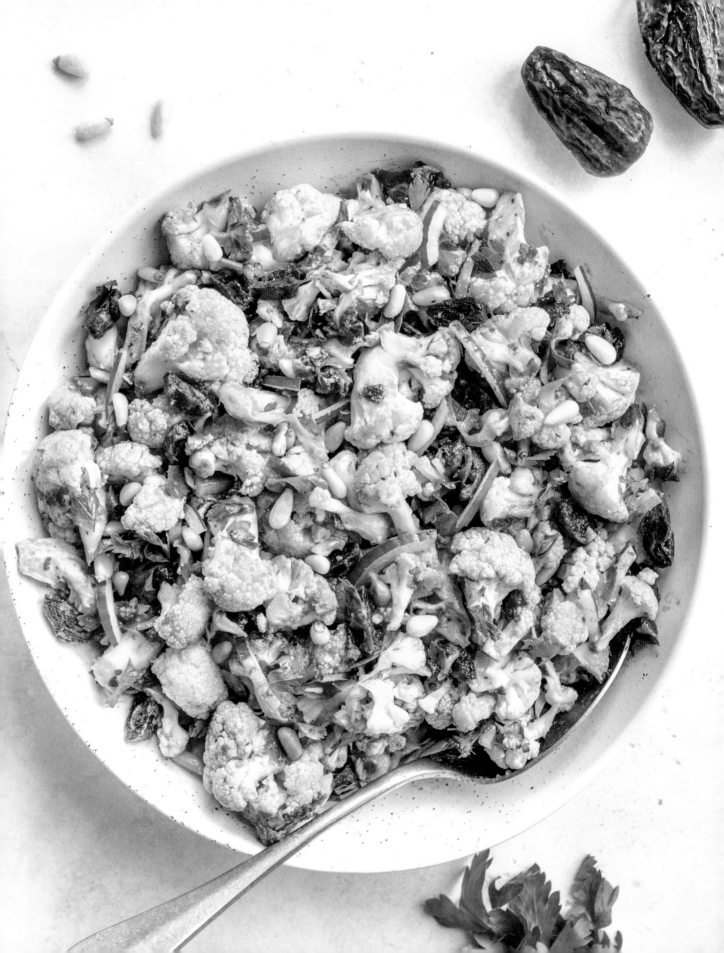

Roasted Butternut Squash & Red Onion Salad with
ORANGE CINNAMON DRESSING

Yield: 4 servings   **Prep Time:** 10 minutes   **Cook Time:** 20 minutes

Have you ever tried adding cinnamon to salad dressing? It adds an unexpected warmth and a bit of spice to the dressing to jazz up even the simplest salad. If you're hesitant to eat raw cauliflower due to tummy concerns, I recommend tossing the cauliflower "couscous" in dressing a few hours in advance; the dressing helps to soften the cauliflower, making it easier to digest.

1 large red onion, cut into thick slices

2 cups cubed butternut squash (about ½-inch cubes)

1½ teaspoons extra-virgin olive oil

1 small head cauliflower

⅓ cup roughly chopped fresh Italian parsley

⅓ cup roughly chopped fresh mint

Orange Cinnamon Dressing

⅓ cup extra-virgin olive oil

1 teaspoon grated orange zest

2 tablespoons freshly squeezed orange juice

1 tablespoon apple cider vinegar

½ teaspoon ground cinnamon

½ teaspoon ground black pepper

¼ teaspoon salt

1. Preheat the oven to 425°F.

2. Place the red onion and butternut squash on a sheet pan. Drizzle with the oil and roast for 20 minutes, or until the squash is tender.

3. While the veggies are roasting, cut the cauliflower into large chucks and place in a food processor. Pulse for about 10 seconds, until it is all broken down to a uniform size and resembles couscous. (You should have 3 to 3½ cups.) Transfer the couscous to a salad bowl.

4. To make the dressing, whisk together the oil, orange zest, orange juice, vinegar, cinnamon, pepper, and salt in a small bowl.

5. Transfer the roasted butternut squash and red onion to the salad bowl with the cauliflower "couscous." Add the parsley and mint and toss the salad in the dressing before serving.

MAKE AHEAD/STORAGE: *The salad can be made and dressed up to 2 hours before serving for the best results. Leftovers can be stored in the fridge for up to 2 days.*

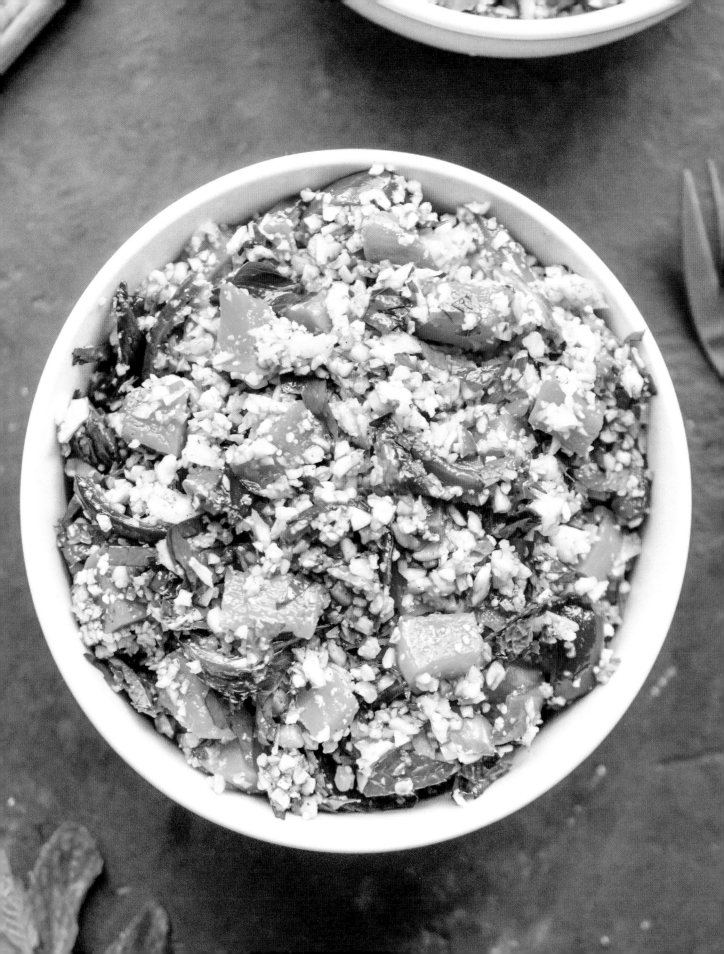

Make ahead

Chipotle Butternut
SQUASH SALAD

Yield: 4 servings **Prep Time:** 20 minutes **Cook Time:** 20 minutes

Baked butternut squash is a fantastic base for a Mexican-inspired salad because it adds a slightly sweet flavor without overpowering the rest of the ingredients. This salad holds up well over a few days, so it's a great make-ahead dish to bring to a summer cookout or potluck. Everyone always goes crazy for the creamy three-ingredient dressing, which packs a lot of flavor.

4 cups cubed butternut squash (about 1½ pounds squash)

2 tablespoons extra-virgin olive oil

1 tablespoon ground cumin

1 teaspoon paprika

½ teaspoon salt

1 red onion, diced

1 red bell pepper, diced

1 cup chopped tomatoes

¾ cup chopped scallions, plus more for serving

½ cup roughly chopped fresh cilantro

1 to 2 jalapeño peppers, thinly sliced

Dressing

½ cup mayonnaise

1½ tablespoons freshly squeezed lime juice

2 teaspoons chipotle chili powder, or 1½ teaspoons chipotle paste

¼ teaspoon salt

1. Preheat the oven to 350°F.

2. Peel the butternut squash, then cut it into ½-inch cubes; you should have about 4 cups. Place the squash in a bowl and toss it with the oil, cumin, paprika, and salt. Spread out the squash on a sheet pan and bake for 20 minutes, or until the butternut squash is tender (but not mushy). Remove from the oven and allow to cool.

3. To make the dressing, whisk together the mayonnaise, lime juice, chipotle chili powder, and salt in a small bowl.

4. In a salad bowl, gently toss the roasted butternut squash, red onion, bell pepper, tomatoes, scallions, cilantro, jalapeño, and dressing. Sprinkle with chopped scallions before serving.

SUBSTITUTIONS: *Skip the onion to make this salad low-FODMAP.*

MAKE AHEAD/STORAGE: *The dressing and salad can be made a day in advance but should be stored separately. Once tossed with the dressing, the salad will last in the fridge for up to 3 days.*

SCD BASICS
Chipotle Paste (page 34)
Easy 3-Minute Mayonnaise (page 42)

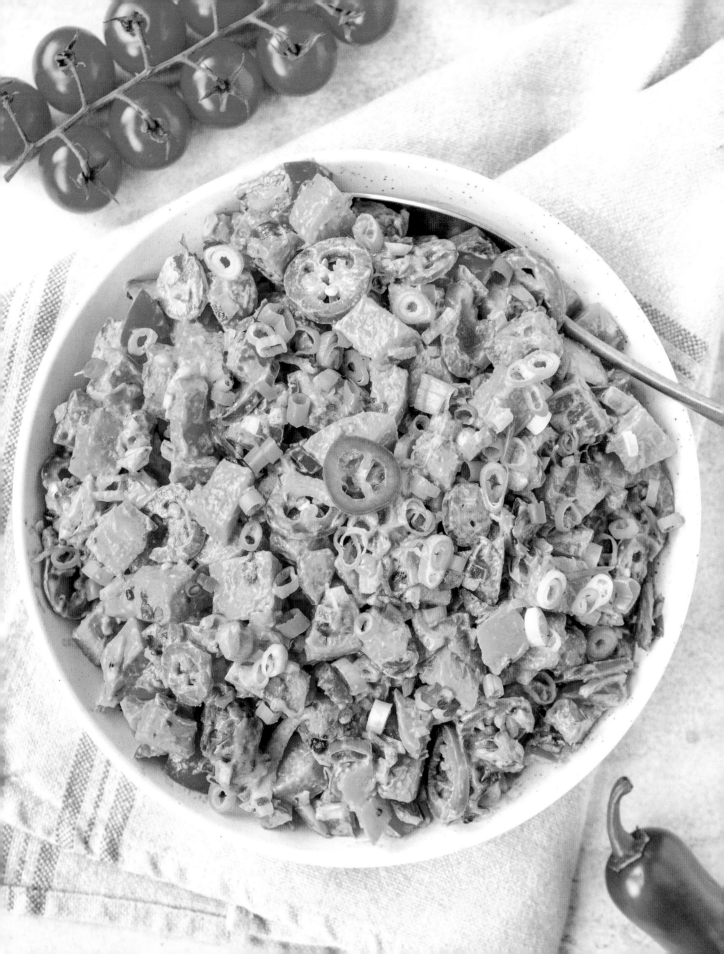

KETO
LOW-FODMAP
PALEO
VEGAN
VEGETARIAN
DAIRY-FREE
EGG-FREE
NUT-FREE

Make ahead

Roasted Pepper, TOMATO & BASIL SALAD

Yield: 4 servings   **Prep Time:** 20 minutes   **Cook Time:** 35 minutes

This salad is my spin on peperonata, an Italian dish made with stewed (or in this case oven-roasted) bell peppers, which are tossed with fresh vegetables and a light garlicky dressing. It's a fantastic summer dish that you can leave in the fridge and enjoy over a few days. Although you don't have to use a variety of bell peppers, the three vibrant colors really make this dish pop.

1 red bell pepper

1 orange bell pepper

1 yellow bell pepper

1½ teaspoons extra-virgin olive oil

1 cup halved cherry tomatoes

⅓ cup pitted Kalamata olives, quartered

3 tablespoons pine nuts, toasted

½ medium red onion, thinly sliced

⅓ cup shredded fresh basil, plus more for garnish

Dressing

1 tablespoon extra-virgin olive oil

1 teaspoon capers, drained and roughly chopped

1 teaspoon red wine vinegar

1 clove garlic, minced

½ teaspoon ground black pepper

Vitamin C
Gram for gram, red bell peppers contain three times the amount of vitamin C as oranges.

1. Preheat the oven to 400°F.

2. Place the bell peppers on a sheet pan, drizzle with the oil, and roast for 35 minutes, flipping halfway through, until they are blistered and slightly charred on all sides.

3. Remove the pan from the oven, invert a bowl over the charred bell peppers, and let rest for 10 minutes. (The trapped steam will make peppers much easier to peel.)

4. To make the dressing, whisk together the oil, capers, vinegar, garlic, and black pepper in a small bowl. Set aside.

5. Peel the skin off the peppers, slice them in half, and remove the stems and seeds. Cut the peppers into thin strips.

6. Place the sliced bell peppers, tomatoes, olives, pine nuts, onion, and basil in a salad bowl. Drizzle the dressing over the top, toss until well mixed, and then garnish with a sprinkle of basil.

SUBSTITUTIONS: *To make the salad low-FODMAP, skip the garlic and onion and replace the extra-virgin olive oil in the dressing with garlic-infused oil. For nut-free, swap the pine nuts for sunflower seeds.*

STORAGE: *Leftovers will last in the fridge for up to 3 days.*

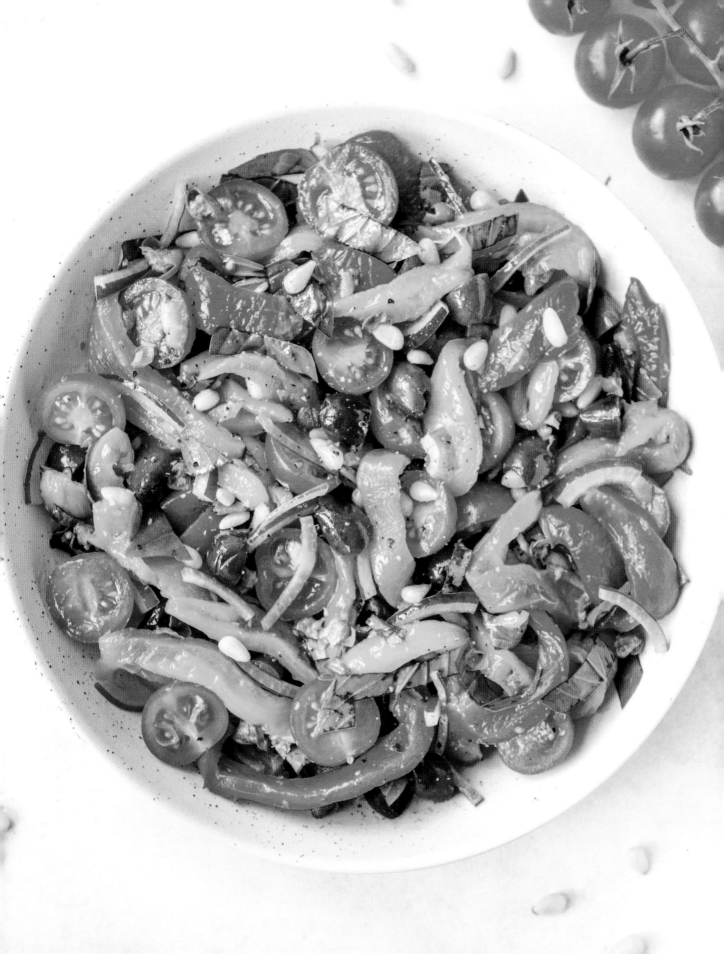

KETO
PALEO
VEGAN
VEGETARIAN
DAIRY-FREE
EGG-FREE
NUT-FREE

Smashed
CUCUMBER SALAD

Yield: 2 servings **Prep Time:** 10 minutes, plus 10 minutes to rest **Cook Time:** —

This incredibly quick-and-easy recipe is an updated spin on a classic Chinese salad. I use the term salad loosely because it's really a cross between a fresh salad and briny pickle. You can divide it as two servings for a light lunch or make four servings as an accompaniment to a spicy dish like Kung Pao Chicken (page 180) or Dan Dan Noodles (page 226). When you smash the cucumber, it becomes tender and absorbs the flavor of the vinegar and garlic dressing quickly.

1 large English cucumber

½ teaspoon salt

2 tablespoons apple cider vinegar

1 tablespoon toasted sesame oil

3 cloves garlic, minced

⅓ cup sliced scallions

¼ cup chopped roasted and salted peanuts or cashews

3 tablespoons chopped fresh cilantro

1 teaspoon black sesame seeds, plus more for garnish if desired

1 teaspoon red pepper flakes

1. Place the cucumber on a cutting board and use a rolling pin or meat pounder to hit the cucumber on all sides until it begins to split and flatten.

2. Using your hands, break the smashed cucumber into small bite-sized pieces and place in a colander. Sprinkle with the salt and allow to rest for 10 minutes to draw out some of the water.

3. In a bowl, whisk together the vinegar, sesame oil, and garlic. Transfer the smashed cucumber to a serving bowl and top with the scallions, peanuts, cilantro, sesame seeds, and red pepper flakes. Toss with the dressing and garnish with additional sesame seeds (if desired) before serving.

SUBSTITUTIONS: *Use almonds for keto; swap the cashews or peanuts for pepitas to make this salad nut- and legume-free.*

STORAGE: *This salad will last in the fridge for up to a day. (The cucumbers will become watery when kept longer than a day and will need to be drained.)*

Water Content

Cucumber has one of the highest water contents of all vegetables (roughly 96 percent). Whenever you're using grated or smashed cucumber in a recipe (such as tzatziki), be sure to salt it first to draw out some of the water so you don't end up with a final dish with lots of excess liquid.

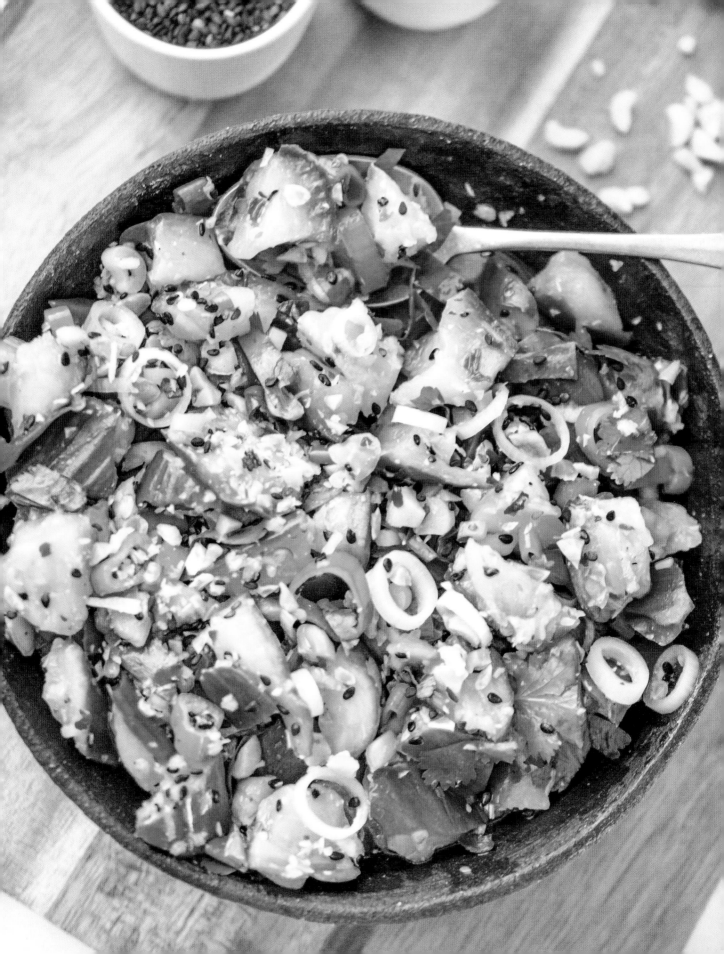

Crunchy
ASIAN SLAW

Yield: 4 servings   **Prep Time:** 20 minutes   **Cook Time:** —

This crunchy Asian slaw is always a crowd-pleaser thanks to the creamy dressing, which I could happily drink through a straw. Make four servings for a side salad or top it with grilled chicken or shrimp to make it a filling meal for two.

Dressing

3 tablespoons toasted sesame oil

2½ tablespoons apple cider vinegar, plus more if needed

2 tablespoons unsweetened, unsalted almond butter

2 tablespoons coconut aminos

1 (1½-inch) piece ginger, peeled, plus more if needed

3 cups finely shredded Napa cabbage

3 cups finely shredded red cabbage

1 cup thinly sliced scallions

½ cup shredded fresh mint leaves, plus more for garnish

½ cup shredded fresh cilantro leaves

½ cup chopped roasted cashews, plus more for garnish

SPECIAL EQUIPMENT
High-powered blender

1. Put the dressing ingredients in a high-powered blender and blend until smooth. (If you're using a regular blender, I recommend roughly chopping the ginger before adding it into the blender to ensure that it blends into a smooth consistency.) Taste and add more vinegar or ginger as desired.

2. Place all of the salad ingredients in a salad bowl. When ready to serve, drizzle the dressing over the top and toss to combine. Garnish with the roasted cashews and extra shredded mint.

SUBSTITUTIONS: *For keto, use almonds in place of the cashews. To make this salad nut-free, use tahini in place of almond butter and swap out the cashews for pepitas or peanuts.*

STORAGE: *Leftovers will last in the fridge for up to 4 days. If it begins to dry out, drizzle 1½ teaspoons of apple cider vinegar and 1½ teaspoons of coconut aminos over the top and toss before serving.*

SCD BASICS
Coco-not Aminos (page 47)

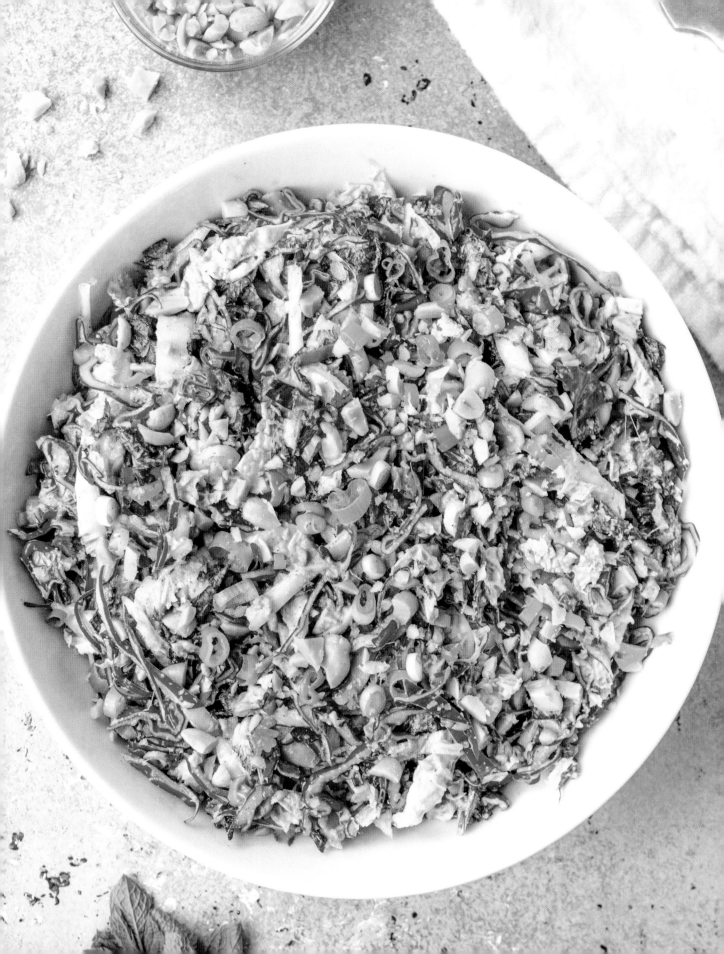

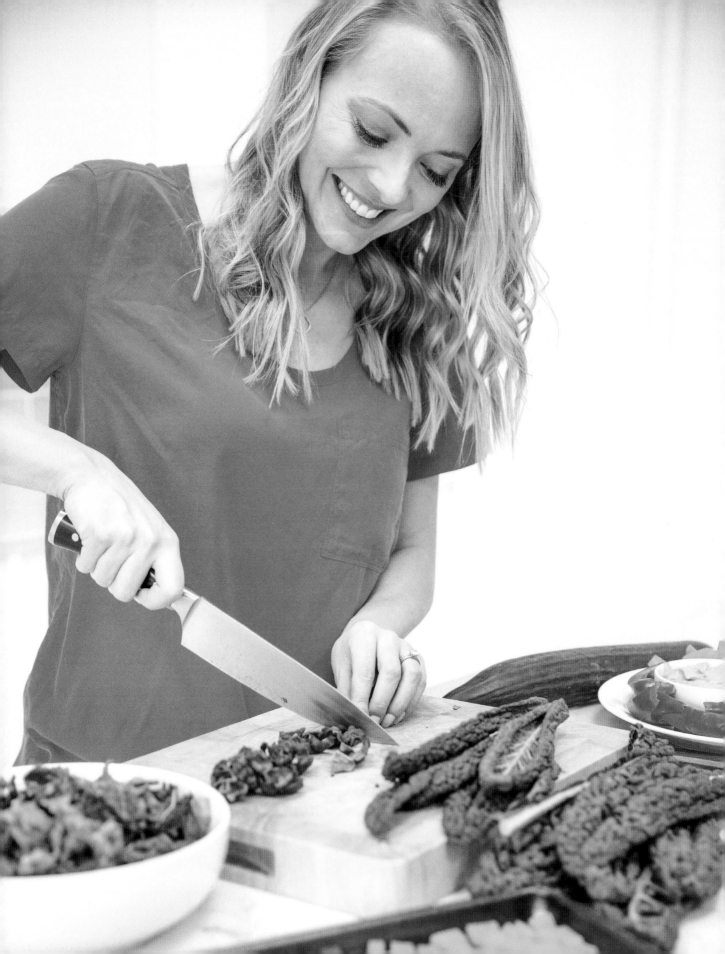

Soups

AIP
KETO
LOW-FODMAP
PALEO
DAIRY-FREE
EGG-FREE
NUT-FREE

Quick Vietnamese
BEEF PHO

Yield: 2 servings **Prep Time:** 10 minutes **Cook Time:** 25 minutes

The secret to a good pho is the broth and the combination of spices used to infuse it with rich flavor. Although authentic pho requires hours of simmering, in this shortcut version I've upped the spice quantities to give it maximum flavor with just 20 minutes of cooking, which makes it a weeknight-friendly recipe. I like to fill the bowls with the noodles, broth, and sliced beef, and I put the herbs, lime, and jalapeño on a large plate to serve on the side so each person can garnish as desired. I love using daikon radish as a noodle in this soup, but zucchini noodles also work well.

1 teaspoon light olive oil

4 cloves garlic, smashed with the side of a knife

1 (2-inch) piece fresh ginger, peeled and thinly sliced

2 star anise

4 whole cloves

1 teaspoon coriander seeds

2 cinnamon sticks

6 cups beef stock

1 tablespoon fish sauce

1 (9-ounce) boneless sirloin steak

1 (2-pound) daikon radish

1 medium yellow onion, cut into eighths

½ cup sliced scallions (1-inch pieces)

¼ cup fresh Thai basil leaves

¼ cup fresh cilantro leaves

1 jalapeño pepper, thinly sliced

For Garnish

1 lime, cut into wedges

Red pepper flakes (optional)

Chili oil (optional)

SCD BASICS
Beef Stock (page 52)

1. Heat the oil in a large pot over high heat, then add the garlic, ginger, star anise, cloves, coriander seeds, and cinnamon sticks. Sauté for 3 to 4 minutes, until fragrant, then pour the stock and fish sauce into the pot. Reduce the heat to medium and simmer for 15 minutes.

2. While the broth is simmering, place the steak in the freezer to firm it up, which will make it easier to slice. Cut both ends off the daikon radish. Use a julienne peeler or spiral slicer to cut long thin noodles; you should get 5 to 6 cups of noodles.

3. After the broth has simmered for 15 minutes, use a small strainer or slotted spoon to remove the star anise, cloves, coriander seeds, and cinnamon sticks. Stir in the onion and simmer for 5 minutes, or until the onion begins to soften. Then add the daikon noodles and cook for 2 more minutes.

4. Remove the beef from the freezer and cut it into paper-thin slices using a sharp knife.

5. Use tongs to remove the noodles and onions from the broth and divide them between 2 bowls. Top the noodles with the thinly sliced beef, scallions, basil, cilantro, and jalapeño, then ladle the hot broth over the top. Garnish with the lime wedges, and, if using, the red pepper flakes and chili oil. Alternatively, divide the noodles, onion, broth, and beef between 2 bowls and serve all of the garnishes on the side.

SUBSTITUTIONS: *For AIP, leave out the star anise, coriander seeds, and jalapeño. To make this pho low-FODMAP, omit the garlic, onions, and scallions and replace the extra-virgin olive oil with an equal amount of garlic-infused oil.*

STORAGE: *Leftovers will last in the fridge for up to 3 days but should not be frozen.*

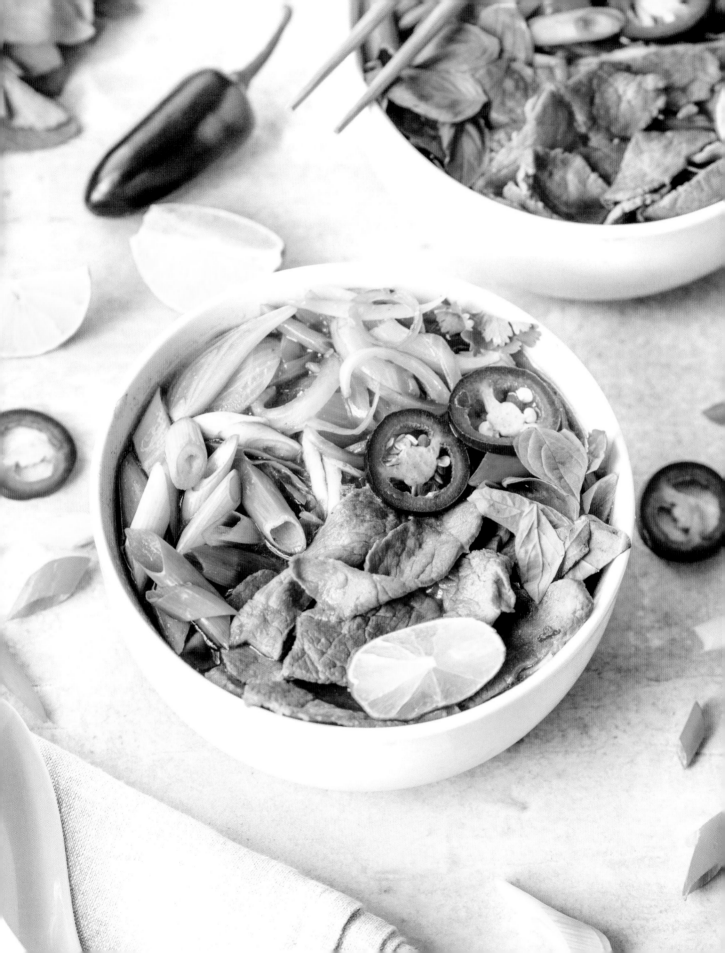

AIP
KETO
LOW-FODMAP
PALEO
DAIRY-FREE
EGG-FREE
NUT-FREE

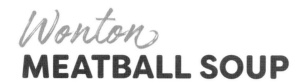

Wonton MEATBALL SOUP

Yield: 4 servings   **Prep Time:** 25 minutes   **Cook Time:** 20 minutes

When you roll wonton filling into meatballs and skip the wrappers, you get all of the flavors of traditional wonton soup with a lot less fuss. The meatballs become really plump and juicy in this soup because they absorb the flavorful broth. Have extra meatballs? Serve them on cauliflower rice and drizzle with chili oil, such as the one used in the Dan Dan Noodles (page 226).

Meatballs

10 ounces medium shrimp, peeled and deveined

1 pound ground pork

⅔ cup thinly sliced scallions

⅓ cup fresh cilantro leaves, roughly chopped

1 (1-inch) piece fresh ginger, peeled and finely diced

1½ tablespoons coconut aminos

1½ tablespoons toasted sesame oil

¼ teaspoon ground white pepper

¼ teaspoon salt

Soup

1 tablespoon toasted sesame oil

1 tablespoon peeled and finely chopped fresh ginger

2 cloves garlic, minced

6 cups chicken stock

1 large carrot, cut into thin half-moons

½ teaspoon ground white pepper

1 bunch bok choy, thinly sliced

⅓ cup sliced scallions

1. Preheat the oven to 350°F.

2. Chop the shrimp into small pieces. Place in a large bowl and add the remaining ingredients for the meatballs. Use your hands to mix until everything is well combined.

3. Using your hands, form the mixture into 24 meatballs (about 1½ inches in diameter) and lay them out evenly on a sheet pan. If the mixture is sticky, wet your hands to prevent it from sticking. Bake the meatballs for 20 minutes, flipping them over halfway through cooking to ensure that they brown evenly on all sides.

4. While the meatballs are baking, place the sesame oil, ginger, and garlic in a large pot over medium-high heat and sauté for 1 minute, until fragrant. Add the stock, carrot, and pepper and simmer for 5 minutes, until the carrots begin to soften.

5. Remove the cooked meatballs from the oven and transfer them to the pot; stir in the bok choy, scallions, and any liquid from the sheet pan. Allow to simmer for another minute before serving. Divide the meatballs and broth evenly among 4 bowls and serve.

SUBSTITUTIONS: *Omit the white pepper and sesame oil to make the soup AIP. For keto, skip the carrot. To make it low-FODMAP, omit the garlic and scallions and use garlic-infused oil.*

STORAGE: *This soup will last in the fridge for up to 3 days. You can store the cooked meatballs in the freezer for up to 2 months.*

SCD BASICS
Coco-not Aminos (page 47)
Chicken Stock (page 53)

Switch It Up

You can substitute ground chicken or turkey for the pork. Also, feel free to use other vegetables such as sliced shiitake mushrooms, shredded Napa cabbage, snow peas, or broccoli.

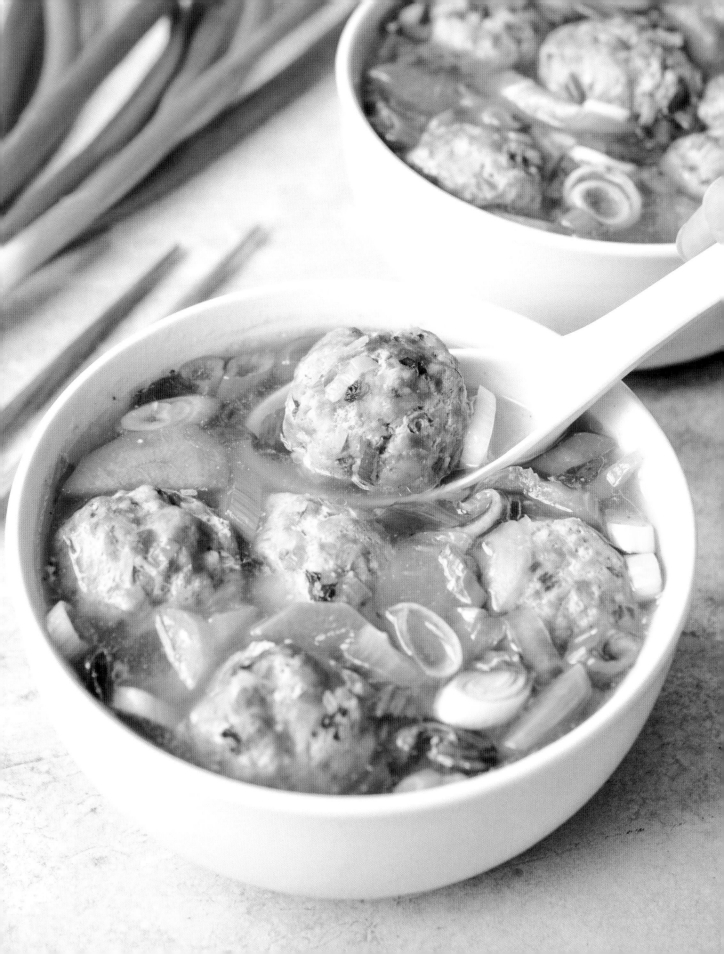

AIP
KETO
PALEO
VEGAN
VEGETARIAN
DAIRY-FREE
EGG-FREE
NUT-FREE

<30 min

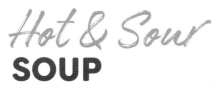

Hot & Sour
SOUP

Yield: 4 servings   **Prep Time:** 10 minutes   **Cook Time:** 16 minutes

The flavors in this soup are extra bold and perfect for warming you from the inside out on a cold day. This recipe is easily customizable to your taste if you want it to be spicier or more sour. Add chicken or shrimp to have extra protein. You can really make this soup your own.

3 cloves garlic, peeled

1 (2-inch) piece fresh ginger, peeled and finely chopped

1 to 2 thinly sliced red chili peppers, such as Fresno

1 tablespoon toasted sesame oil

7 ounces sliced shiitake mushrooms (about 3 cups)

2 cups shredded green cabbage

6 cups chicken or vegetable stock

¼ cup apple cider vinegar

2 tablespoons coconut aminos

½ teaspoon ground white pepper

½ cup sliced scallions, plus more for garnish

1. In a mini food processor or using a pestle and mortar, blend the garlic, ginger, and desired amount of sliced red chili pepper until the mixture is minced.

2. Heat the sesame oil in a large pot over medium heat. Add the mushrooms and sauté for 3 to 4 minutes until they begin to soften. Add the garlic and ginger mince and the cabbage and cook for 3 minutes, or until the cabbage begins to soften.

3. Pour the stock, vinegar, and coconut aminos into the pot and season with the pepper; reduce the heat to medium-low and simmer for 10 minutes. A minute or two before serving, stir in the scallions. Divide the soup evenly among 4 bowls and garnish with sliced scallions.

SUBSTITUTIONS: *Omit the white pepper and red chili pepper to make this soup AIP.*

STORAGE: *The soup will last in the fridge for up to 3 days.*

SCD BASICS

Coco-not Aminos (page 47)

Chicken or Vegetable Stock (page 53)

Chili Peppers
Freeze leftover chilies that are starting to soften. You can grate the frozen chilies into soups, sauces, or stir-fries for a kick of spice.

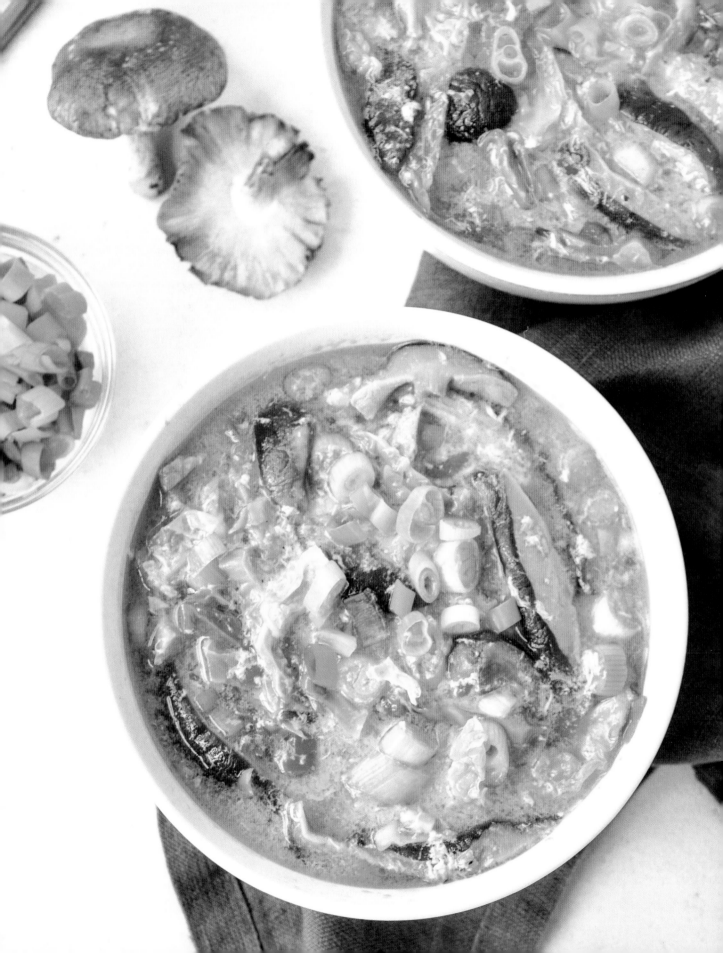

Zuppa TOSCANA

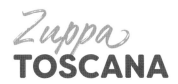

Yield: 6 servings   **Prep Time:** 10 minutes   **Cook Time:** 25 minutes

Zuppa Toscana is an Italian soup that's traditionally made with cubes of potato, spicy sausage, and a cream-based broth. In this version, a handful of herbs and spices turn ground pork (or ground chicken or turkey, if you prefer) into "hot sausage," and cauliflower florets make a chunky replacement for the potatoes. This recipe uses coconut milk in place of the traditional cream, but don't worry about the soup having a coconut flavor; the bold spices completely overpower the coconut milk, and you still get all of the creaminess you expect from this soup.

5 strips thick-cut bacon

1 pound ground pork

2 teaspoons paprika

1 teaspoon fennel seeds

1 teaspoon dried oregano leaves

1 teaspoon dried thyme leaves

1 teaspoon ground black pepper

½ teaspoon red pepper flakes, plus more for garnish if desired

½ teaspoon salt

1 medium yellow onion, finely diced

2 cloves garlic, minced

5 cups chicken stock

⅔ cup canned full-fat coconut milk

1 medium head cauliflower, cut into florets (about 3 cups)

3 cups shredded Tuscan ("dino") kale

1. In a large pot over medium-high heat, cook the bacon for 6 to 8 minutes, until browned and crisp. Remove the bacon from the pot and set aside on a paper towel–lined plate, leaving the excess bacon grease in the pot.

2. Add the ground pork, paprika, fennel seeds, oregano, thyme, pepper, red pepper flakes, and salt. Use a wooden spoon to break the pork into small pieces. Add the onion and garlic and continue to cook until the onion has become translucent and the pork is cooked through, 5 to 6 minutes.

3. Pour the chicken stock and coconut milk into the pot, then add the cauliflower florets and kale. Reduce the heat to medium and simmer for 8 to 10 minutes, until the cauliflower florets are tender.

4. Before serving, roughly chop the bacon and stir it into the soup. Garnish with additional red pepper flakes, if desired.

SUBSTITUTIONS: *Skip the onion and garlic and swap the cauliflower florets for diced potato to make this soup low-FODMAP.*

STORAGE: *This soup will last in the fridge for up to 4 days or in the freezer for up to 3 months.*

SCD BASICS
Chicken Stock (page 53)

Freezing the Soup

If you're making this soup to be frozen, reduce the cook time after adding the cauliflower and kale to 5 minutes. The vegetables will continue to cook when the soup is thawed and reheated, so undercooking them will ensure they are tender without becoming mushy.

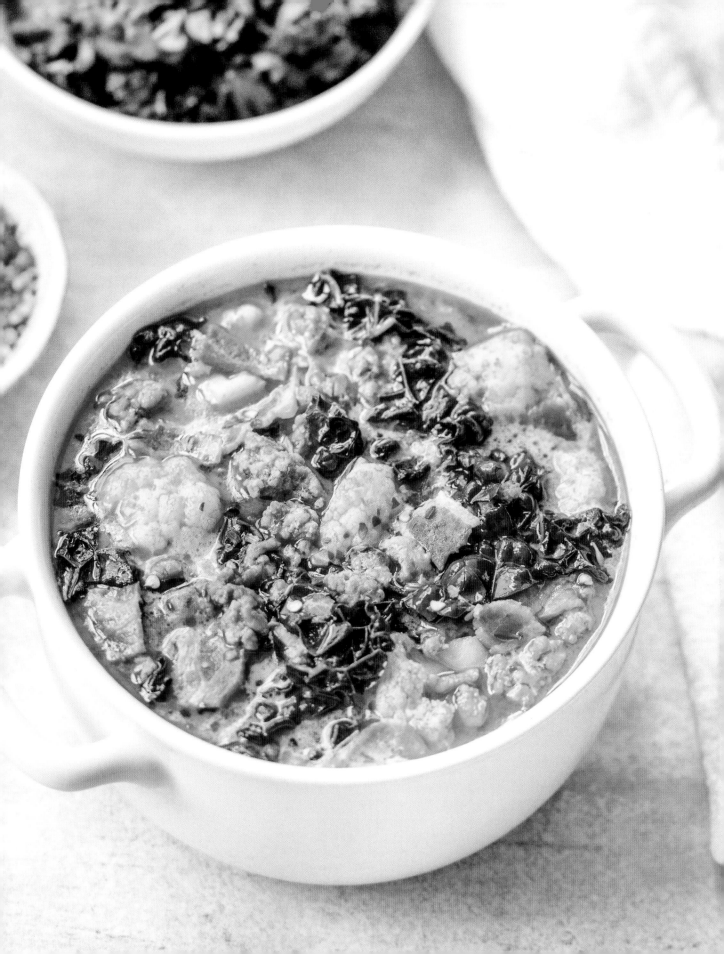

Southwest Chicken &
BACON CHOWDER

Yield: 6 servings   **Prep Time:** 10 minutes   **Cook Time:** 40 minutes

Although most chowders get their creaminess from a dairy product or roux, the creaminess in this recipe is thanks to a secret vegetable—cauliflower! This chunky chowder is packed with chicken, bacon, veggies, and a lot of spice, which makes it feel more substantial than your average soup. You can adjust the amount of cayenne pepper and jalapeños to reach your preferred level of spiciness.

1 large head cauliflower, cut into florets (about 4 cups)

4 cups chicken stock, divided

1 cup unsweetened almond milk, plus more as desired

1 teaspoon olive oil

6 strips thick-cut bacon

1 medium yellow onion, diced

2 jalapeño peppers, finely diced

3 cloves garlic, minced

1 large carrot, diced

1 red bell pepper, diced

6 ounces boneless, skinless chicken breast, cooked and cubed (about 2 cups)

2 teaspoons cayenne pepper

1½ teaspoons ground cumin

½ teaspoon salt

½ teaspoon ground black pepper

⅓ cup sliced scallions, plus 1 tablespoon for garnish if desired

3 tablespoons chopped fresh cilantro, for garnish (optional)

Bacon Is Optional

If you prefer to leave out the bacon, increase the salt to 1 teaspoon.

SCD BASICS
Chicken Stock (page 53)

1. Place the cauliflower florets in a large pot over medium heat and cover with 2 cups of the stock (or enough to cover the florets). Simmer for 15 minutes, or until the florets are very tender.

2. Transfer the cauliflower and any liquid in the pot to a blender, pour in the almond milk and 1 cup of the remaining stock, and blend until completely smooth. Rinse the pot and wipe it to dry it completely.

3. Warm the oil in the pot over medium-high heat, then add the bacon and cook for 8 minutes, or until crispy. Transfer the cooked bacon to a paper towel–lined plate and set aside. Drain all but 1 tablespoon of bacon grease from the pot.

4. Add the onion, jalapeños, and garlic to the pot and cook for about 5 minutes, until the onion softens. Then add the carrot, bell pepper, and the remaining 1 cup of stock and simmer for 5 minutes, or until the vegetables become tender.

5. Reduce the heat to medium and pour the cauliflower puree into the pot, then stir in the cooked chicken, cayenne pepper, and cumin. Roughly chop the bacon and add three-quarters of it to the pot, reserving the remainder for garnish. Season the soup with the salt and black pepper and simmer for 5 minutes to allow the flavors to meld. If the soup is thicker than you like, add more almond milk until it reaches the desired consistency.

6. Just before serving, stir in the scallions. Ladle the soup into 6 bowls and garnish with the remaining chopped bacon and the scallions and cilantro, if using.

SUBSTITUTIONS: *Omit the carrot to make this soup keto. Use coconut milk in place of almond milk to make it nut-free.*

STORAGE: *Leftovers will last in the fridge for up to 4 days or in the freezer for up to 3 months.*

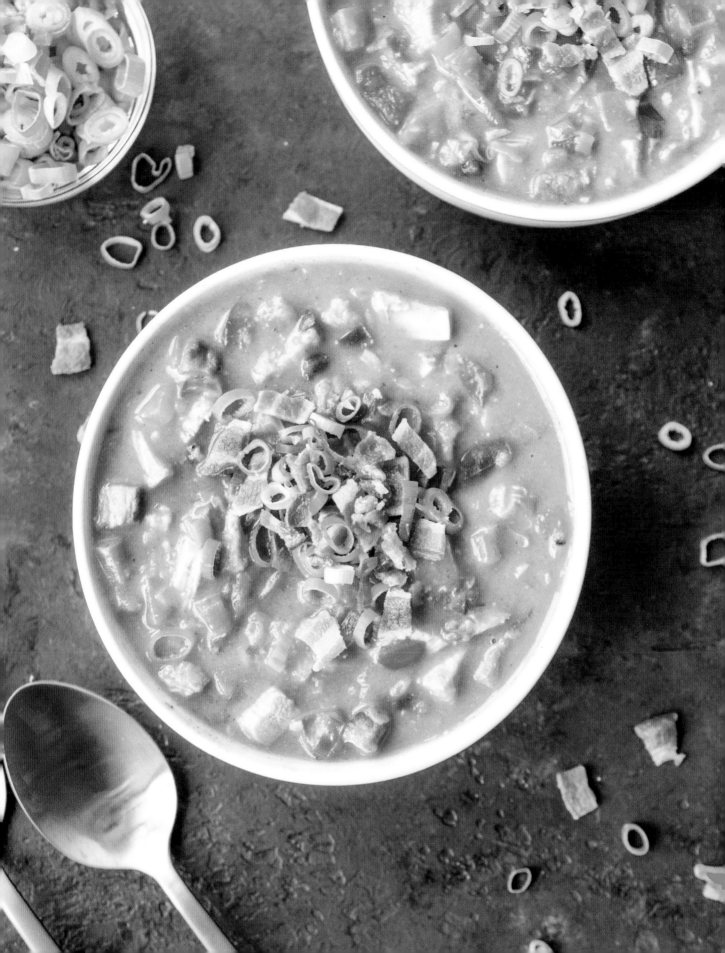

AIP
KETO
PALEO
VEGAN
VEGETARIAN
DAIRY-FREE
EGG-FREE
NUT-FREE

Mom's Feel-Better
CHICKEN & RICE SOUP

Yield: 6 servings **Prep Time:** 10 minutes **Cook Time:** 32 minutes

Everyone needs one simple chicken soup recipe to make quickly when someone isn't feeling well. It doesn't need to be fancy or require hours of simmering. It should just be comforting, tasty, and nutritious. This is a grain-free version of the soup that my mom used to make whenever I was getting sick. Within minutes of detecting a sniffle or cough, she would have it boiling on the stove, and it always seemed to do the trick. This soup is packed with so many vegetables that it's almost a stew. It reheats well, so you can make a big batch to eat through the week until you get back on your feet.

1 tablespoon extra-virgin olive oil

1 medium yellow onion, diced

2 tablespoons peeled and chopped fresh ginger

3 cloves garlic, minced

1 cup chopped carrots

1 cup chopped celery

8 cups chicken stock

1½ tablespoons freshly squeezed lemon juice

1 pound boneless, skinless chicken breasts (see tip)

3 cups fresh or frozen riced cauliflower

2 cups roughly chopped curly kale

½ teaspoon ground black pepper

1 cup fresh spinach

1. In a large pot, heat the oil over medium heat. Add the onion, ginger, and garlic and sauté for 2 minutes, then add the carrots and celery and cook for 5 more minutes, until the carrots begin to soften.

2. Pour the stock and lemon juice into the pot and add the chicken breasts. Simmer on medium heat until the chicken breasts are cooked through, about 20 minutes.

3. Transfer the chicken breasts from the pot to a cutting board to cool slightly; shred them into small pieces.

4. Return the shredded chicken to the pot and stir in the riced cauliflower, kale, and pepper. Simmer for 3 to 4 minutes, or until the cauliflower is tender.

5. Right before serving, stir in the spinach and simmer for a few minutes until it wilts. Divide the soup among 6 bowls.

Shorten the Cook Time
You can reduce the cook time for this soup to 15 minutes by using rotisserie or leftover cooked chicken and simmering the soup for just 2 minutes in Step 2. Alternatively, cut the raw chicken breasts in half and reduce the cook time in Step 2 to 10 minutes.

SUBSTITUTIONS: *Skip the black pepper to make it AIP. Omit the carrot to make it keto. Make this soup vegetarian or vegan by using vegetable stock in place of the chicken stock and swapping the shredded chicken for mushrooms.*

STORAGE: *Leftovers will last in the fridge for up to 4 days. You can freeze it for up to 2 months, although you will likely have to add 1 cup of chicken stock to the soup after thawing to thin it.*

SCD BASICS
Chicken Stock (page 53)

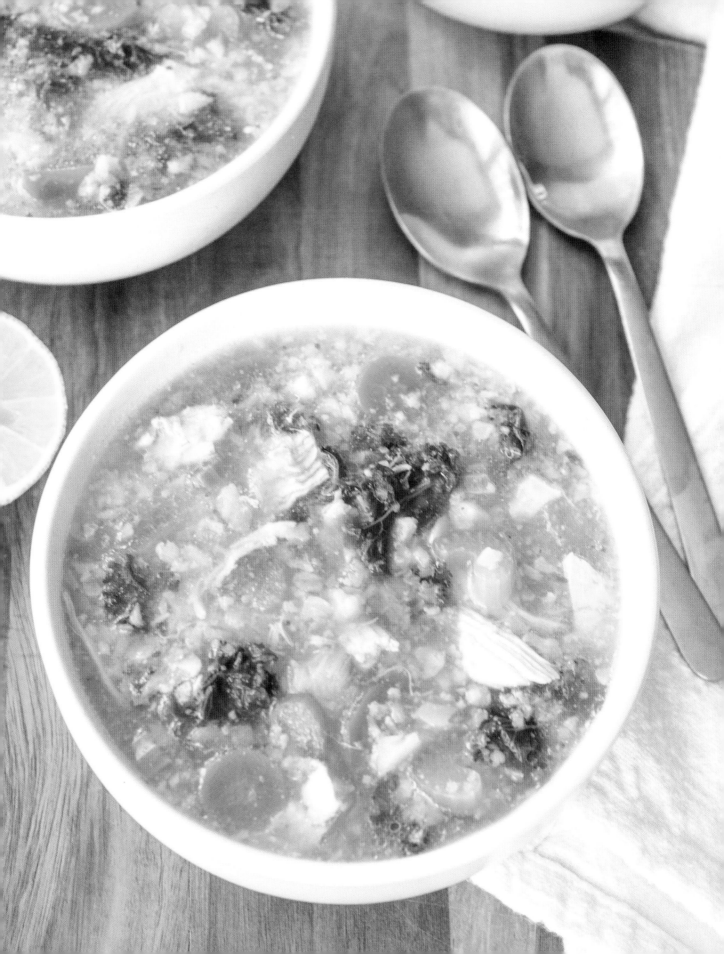

AIP
KETO
PALEO
DAIRY-FREE
EGG-FREE
NUT-FREE

Chicken Pot Pie
SOUP

Yield: 4 servings   **Prep Time:** 10 minutes   **Cook Time:** 20 minutes

This soup is truly comfort in a bowl. It's deliciously creamy and perfect for those cold winter days when you crave something warm and hearty. Readers of my blog have given this soup glowing reviews; they say that it's absolutely to die for and a family favorite that everyone always devours.

1 medium head cauliflower, cut into florets (about 3 cups)

3 cups chicken stock, divided, plus more as needed

1 cup unsweetened almond milk

1 tablespoon extra-virgin olive oil

1 medium yellow onion, finely diced

1 cup finely diced celery (about 2 medium stalks)

1 cup finely diced carrots (about 1 large carrot)

2 cloves garlic, minced

1 teaspoon dried rosemary leaves

1 teaspoon dried thyme leaves

½ teaspoon ground black pepper

¼ teaspoon salt

1 cup frozen peas

6 ounces boneless, skinless chicken breasts or thighs, cooked and diced (about 2 cups)

1 tablespoon chopped fresh Italian parsley, for garnish (optional)

1. Place the cauliflower florets in a large pot over medium heat with 1 cup of the stock; the florets should be almost covered, so use more stock if necessary. Cover with a lid and steam for 6 minutes, or until the cauliflower is tender and can be easily pierced with a fork.

2. Transfer the cauliflower and any liquid in the pot to a blender. Pour the almond milk and 1 cup of the remaining stock into the blender and blend until completely smooth. Set aside.

3. Place the oil in the large pot over medium-high heat and add the onion, celery, carrots, and garlic and cook for 4 to 5 minutes, until the onion is translucent. Stir in the rosemary, thyme, pepper, salt, and the remaining 1 cup of chicken stock. Simmer for 8 to 10 minutes, until the carrots become tender.

4. Stir in the peas, cubed chicken, and cauliflower puree and cook for another 5 minutes, or until everything is warm. If the soup is too thick, add more stock until it reaches the desired consistency.

5. Divide the soup among 4 bowls and garnish with fresh parsley before serving, if desired.

SUBSTITUTIONS: *To make this soup nut-free and AIP, use coconut milk in place of almond milk. For keto, skip the carrots and replace the frozen peas with 1 cup of green beans, cut into small pieces.*

STORAGE: *Leftovers will last in the fridge for up to 4 days or in the freezer up to 4 months.*

SCD BASICS
Chicken Stock (page 53)

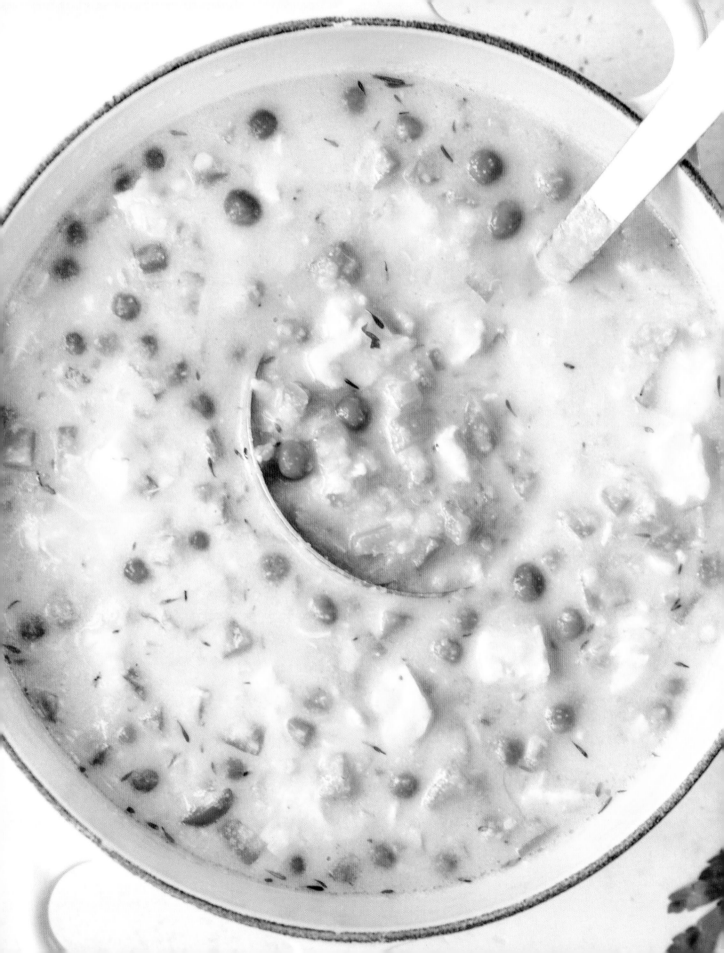

Greek
AVGOLEMONO SOUP

Yield: 4 servings **Prep Time:** 5 minutes **Cook Time:** 15 minutes

I'm always looking for easy soup recipes, and my friend Jordan (the source of many great recipe ideas) suggested I try avgolemono, a lemony egg drop soup with Greek origins. It has become one of my favorite quick weeknight soups that I can make in less than 20 minutes. The broth has a silky, creamy consistency that is both comforting and refreshing thanks to a lovely kick of lemon. Be sure to temper the eggs before adding them to the soup so that you don't end up with scrambled egg soup.

1 tablespoon extra-virgin olive oil

1 large yellow onion, diced

¼ teaspoon salt

6 cups chicken stock

2 (3-ounce) boneless, skinless chicken breasts or thighs, cooked and cubed (about 2 cups)

4 medium eggs, at room temperature

5 tablespoons freshly squeezed lemon juice

3 cups fresh or frozen riced cauliflower

For Garnish

2 tablespoons chopped fresh Italian parsley

½ teaspoon ground black pepper

½ lemon, thinly sliced

1. Heat the oil in a large pot over medium heat, then add the onion and salt. Sauté for 3 to 4 minutes, until the onion is translucent.

2. Pour the stock into the pot and add the cooked chicken. Reduce the heat to medium-low and simmer for 5 minutes.

3. While the soup is simmering, crack the eggs into a medium-sized bowl and whisk until light and frothy, then add the lemon juice and whisk for another 10 seconds. Slowly pour a ladle of broth from the pot into the bowl, whisking continuously to ensure that the eggs do not curdle. Repeat with two more ladles of broth, whisking continuously as you pour in the broth.

4. Add the riced cauliflower to the soup and simmer for 3 minutes, or until it's al dente (tender but not mushy), then slowly pour the egg and lemon mixture into the pot as you continuously whisk the soup.

5. Divide the soup among 4 bowls and garnish with the parsley, pepper, and lemon slices before serving.

SUBSTITUTIONS: *To make this soup vegetarian, omit the chicken breasts and use vegetable stock in place of chicken stock.*

STORAGE: *This soup will last in the fridge for up to 2 days but should not be frozen.*

Juicing Citrus

To get the maximum amount of juice out of citrus fruit, microwave them! Place the fruit in the microwave for 15 seconds, and then allow to cool for a few minutes before cutting in half and juicing. Even old, rock-hard limes and lemons that have been sitting in your fruit bowl for too long will release more juice when you use this method.

SCD BASICS
Chicken Stock (page 53)

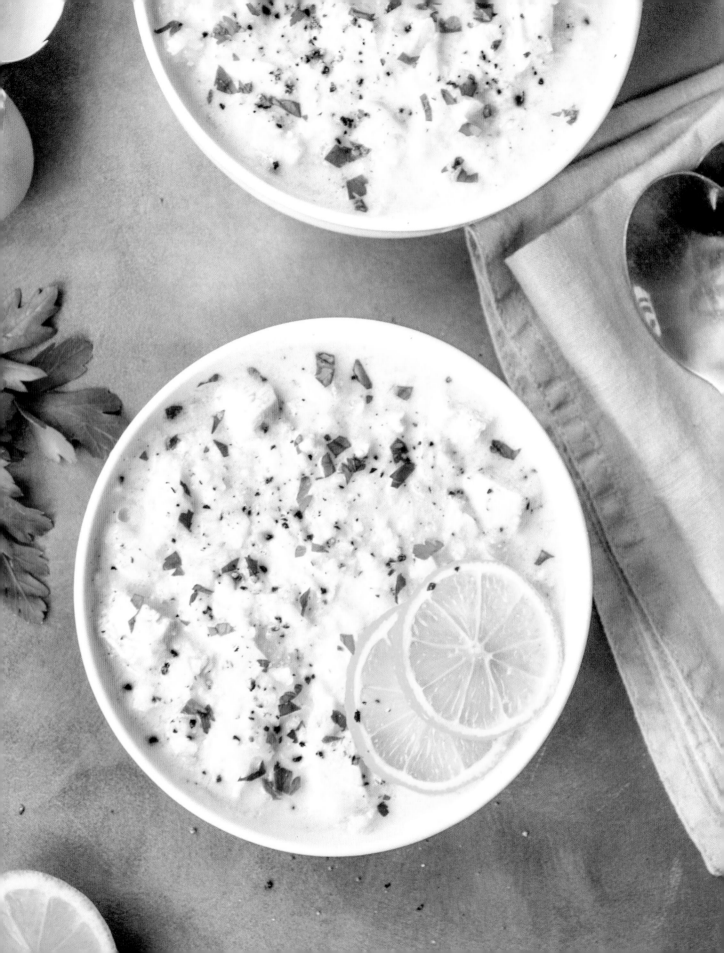

KETO
LOW-FODMAP
PALEO
VEGAN
VEGETARIAN
DAIRY-FREE
EGG-FREE

Cheesy BROCCOLI SOUP

Yield: 6 servings   **Prep Time:** 10 minutes   **Cook Time:** 23 minutes

This soup is rich, creamy, and delicious. I love a smooth soup, but you can adjust the texture to your liking by blending it for just a few seconds to get small bits of broccoli, or skip the blending step altogether for a chunkier soup. I'm happy to report that using nutritional yeast gives the same cheesy flavor as cheddar, so you won't feel like you're missing out if you go with the dairy-free option.

1 tablespoon extra-virgin olive oil

1 medium yellow onion, finely diced

1 stalk celery, diced

⅓ cup finely diced carrots (about 1 small carrot)

3 cloves garlic, minced

2 pounds broccoli, cut into florets (about 4 cups florets)

2½ cups chicken or vegetable stock

¾ cup cashews, soaked in boiling water for 10 minutes and drained

1 cup unsweetened almond milk

1 teaspoon Dijon mustard

¾ cup shredded cheddar cheese

1 teaspoon salt

½ teaspoon ground black pepper

½ teaspoon paprika

¼ cup cooked and roughly chopped bacon, for garnish (optional)

1 tablespoon chopped fresh chives, for garnish (optional)

SPECIAL EQUIPMENT
High-powered blender
Immersion blender

1. Heat the oil in a large pot over medium-high heat. Add the onion, celery, carrots, and garlic and sauté for 5 minutes, or until the onion is translucent.

2. Stir in the broccoli florets and stock, cover the pot with a lid, and simmer for 8 minutes, until the broccoli is fork tender.

3. While the broccoli is cooking, place the cashews in a high-powered blender with the almond milk and mustard and blend until completely smooth.

4. Remove 2 or 3 broccoli florets from the pot to reserve for garnish. Place an immersion blender into the pot and blend the broccoli and broth mixture to your desired consistency.

5. Pour the cashew mixture into the soup and stir in the cheddar cheese, salt, pepper, and paprika. Bring the soup to a gentle simmer and cook for 5 to 10 minutes to develop the flavors. Cut the reserved broccoli florets into 6 pieces.

6. Divide the soup among 6 bowls and garnish with the broccoli florets and, if desired, the chopped bacon and chives.

SUBSTITUTIONS: *You can use macadamia nuts in place of cashews for low-FODMAP and to reduce the carbs for keto. Replace the cheddar cheese with ⅓ cup of nutritional yeast to make this soup dairy-free and Paleo; also use vegetable stock for vegan.*

STORAGE: *Leftovers will last in the fridge for up to 4 days or in the freezer for up to 4 months.*

SCD BASICS
Chicken or Vegetable Stock
(page 53)

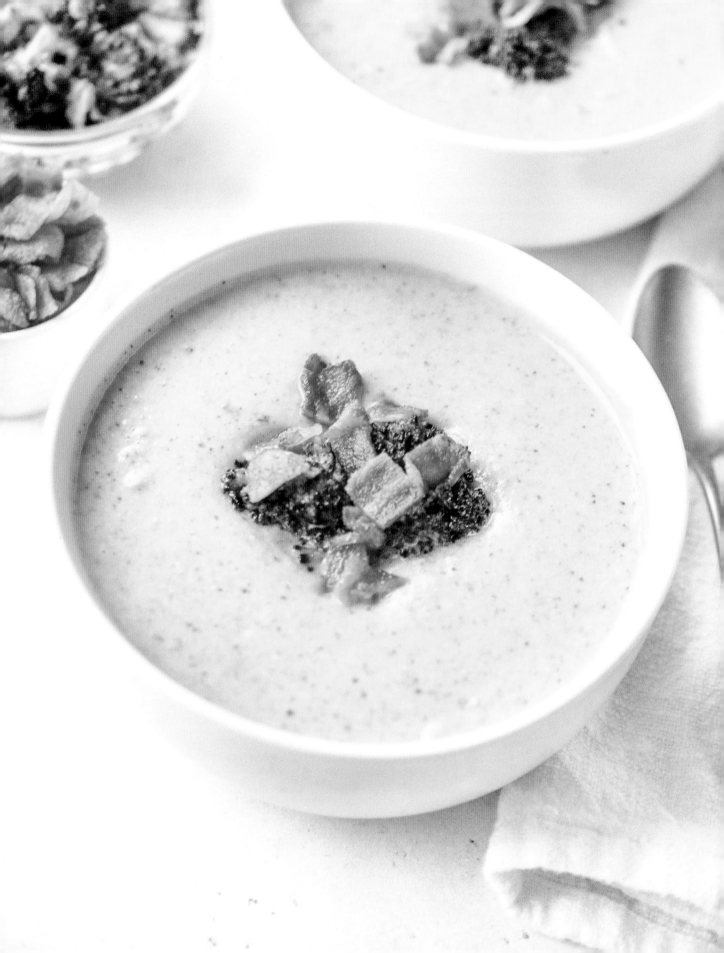

AIP
PALEO
VEGAN
VEGETARIAN
DAIRY-FREE
EGG-FREE
NUT-FREE

Butternut Squash, LEEK & APPLE SOUP

Yield: 4 servings **Prep Time:** 10 minutes **Cook Time:** 35 minutes

This silky smooth soup is perfect for a cold winter day. Baking the butternut squash gives the soup a deliciously rich roasted flavor, which is balanced out with a hint of sweetness from the apple and leeks. Don't skip the nutmeg—it may seem unnecessary, but it really enhances the flavor of the soup.

1 large leek, halved lengthwise and thinly sliced

1 medium apple, such as McIntosh, Pink Lady, or Braeburn

1 medium butternut squash (about 3 pounds), peeled and cut into cubes

4 cloves garlic, unpeeled (but thin, papery skins removed)

2 tablespoons extra-virgin olive oil, divided

1 medium yellow onion, thinly sliced

1 teaspoon salt, divided

4 cups chicken or vegetable stock

½ teaspoon ground black pepper

½ teaspoon ground nutmeg

1½ teaspoons chopped fresh sage

1. Preheat the oven to 350°F. Place the leek slices in a bowl of water and leave them submerged for 5 minutes to loosen any dirt from between the leaves. Use a slotted spoon to transfer the leek to a paper towel–lined plate to drain while you prep the sheet pan.

2. Cut the apple into quarters and remove the core. Place the apple wedges, butternut squash cubes, and garlic cloves on a sheet pan. Drizzle with 1 tablespoon of the oil and roast for 30 minutes, or until the squash is tender.

3. While the squash is roasting, heat the remaining 1 tablespoon of oil in a large pot over low heat and add the leek and onion. Season with ½ teaspoon of the salt and cook for 20 minutes, or until the leek and onion are soft and beginning to turn golden.

4. Transfer the roasted butternut squash and apple to a blender. Squeeze the garlic cloves out of their skins and into the blender, then add the sautéed leek and onion and the stock. Blend until completely smooth.

5. Pour the soup back into the pot. Season with the pepper, nutmeg, and remaining ½ teaspoon of salt and simmer for 5 minutes.

6. Divide the soup among 4 bowls and garnish with the sage.

SUBSTITUTIONS: *Omit the nutmeg and pepper to make this soup AIP.*

STORAGE: *Leftovers will last in the fridge for up to 4 days or in the freezer for up to 4 months.*

Freezing Soup

When freezing soup in containers, fill them 80 percent full so there is enough room for the soup to expand once frozen. Not leaving enough space may cause the lid to come off, and more space than needed will equate to more air making contact with the soup and potentially resulting in faster freezer burn.

SCD BASICS
Chicken or Vegetable Stock
(page 53)

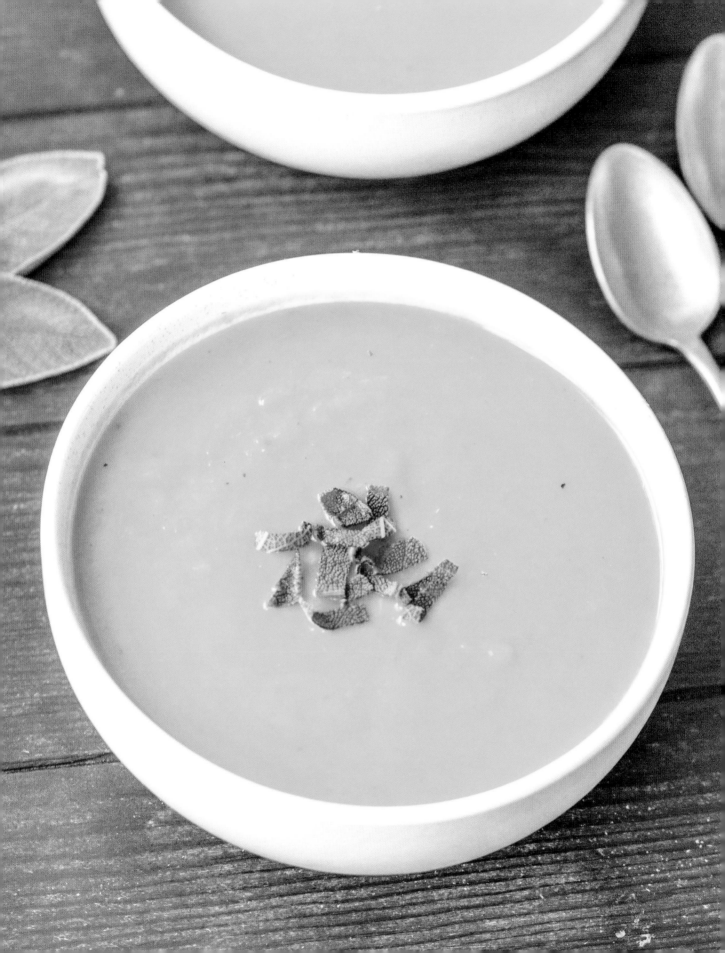

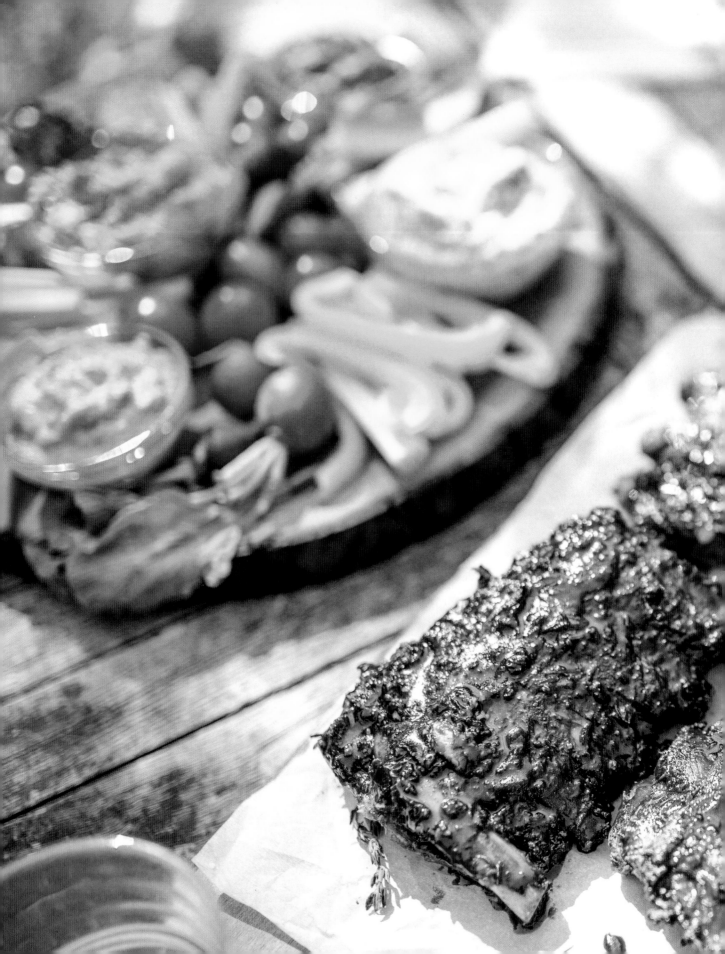

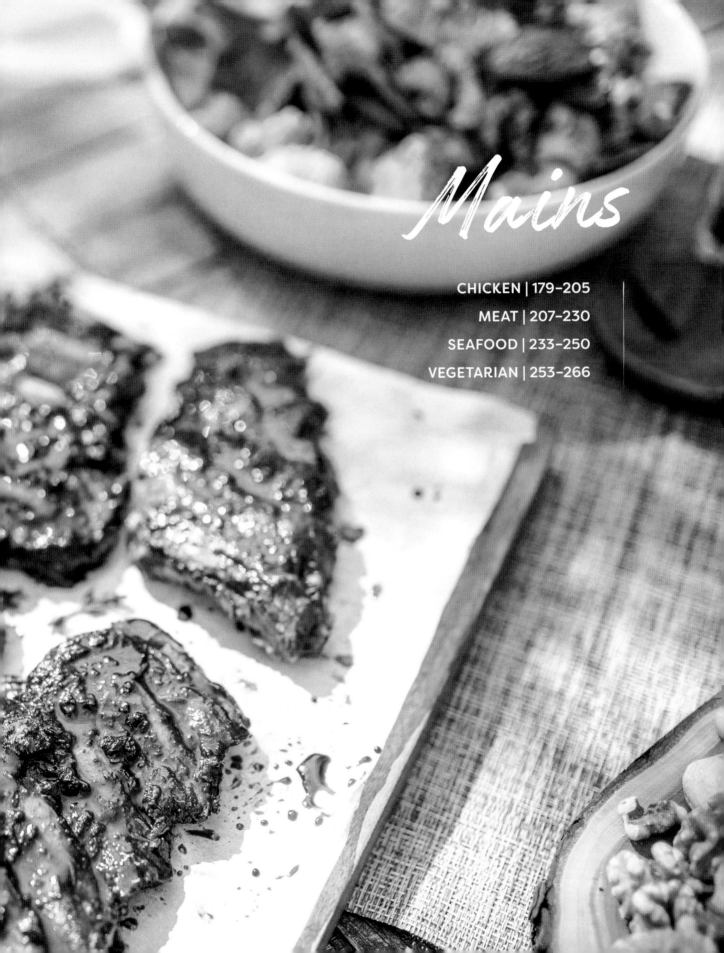

Mains

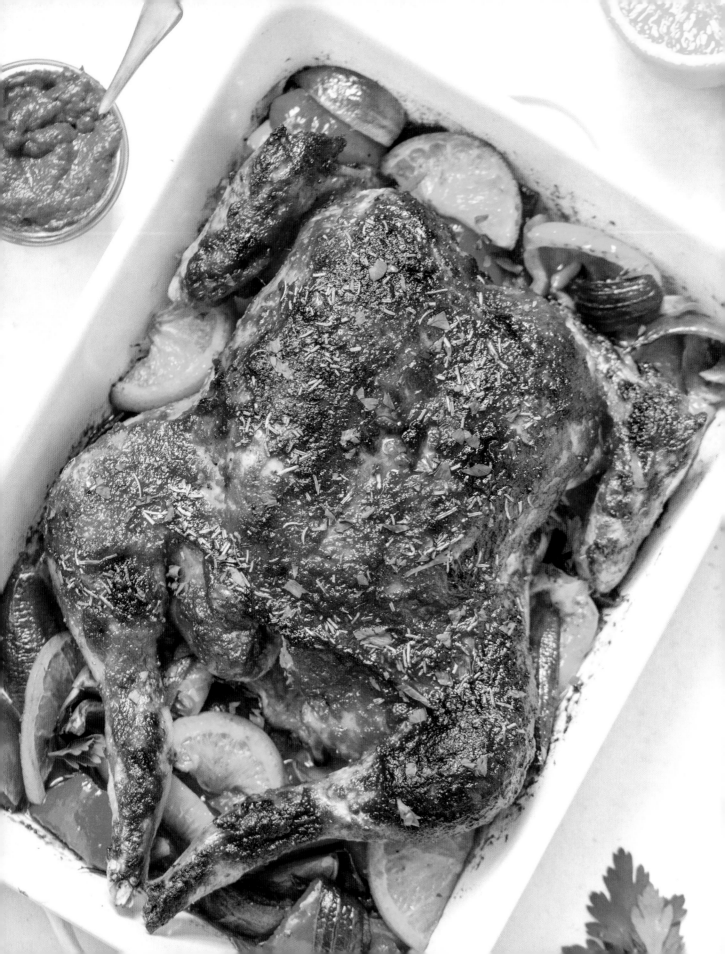

Chicken

Kung Pao
CHICKEN

Yield: 4 servings   **Prep Time:** 20 minutes   **Cook Time:** 15 minutes

Long gone are the days of Chinese takeout, but with recipes like this, you don't have to miss it! This dish is lip-numbingly spicy thanks to the Sichuan peppercorns, which are not to be skipped and can be found at most Asian grocery stores (or online). Serve this dish on a bed of cauliflower rice (like the one on page 272) or spaghetti squash to sop up all of the delicious sauce. Definitely make extra because the leftovers are just as good when reheated the next day.

1½ pounds boneless, skinless chicken breasts, cut into 1-inch cubes

1½ tablespoons apple cider vinegar

1½ tablespoons coconut aminos

2 teaspoons baking soda

¼ teaspoon salt

¼ teaspoon ground black pepper

1 tablespoon avocado oil

1½ teaspoons toasted sesame oil

4 cloves garlic, minced

1½ tablespoons finely chopped fresh ginger

1 teaspoon ground Sichuan peppercorns (see tip)

4 to 5 dried bird's eye chilies, cut into ½-inch pieces

1 red bell pepper, cut into 1-inch pieces

1 green bell pepper, cut into 1-inch pieces

½ cup sliced scallions (1-inch pieces)

½ cup peanuts or cashews

Sauce

¼ cup coconut aminos

2 tablespoons apple cider vinegar

2 tablespoons aged balsamic vinegar

2 tablespoons chicken stock

1½ tablespoons honey

1. Place the cubed chicken, apple cider vinegar, coconut aminos, baking soda, salt, and pepper in a bowl. Stir well, making sure that the chicken pieces are all well coated; set aside to marinate for 10 minutes.

2. To prepare the sauce, pour all of the sauce ingredients into a saucepan over medium heat. Simmer for about 8 minutes, until the liquid has reduced by two-thirds and has become a thick sauce. Once thickened, remove the pan from the heat.

3. Meanwhile, heat the avocado oil in a large skillet over high heat. Add the marinated chicken and the marinade and cook for about 6 minutes, until it's seared on all sides and cooked through. Use a slotted spoon to transfer the chicken to a plate and set aside.

4. Lower the heat to medium and pour the sesame oil into the skillet. Stir in the garlic, ginger, Sichuan peppercorns, and dried chilies and cook for 1 minute until fragrant. Add the bell peppers to the skillet and sauté for 4 minutes, until they begin to soften.

5. Return the chicken to the skillet and add the sauce, scallions, and peanuts. Toss to coat everything in the sauce and cook for another 2 minutes, until the chicken is warmed through.

SUBSTITUTIONS: *For keto, skip the honey and omit the cashews. For legume- or nut-free, omit the peanuts or cashews.*

STORAGE: *Leftovers will last in the fridge for up to 4 days.*

TIP: *Sichuan peppercorns are most commonly sold as whole peppercorns. Use a mortar and pestle or coffee grinder to grind them.*

SCD BASICS: SCD Balsamic Vinegar (page 46), **Coco-not Aminos** (page 47), **Chicken Stock** (page 53)

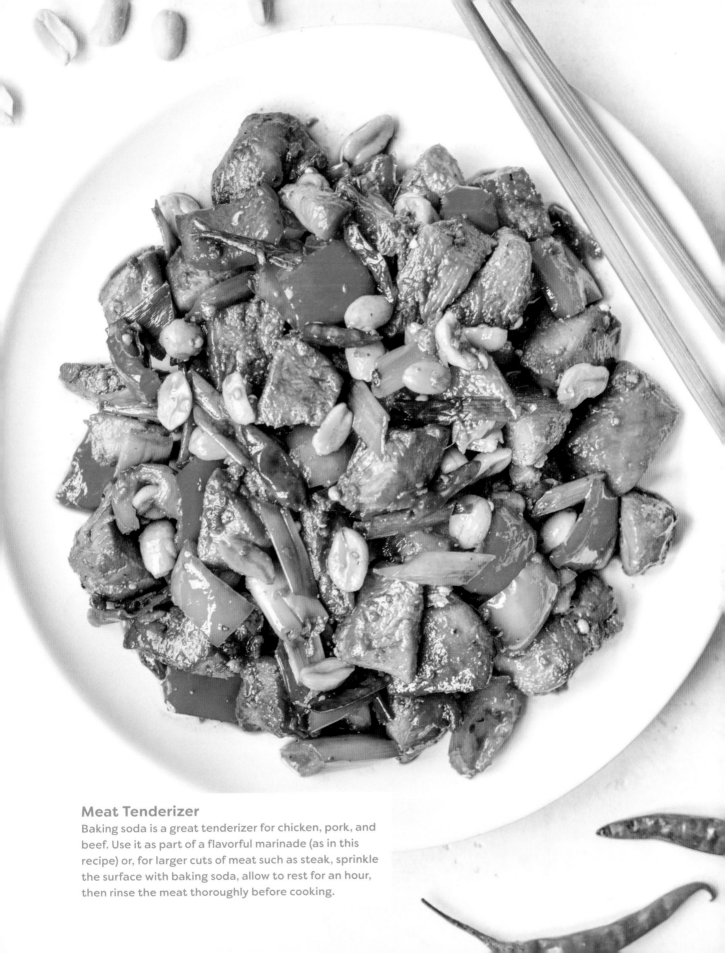

Meat Tenderizer

Baking soda is a great tenderizer for chicken, pork, and beef. Use it as part of a flavorful marinade (as in this recipe) or, for larger cuts of meat such as steak, sprinkle the surface with baking soda, allow to rest for an hour, then rinse the meat thoroughly before cooking.

LOW-FODMAP
PALEO
VEGAN
VEGETARIAN
DAIRY-FREE
EGG-FREE

Peanut Chicken
NOODLE BOWL

Yield: 2 servings **Prep Time:** 10 minutes **Cook Time:** 15 minutes

This dish is a healthy spin on one of my favorite Thai-style noodle dishes. With a start-to-finish cook time of less than 30 minutes, it's an easy weeknight dinner to make with ingredients that you likely already have in your kitchen. This is a recipe you will definitely want to double because the leftovers are delicious eaten warm or cold.

Sauce

¼ cup unsweetened, unsalted peanut or almond butter

⅓ cup unsweetened almond milk

2 tablespoons coconut aminos

2 tablespoons apple cider vinegar

1 (1-inch) piece fresh ginger, peeled and roughly chopped

1 clove garlic, peeled

8 ounces boneless, skinless chicken breasts, cut into 1-inch cubes

¼ teaspoon salt

¼ teaspoon ground black pepper

1 tablespoon toasted sesame oil

1 red bell pepper, sliced into thin strips

12 ounces packaged butternut squash noodles (see tip)

3 cups chopped spinach

½ cup chopped scallions

For Garnish

⅓ cup chopped roasted cashews

2 tablespoons chopped fresh cilantro

2 tablespoons sliced scallions

Lime wedges

1. To make the sauce, place the peanut butter, almond milk, coconut aminos, vinegar, ginger, and garlic in a blender and blend until completely smooth. Set aside.

2. Season the cubed chicken with the salt and pepper. Heat the oil in a large skillet over medium heat, then add the seasoned chicken and sauté until cooked through, about 6 minutes. Remove from the skillet and set aside.

3. Add the bell pepper strips to the skillet and cook for 3 minutes, until they begin to soften, then add the butternut squash noodles and cook for 2 to 3 minutes. Be gentle with the noodles to ensure that they don't break as you stir. Next return the cooked chicken to the pan and add the spinach, scallions, and peanut sauce and gently toss with tongs to ensure everything is well coated in the sauce. Cook for another minute until the spinach begins to wilt and the noodles are al dente. Garnish each serving with some chopped cashews, cilantro, scallions, and a lime wedge.

SUBSTITUTIONS: *For low-FODMAP, omit the garlic, scallions, and cashews. For Paleo, use almond butter instead of peanut butter. Swap the chicken for shiitake mushrooms to make the dish vegan/vegetarian.*

STORAGE: *Leftovers will last in the fridge for up to 3 days.*

TIPS: *If you can't find precut butternut squash noodles at the store, cut the long neck off of 1 medium butternut squash and peel it. Use a julienne peeler or spiral slicer to cut the noodles. If you find it difficult to cut the butternut squash into noodles because of its firm flesh, you can bake it for 10 minutes in a preheated 350ºF oven to soften it a bit. Allow the squash to cool before spiral slicing.*

SCD BASICS
Coco-not Aminos (page 47)

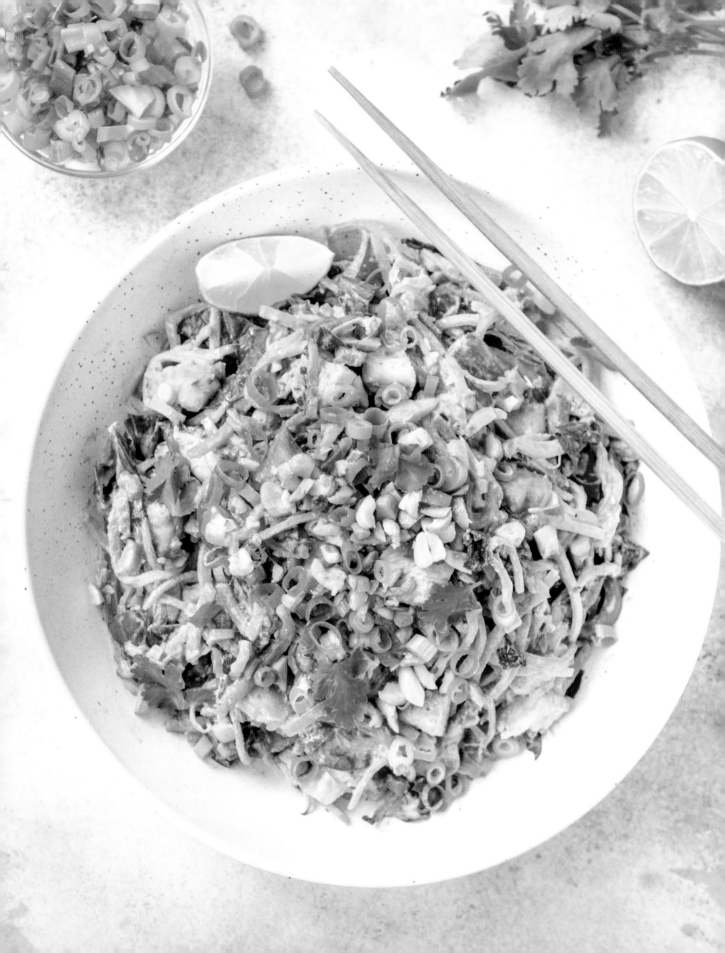

Make ahead

Hawaiian
CHICKEN SKEWERS

Yield: 8 skewers   **Prep Time:** 10 minutes, plus 1 hour to marinate chicken   **Cook Time:** 15 minutes

If you're a fan of Hawaiian pizza, then you will love these easy-to-make skewers. The vibrant veggies, pineapple, bacon, and chicken are slathered in a deliciously sweet and sticky teriyaki sauce that also acts as a marinade for the chicken to make it extra tender and flavorful. The skewers are a great make-ahead dish for a summer cookout, or you can cut the recipe in half to serve them as a fun appetizer with extra sauce on the side for dipping.

Marinade

¼ cup no-sugar-added pineapple juice

¼ cup coconut aminos

¼ cup honey

1 (1-inch) piece fresh ginger, roughly chopped

2 cloves garlic, peeled

12 ounces boneless, skinless chicken breasts, cut into 2-inch cubes

1 medium pineapple, or 3 cups precut fresh pineapple cubes

1 large red onion

1 red bell pepper

1 yellow bell pepper

12 strips bacon, cut in half crosswise

Chopped fresh Italian parsley, for garnish

SPECIAL EQUIPMENT
8 stainless steel or wooden skewers (see tip)

1. To make the marinade, put the pineapple juice, coconut aminos, honey, ginger, and garlic in a blender and blend until smooth. Place the cubed chicken in a bowl and pour half of the marinade over the top; reserve the other half for basting and serving. Allow the chicken to marinate for about an hour in the fridge.

2. While the chicken is marinating, cut the pineapple into 2-inch cubes and the onion and bell peppers into 2-inch pieces.

3. Heat a grill to medium-high heat. Thread the marinated chicken, pineapple, onion, bell peppers, and bacon onto the skewers, alternating among each until the skewers are filled. For the bacon, fold each half slice three times before threading it on the skewer.

4. Place the skewers on the grill and brush with some of the reserved sauce. Grill for 15 minutes, turning the skewers and brushing with more sauce every 5 minutes, until the chicken is cooked through and golden, and the bacon is cooked.

5. Transfer the skewers to a platter or tray, brush them with some of the leftover sauce, and sprinkle with chopped parsley before serving.

MAKE AHEAD/STORAGE: *You can marinate the chicken and thread it on the skewers with the other ingredients a day before grilling. Leftover skewers and sauce can be stored in the fridge for up to 3 days. Reserve a bit of sauce to brush over the skewers before reheating; it really brings the leftover skewers back to life.*

Wooden Skewers
If you're using wooden skewers, soak them in water for a minimum of 30 minutes to ensure that they don't burn on the grill. Putting the skewers in a tall bottle or vase filled with water will help keep them fully submerged.

SCD BASICS
Coco-not Aminos (page 47)

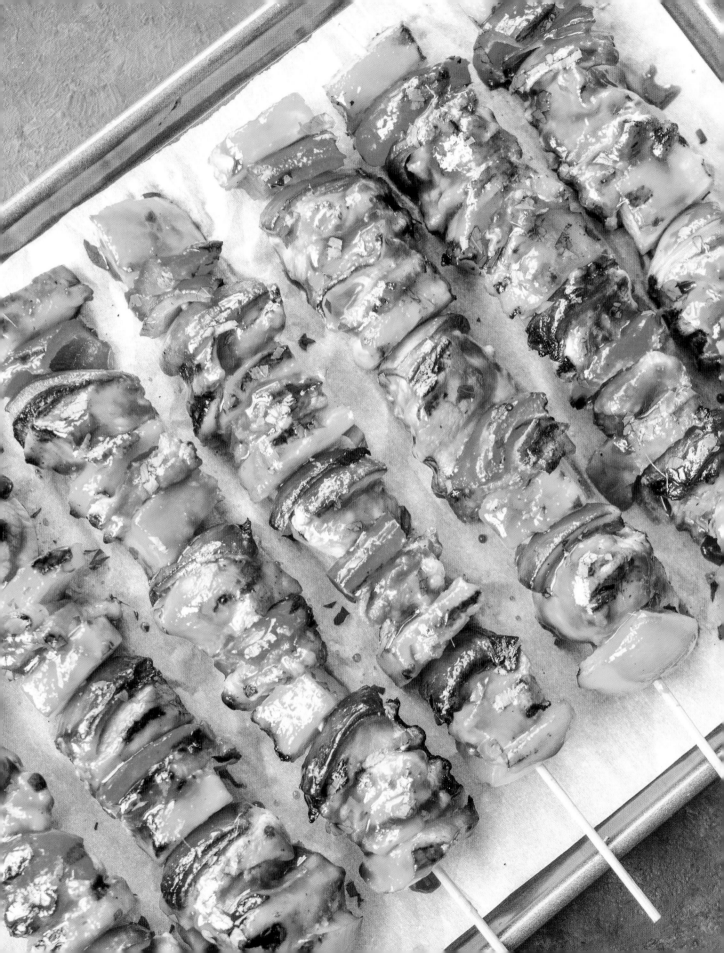

Make ahead

Harissa & Orange
SPATCHCOCK ROAST CHICKEN

Yield: 6 servings   **Prep Time:** 15 minutes, plus 10 minutes resting time   **Cook Time:** 40 minutes

Roast chicken was regularly on the menu for Sunday night dinner when I was growing up. I remember always standing close to my dad while he carved the chicken so that I could sneak pieces of the crispy skin when no one was looking. (I confess that I still do that now.) Spatchcocking a chicken (a simple four-minute task that involves removing the backbone to lay the chicken flat) reduces the cooking time, helps to ensure the whole bird cooks evenly, and increases the amount of delicious crispy skin. Intimidated by the process? You can ask your butcher to do it for you; alternatively, use a combination of skin-on, bone-in thighs, legs, and breasts, but reduce the oven temperature and time to 350°F for 30 minutes.

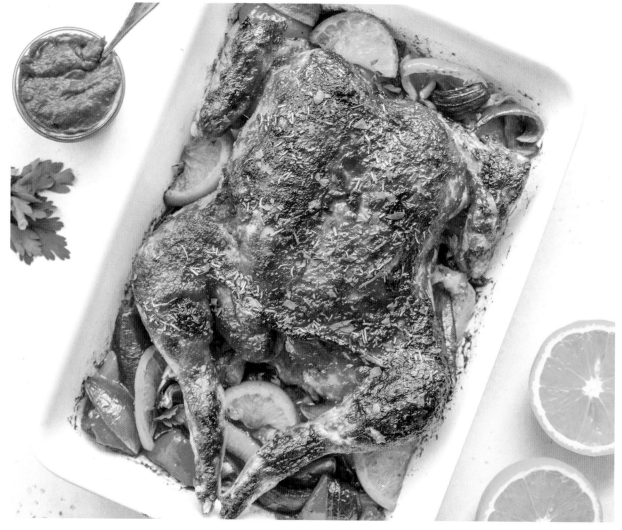

1 (4- to 4½-pound) whole chicken

Harissa Orange Paste

1½ tablespoons harissa

2 tablespoons softened ghee or unsalted butter

1 teaspoon grated orange zest

1 tablespoon freshly squeezed orange juice

1 clove garlic, minced

½ teaspoon paprika

½ teaspoon dried rosemary leaves

¼ teaspoon salt

¼ teaspoon pepper

2 red onions, cut into eighths

1 red bell pepper, cut into 2-inch pieces

1 orange or yellow bell pepper, cut into 2-inch pieces

½ orange, cut into thin half-moons

1 tablespoon harissa

1 tablespoon freshly squeezed orange juice

1 tablespoon extra-virgin olive oil

½ teaspoon paprika

1½ teaspoons chopped fresh Italian parsley

MAKE AHEAD/STORAGE: *You can spatchcock the chicken and leave it to marinate in the harissa orange paste a day in advance of roasting. Leftovers will last in the fridge for up to 4 days. Try cutting up the veggies and chicken and tossing them into salads. Freeze the backbone as well as any of the remaining carcass to make Chicken Stock (page 53).*

SCD BASICS
Harissa (page 33)

1. Preheat the oven to 450°F.

2. Spatchcock the chicken by removing the backbone, flipping the chicken over, and pressing down to flatten it (see the diagram).

3. Place the chicken breast side up in a large roasting pan or baking dish. Place all of the ingredients for the harissa orange paste in a small bowl and use a fork to mix them together until well blended. Smear the paste all over the outside of the chicken, ensuring that the entire bird is covered in the paste.

4. Arrange the onions, bell peppers, and orange slices around the chicken. In a small bowl, whisk together the harissa, orange juice, oil, and paprika and drizzle over the vegetables. Use your hands to gently toss to ensure that the vegetables are all well coated.

5. Roast for 40 minutes or until a meat thermometer inserted into the thickest part of the breast reads 160°F.

6. Allow the chicken to rest for 10 minutes before transferring to a cutting board, garnishing with chopped parsley, and carving.

SUBSTITUTIONS: *For dairy-free, replace the ghee or butter with 1 tablespoon of extra-virgin olive oil.*

How to Spatchcock a Chicken

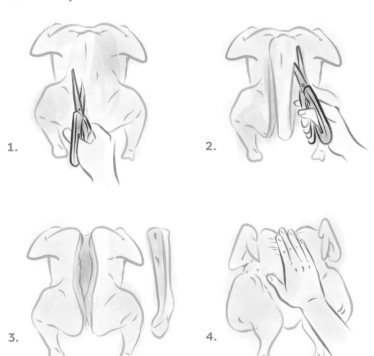

1.   2.

3.   4.

every last bite   187

AIP
KETO
PALEO
DAIRY-FREE
EGG-FREE
NUT-FREE

Balsamic
CHICKEN & GRAPES

Yield: 4 servings **Prep Time:** 10 minutes **Cook Time:** 55 minutes

This one-pan chicken dish is fancy enough to serve to guests but easy enough to make for a weeknight dinner. The combination of chicken, juicy grapes, and a balsamic sauce creates a richly flavored dish that pairs wonderfully with a side of cauliflower mash.

1 tablespoon extra-virgin olive oil

6 bone-in, skin-on chicken thighs

½ teaspoon salt

½ teaspoon ground black pepper

1 medium red onion, thinly sliced

¼ cup finely diced shallots

3 cloves garlic, minced

⅔ cup chicken stock

3 tablespoons aged balsamic vinegar

1½ teaspoons Dijon mustard

1 teaspoon dried rosemary leaves

2 cups seedless red grapes

1. Preheat the oven to 350°F.

2. Heat the oil in a large cast-iron skillet or other ovenproof skillet over medium-high heat. Season the chicken thighs on both sides with the salt and pepper, then place in the skillet skin side down. Cook for 4 minutes or until the skin is golden and crisp; flip and cook for another 4 minutes on the other side. Once the chicken has been seared on both sides, transfer to a plate and set aside. (Don't worry if the thighs aren't cooked through yet.)

3. Lower the heat to medium and place the onion, shallots, and garlic in the skillet; cook for 5 minutes, until the onion begins to soften. Stir in the chicken stock, balsamic vinegar, Dijon mustard, and rosemary and simmer for 8 minutes, until the liquid begins to reduce.

4. Return the chicken thighs to the skillet and arrange the grapes around the chicken. Spoon some of the sauce over the chicken and transfer the skillet to the oven to bake for 30 minutes or until the chicken is cooked through.

SUBSTITUTIONS: *For AIP, omit the mustard and pepper. Replace the grapes with sautéed mushrooms to make it keto.*

Meat Temperatures

A meat thermometer is the easiest and quickest way to ensure that meat is cooked to your liking. Here's a general guide:

Chicken	165°F
Pork (ground)	160°F
Pork (medium)	150°F
Pork (well-done)	160°F
Beef (rare)	115°F
Beef (medium-rare)	120°F
Beef (medium)	130°F
Beef (medium-well)	140°F
Beef (well-done)	150°F
Beef (ground)	150°F

Warming Plates

Warm plates in the oven at 150°F for 10 minutes or in the microwave for 30 seconds before serving. This will keep plated food warmer for longer and reduce the stress of trying to serve a dish before it starts to cool (especially when you're serving guests).

SCD BASICS
SCD Balsamic Vinegar (page 46), **Chicken Stock** (page 53)

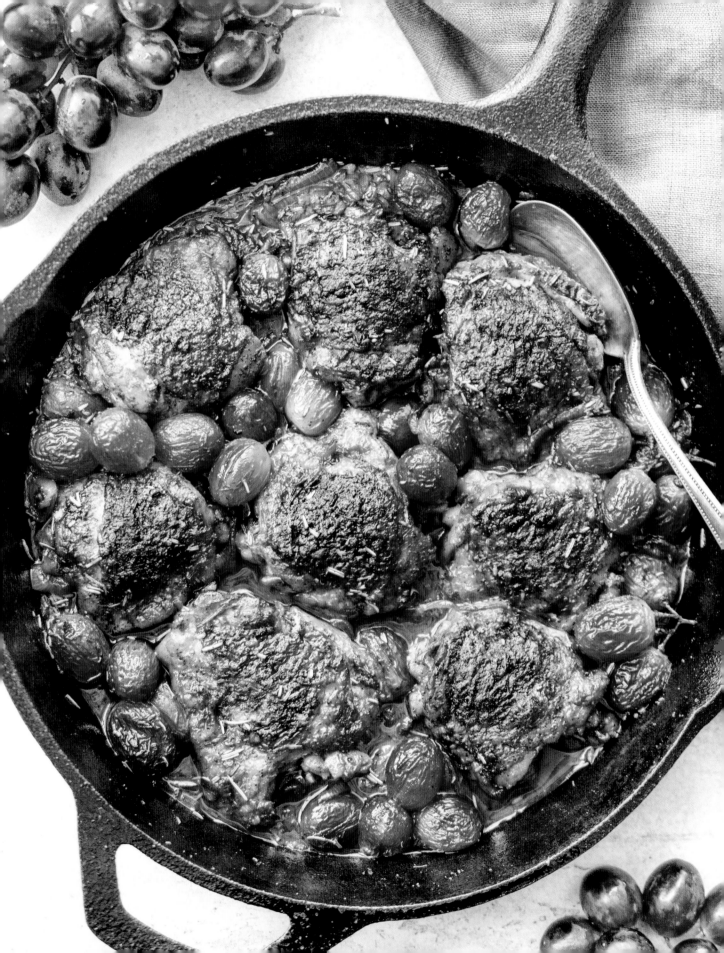

KETO
LOW-FODMAP
PALEO
DAIRY-FREE
EGG-FREE
NUT-FREE

< 30 min

Spicy Honey
UN-FRIED CHICKEN

Yield: 3 servings   **Prep Time:** 10 minutes   **Cook Time:** 20 minutes

This healthier spin on honey fried chicken uses my absolute favorite cut of chicken: boneless, skin-on chicken thighs. You get all of the good flavor from the dark meat of the thighs, plus the crispy skin, but with a shorter cook time and without the hassle of eating around a bone. You don't need to be a butcher to debone thighs. You can do it in minutes with a knife and a pair of kitchen shears. If you prefer, though, you can always ask the butcher to debone the thighs for you.

6 bone-in, skin-on chicken thighs

1½ tablespoons extra-virgin olive oil or avocado oil, divided

½ teaspoon salt

½ teaspoon ground black pepper

½ teaspoon cayenne pepper

Sauce

¼ cup unsalted butter or ghee

2 cloves garlic, minced

1½ tablespoons honey

1 teaspoon smoked paprika

¾ teaspoon cayenne pepper

¼ teaspoon ground black pepper

¼ teaspoon salt

1 red chili pepper, such as Fresno, thinly sliced

1. Preheat the oven to 350°F.

2. To debone a chicken thigh, lay it on a cutting board, skin side down. Run a knife down both sides of the bone in the middle, then pull the bone up with your fingers and use the knife or kitchen scissors to cut the meat away from the bone and joint until the meat is completely detached. Repeat with the remaining thighs.

3. Heat 1 tablespoon of the olive oil in a large ovenproof skillet over medium-high heat. Season the chicken thighs on both sides with the salt, pepper, and cayenne pepper. Place them skin side down in the skillet and cook for about 5 minutes or until the skin is golden and crisp. Flip the chicken and cook for another 2 to 3 minutes until lightly seared.

4. Transfer the skillet to the oven to bake for 10 minutes, or until the chicken is cooked through.

5. While the chicken is baking, make the sauce: Melt the butter in a saucepan over medium-low heat. Add the garlic and heat for 2 minutes, until the garlic is fragrant. (Make sure not to burn it; otherwise, it will become bitter.) Gently whisk in the honey, paprika, cayenne pepper, black pepper, salt, and red chili pepper until the honey has melted and everything is well combined.

6. Transfer the cooked chicken to a large bowl, pour the sauce over the top, and toss until the chicken is well coated.

Save the Bones
Once you have cut the bones from the thighs, store them in a zip-top bag in the freezer until the next time you make Chicken Stock (page 53).

SUBSTITUTIONS: *Skip the honey for keto. For low-FODMAP, use maple syrup in place of the honey and omit the garlic. For dairy-free, use coconut oil in place of the butter or ghee.*

STORAGE: *Leftovers will last in the fridge for up to 3 days. Reheat in the oven on broil to recrisp the skin.*

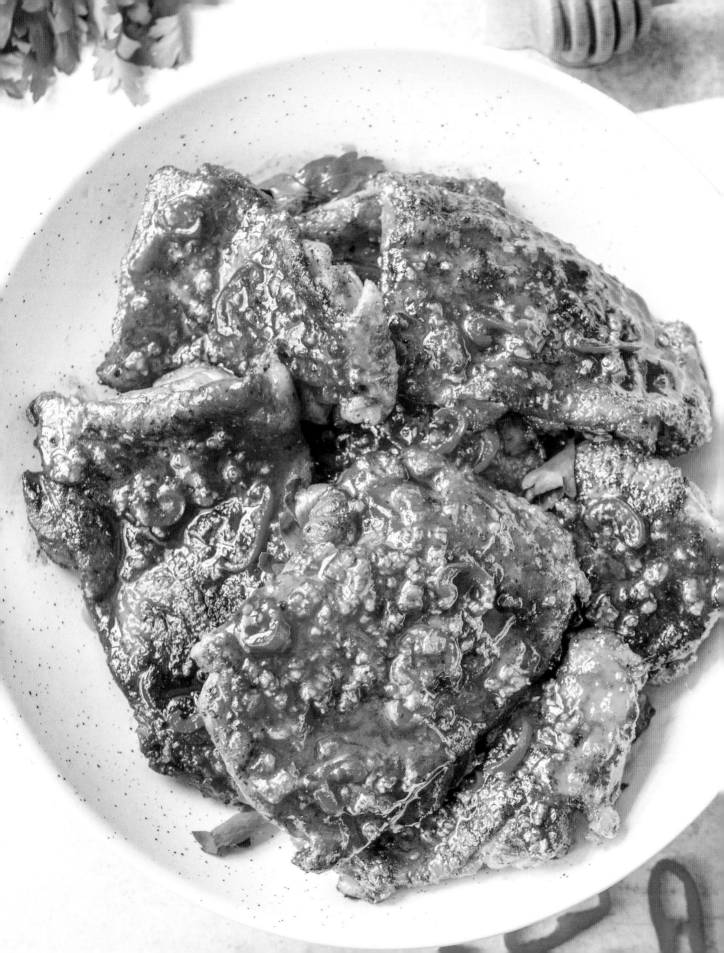

Italian CHICKEN BURGERS

Yield: 6 servings   **Prep Time:** 20 minutes   **Cook Time:** 10 minutes

Ground chicken is my favorite protein to use for burgers. It has less fat and fewer calories than beef, and its mild taste means it's the perfect blank canvas for bold ingredients, like the lemon herb mayonnaise, crispy prosciutto, grilled onion, and sun-dried tomatoes in this Italian-inspired recipe.

Lemon Herb Mayonnaise

½ cup mayonnaise

2 tablespoons chopped fresh basil

1 tablespoon chopped fresh Italian parsley

1 tablespoon freshly squeezed lemon juice

1 clove garlic, minced

Chicken Burgers

1½ pounds ground chicken or turkey

1 medium egg

¼ cup chopped oil-packed sun-dried tomatoes

¼ cup minced red onions

3 tablespoons blanched almond flour

2 tablespoons chopped fresh basil

2 tablespoons chopped fresh Italian parsley

1 teaspoon grated lemon zest

1 tablespoon freshly squeezed lemon juice

3 cloves garlic, minced

1 teaspoon ground black pepper

½ teaspoon salt

1 large red onion, sliced

6 slices prosciutto

2 heads baby romaine lettuce

½ cup oil-packed sun-dried tomatoes

1. To make the lemon herb mayonnaise, whisk together the mayonnaise, herbs, lemon juice, and garlic. Set aside.

2. Place the ground chicken, egg, sun-dried tomatoes, onion, almond flour, herbs, lemon zest and juice, garlic, pepper, and salt in a large bowl and use your hands to mix well. Divide the mixture into 6 equal portions and form each portion into a patty about 1½ inches thick. If the mixture is too sticky, wet your hands before forming the patties.

3. Heat a grill to medium heat or a grill pan over medium heat. Place the burger patties and sliced red onion on the grill. Cook the onion slices for 2 minutes, until they have slightly softened; remove from the heat and set aside. Cook the patties for about 5 minutes per side, until grill marks form and they are cooked through. Place the prosciutto slices on the grill and cook for 2 to 3 minutes, until crisp.

4. To assemble a burger, place 2 lettuce leaves on a plate with the edges partially overlapping. Spread a spoonful of the lemon herb mayonnaise over the leaves, top with 4 or 5 sun-dried tomatoes, some slices of grilled onion, 1 slice of crispy prosciutto, and a burger patty. Place another 2 lettuce leaves on top of the patty, then wrap the burger in parchment paper to make it easy to pick up and eat. Repeat with the remaining burger patties.

SUBSTITUTIONS: *Omit the garlic and onion to make them low-FODMAP. Swap the almond flour for coconut flour to make the burgers nut-free.*

STORAGE: *Leftovers will last in the fridge for up to 4 days or in the freezer for up to 2 months.*

SCD BASICS
Sun-Dried Tomatoes (page 38)
Easy 3-Minute Mayonnaise (page 42)

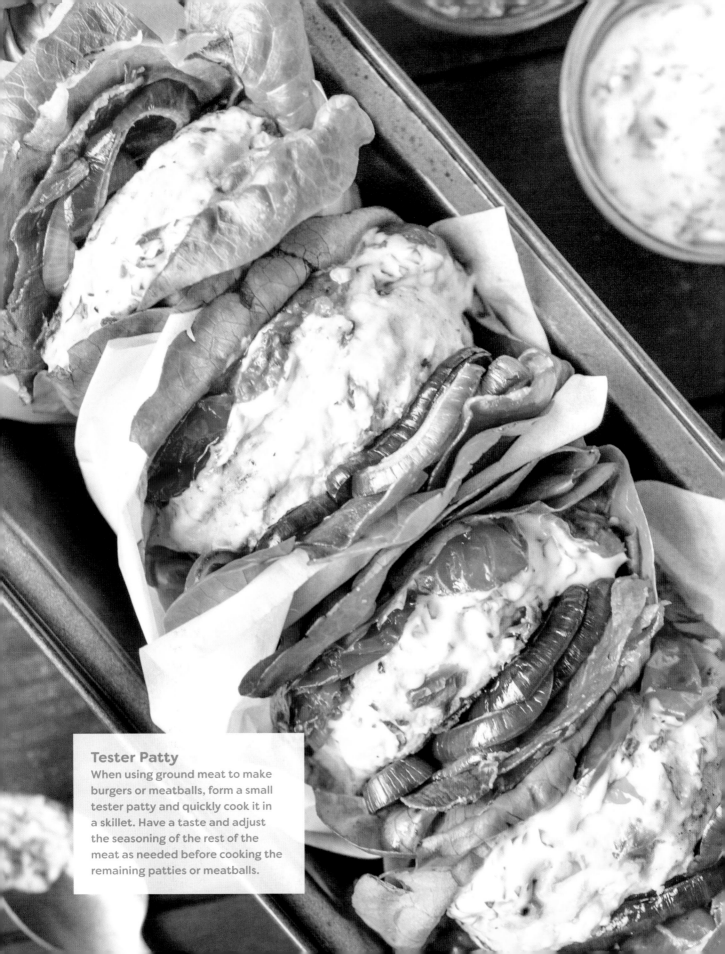

Tester Patty
When using ground meat to make burgers or meatballs, form a small tester patty and quickly cook it in a skillet. Have a taste and adjust the seasoning of the rest of the meat as needed before cooking the remaining patties or meatballs.

Sun-Dried Tomato, Basil & "Goat Cheese" STUFFED CHICKEN BREASTS

Make ahead

Yield: 4 servings   **Prep Time:** 20 minutes   **Cook Time:** 37 minutes

As a fan of fuss-free cooking, I typically try to avoid anything "stuffed" because it usually looks rather complicated to make. These chicken breasts are an exception to my rule because they are not only easy to make but an absolute showstopper of a dish. Whether you are on SCD or a gourmet foodie, this is a fantastic dish to serve when you want to impress.

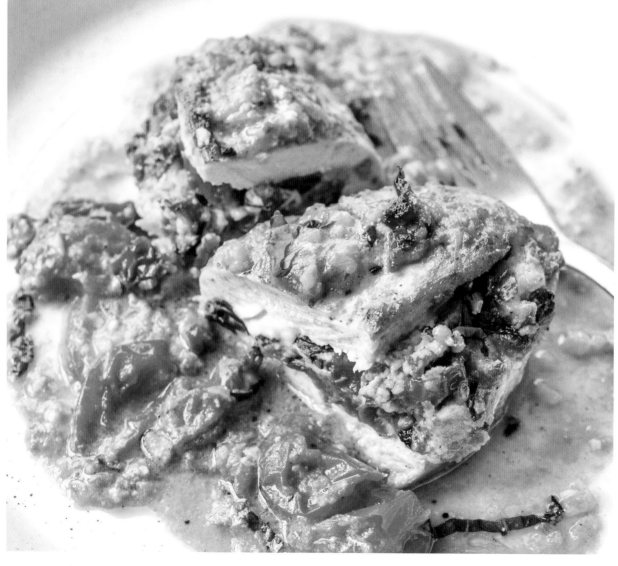

Creamy "Goat Cheese" Filling

⅔ cup raw cashews, soaked in boiling water for 10 minutes and drained

1 tablespoon water

1½ teaspoons freshly squeezed lemon juice

1 clove garlic, peeled

1 teaspoon coconut oil

1 teaspoon apple cider vinegar

4 large boneless, skinless chicken breasts

½ teaspoon dried oregano leaves

½ teaspoon salt

½ teaspoon ground black pepper

⅓ cup chopped sun-dried tomatoes

⅓ cup chopped fresh basil, plus 1 tablespoon for garnish

2 tablespoons light olive oil or avocado oil, divided

¼ teaspoon cayenne pepper

1 medium yellow onion, diced

2 cloves garlic, minced

1 cup unsweetened almond milk

1 cup chicken stock

1 cup halved cherry tomatoes

SPECIAL EQUIPMENT
High-powered blender

1. Preheat the oven to 350°F.

2. To make the filling, place the cashews, water, lemon juice, garlic, coconut oil, and vinegar in a high-powered blender and blend until completely smooth. Set aside.

3. Place a chicken breast on a cutting board and, holding your knife parallel to the cutting board, cut horizontally three-fourths of the way through the thickest part of the breast so that the breast can be opened flat onto the cutting board like a book. Repeat with the remaining chicken breasts.

4. Lay all of the chicken breasts open on a cutting board and season with the oregano, salt, and pepper. On one half of an opened chicken breast, evenly spread 2 tablespoons of the cashew filling. Top with one-quarter of the sun-dried tomatoes and chopped basil, then close the chicken breast by folding the top half of the breast over the filling. Repeat with the remaining breasts.

5. Heat 1 tablespoon of the oil in a large cast-iron or other ovenproof skillet over medium-high heat. Once hot, season the top of the chicken breasts with the cayenne pepper, then place in the skillet to sear for 4 minutes per side. Remove the chicken breasts from the skillet and set aside on a plate. (Don't worry if they aren't cooked through yet; they will finish cooking in the oven.)

6. Heat the remaining 1 tablespoon of the oil in the skillet over medium-high heat, then add the onion and garlic and sauté for 4 minutes, until the onion begins to soften. Increase the heat to high, and stir in the almond milk, chicken stock, and tomatoes. Simmer for 5 minutes, allowing the sauce to thicken.

7. Return the chicken breasts to the skillet, spoon some of the sauce over each breast, and bake for 20 minutes. The chicken is done when a meat thermometer inserted into the thickest part of the breast reads 165°F. Garnish the chicken with chopped basil before serving.

MAKE AHEAD/STORAGE: *The chicken can be stuffed a day in advance. Leftovers will last in the fridge for up to 4 days.*

SCD BASICS
Sun-Dried Tomatoes (page 38)
Chicken Stock (page 53)

KETO
LOW-FODMAP
PALEO
DAIRY-FREE
EGG-FREE
NUT-FREE

Chicken ENCHILADAS

Yield: 10 enchiladas **Prep Time:** 15 minutes **Cook Time:** 45 minutes

When trying to decide which recipes from my website to include in this book, I asked my Instagram followers which dishes were their favorites. These chicken enchiladas won by a landslide! Although they look elaborate, they are very easy to make and really satisfy a Mexican food craving. The enchiladas reheat well, so make extra to enjoy throughout the week. You can serve them topped with anything from salsa and guacamole to extra cheese, sliced radishes, jalapeños, or scallions.

Enchilada Sauce

1 large yellow onion, quartered

2 jalapeño peppers

5 cloves garlic, peeled

1½ teaspoons extra-virgin olive oil

3½ cups fresh chopped tomatoes (about 2½ pounds tomatoes)

1¼ cups chicken stock

1 tablespoon ground cumin

½ teaspoon cayenne pepper

¼ teaspoon salt

Enchiladas

1½ pounds boneless, skinless chicken breasts, cooked and shredded (about 3 cups)

2 large zucchini (see the tip)

½ cup plus 2 tablespoons shredded cheddar cheese (optional), plus more for the top as desired

Toppings (Optional)

1 tablespoon chopped fresh cilantro

1 small avocado, chopped

¼ cup chopped tomatoes

1 jalapeño pepper, thinly sliced

1 radish, thinly sliced

4 lime wedges

1. Preheat the oven to 350°F.

2. Place the onion, jalapeño peppers, and garlic in a food processor and blend until everything has broken into a fine mince.

3. Heat the oil in a medium-sized skillet over medium heat. Transfer the onion mixture to the skillet and sauté for 4 minutes, until the onion begins to soften, then add the remaining ingredients for the enchilada sauce. Allow to simmer for 20 minutes, stirring every few minutes until the sauce has thickened.

4. Taste the sauce and adjust the seasoning by adding more cumin, cayenne pepper, or salt. Place the shredded chicken in a bowl, pour half of the sauce over the chicken, and stir so that it's well coated. Set aside.

5. Trim the ends off the zucchini, and cut them in half lengthwise, then lay the zucchini halves cut side up on the cutting board. Use a vegetable peeler to cut thin broad ribbons off the zucchini. You should get 8 ribbons from each half.

6. Lay 3 ribbons of zucchini on a cutting board, putting the longest ribbon down first with the other two ribbons on either side with edges slightly overlapping.

7. Place about 2 large tablespoonfuls of the chicken mixture on the set of zucchini ribbons. Sprinkle with 2 tablespoons of the shredded cheddar, if using. Pressing firmly, roll the zucchini over the chicken mixture and place in an 11 by 7-inch baking dish with the seam side down. Repeat with the remaining zucchini ribbons until the dish is tightly packed with enchilada rolls.

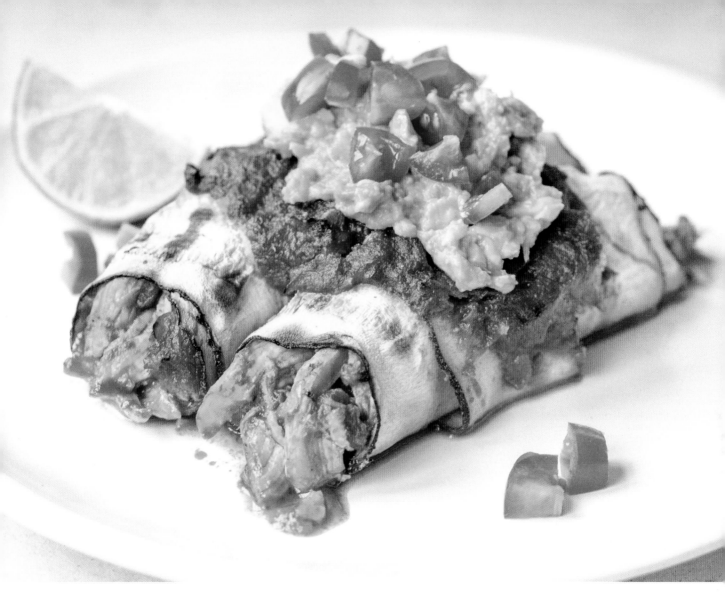

SUBSTITUTIONS: *For low-FODMAP, omit the onion and garlic. For Paleo or dairy-free, omit the cheese.*

STORAGE: *Leftovers will last in the fridge for up to 4 days. Although the enchiladas can be frozen after baking, they will release water when thawed and may need to be drained after baking.*

TIP: *Long, thin zucchini work best for producing the strips you need to wrap the enchiladas.*

SCD BASICS
Chicken Stock (page 53)

8. Spoon the remaining enchilada sauce over the rolls, then bake for 20 minutes, until the zucchini is tender. If you would like a bit more cheese, you can add it to the top of the enchiladas about 5 minutes before they are done; then bake until the cheese is melted.

9. Remove the dish from the oven. If there is a lot of liquid at the bottom of the dish from the zucchini, use a baster or spoon to remove it from the dish. Before serving, sprinkle the enchiladas with your toppings of choice.

Shredded Chicken
The fastest way to make shredded or diced chicken for a recipe is to place raw chicken breasts in a pot filled with just enough water to cover the chicken. Bring to a simmer and cook for 20 minutes. Cut the chicken to ensure it is cooked all the way through before shredding it with two forks.

One-Pan Spanish
CHICKEN & RICE

Yield: 4 servings **Prep Time:** 10 minutes **Cook Time:** 30 minutes

I love the ease of a one-pan meal; there's no need to worry about side dishes, and you have only one pan to wash (because no one enjoys washing dishes). The riced cauliflower takes on a paella-esque flavor thanks to the saffron (which you can find in the spice aisle of most stores), paprika, and lemon. Chorizo adds a nice kick of spice; if you're unable to find an SCD-legal brand, check out my easy recipe on page 50.

6 boneless, skinless chicken thighs

1½ teaspoons paprika, divided

¼ teaspoon ground coriander

¼ teaspoon cayenne pepper

¼ teaspoon salt

¼ teaspoon ground black pepper

1 tablespoon extra-virgin olive oil

2 cloves garlic, minced

1 medium yellow onion, diced

1 red bell pepper, diced

5 ounces ground chorizo

¾ cup chicken stock

1½ tablespoons white wine vinegar

¾ cup chopped tomatoes

½ cup pitted green olives, cut in half

⅓ cup frozen peas

½ teaspoon saffron threads

3½ cups fresh riced cauliflower

½ lemon, cut into thin half-moons

2 tablespoons chopped fresh Italian parsley, for garnish

1. Preheat the oven to 375°F.

2. Season the chicken thighs on both sides with 1 teaspoon of the paprika, the coriander, cayenne pepper, salt, and black pepper. Heat the oil in a large ovenproof skillet over medium-high heat and cook the chicken for 4 to 5 minutes per side, until golden. Remove the chicken from the skillet and set aside.

3. Lower the heat to medium, add the garlic to the skillet, and scrape the skillet with a wooden spoon to loosen any bits of chicken (extra flavor!). Cook the garlic for a minute until it becomes fragrant, then add the onion, red pepper, and chorizo. Cook for 5 minutes, using a wood spoon to break up the chorizo, until the pepper begins to soften and the meat is cooked through.

4. Add the chicken stock, vinegar, tomatoes, olives, peas, the saffron, and the remaining ½ teaspoon of paprika and stir to combine. Add the riced cauliflower to the skillet and stir thoroughly so that everything is well mixed together.

5. Arrange the chicken thighs on top of the riced cauliflower and scatter 5 or 6 lemon slices around the skillet, cover with aluminum foil, and transfer to the oven to bake for 15 minutes, until the cauliflower is tender and most of the liquid in the skillet has been absorbed. Garnish with the chopped parsley before serving.

SCD BASICS
Chorizo (page 50)
Chicken Stock (page 53)

SUBSTITUTIONS: *Omit the frozen peas for keto.*

STORAGE: *Leftovers will last in the fridge for up to 4 days.*

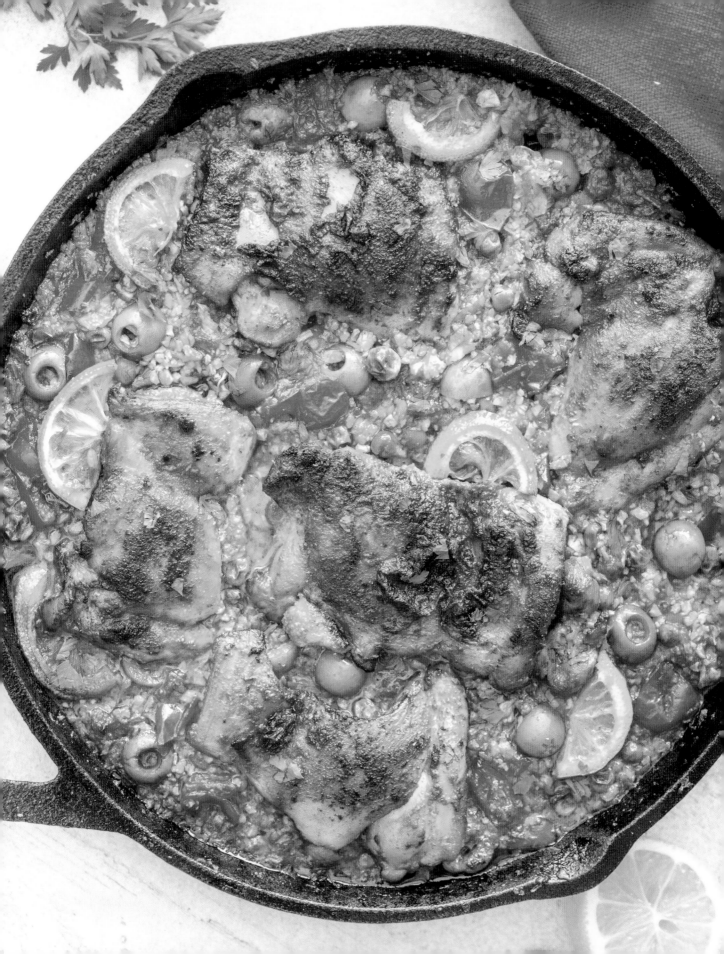

Sheet Pan
GREEK CHICKEN

Yield: 4 servings   **Prep Time:** 10 minutes   **Cook Time:** 35 minutes

This dish is the most popular recipe on my blog, so I knew it had to be included in this cookbook. It's an incredibly simple recipe that requires minimal effort but results in a really flavorful one-pan meal. When it comes to foolproof dishes, this one is a hard one to beat. Feta is an "advanced" SCD food that you should eat only after being in remission for six months or more, so add it only if you are ready. You can swap salmon for the chicken if you are pescatarian, but don't add the salmon until you add the basil and feta to the pan so that the fish doesn't overcook.

1 red bell pepper, cut into strips

1 yellow bell pepper, cut into strips

1 large red onion, cut into eighths

14 ounces cherry tomatoes (about 2 cups)

⅔ cup pitted Kalamata olives

½ cup artichoke hearts

1 lemon, cut into wedges

¼ cup extra-virgin olive oil

1½ tablespoons aged balsamic vinegar, or 2 teaspoons red wine vinegar

2 cloves garlic, minced

1 teaspoon dried oregano leaves

½ teaspoon smoked paprika

½ teaspoon ground black pepper

¼ teaspoon salt

6 boneless, skinless chicken thighs

¼ cup chopped feta (optional)

3 tablespoons chopped fresh basil, divided

1. Preheat the oven to 400°F.

2. Place the bell peppers, onion, tomatoes, olives, artichoke hearts, and lemon wedges on a sheet pan or in a large baking dish.

3. In a bowl, whisk together the oil, vinegar, garlic, oregano, and smoked paprika. Pour one-third of the sauce over the veggies, sprinkle with the pepper and salt, and toss until well coated. Place the chicken thighs on top of the veggies and brush the chicken with more of the sauce from the bowl. Roast for 25 minutes.

4. Remove the pan from the oven and sprinkle the feta (if using) and 2 tablespoons of the basil on top. Pour the remaining sauce over the veggies and chicken and return to the oven for another 5 to 10 minutes, until the chicken is cooked through.

5. Before serving, garnish with the remaining 1 tablespoon of basil.

SUBSTITUTIONS: *Omit the red onion, garlic, and artichokes for low-FODMAP. Omit the feta if you are Paleo, dairy-free, or new to SCD.*

STORAGE: *Leftovers will last in the fridge for up to 4 days and are great added into salad.*

Roasting Veggies

When roasting veggies, place a sheet pan in the oven while it preheats. When you put the seasoned vegetables on the hot pan, they will immediately start cooking, reducing cooking time. This method also helps the veggies cook evenly on both sides.

SCD BASICS
SCD Balsamic Vinegar (page 46)

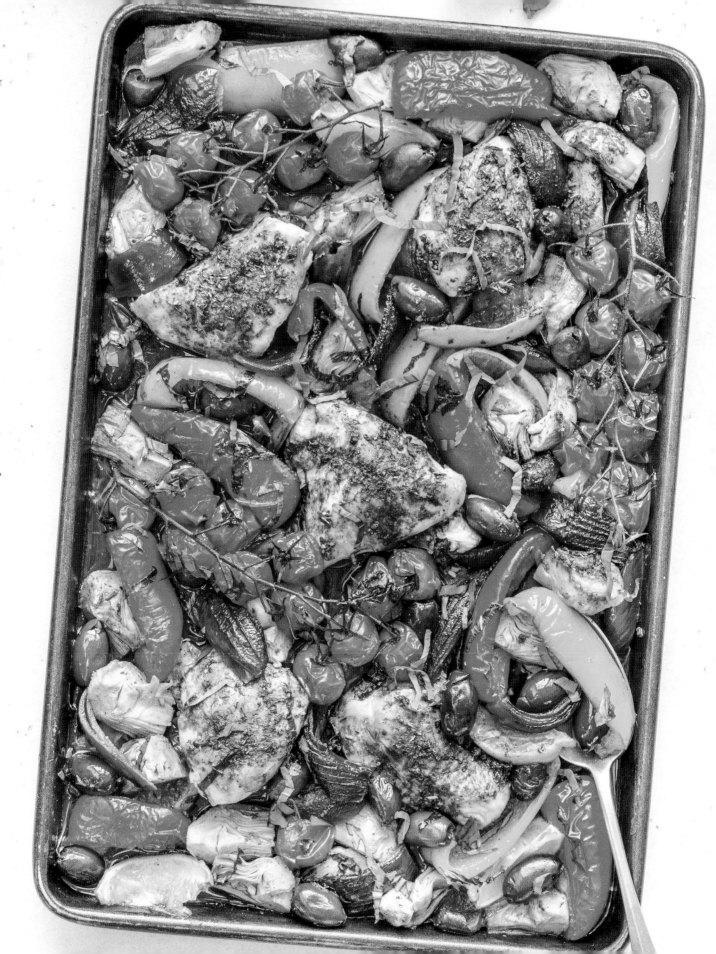

KETO
LOW-FODMAP
PALEO
DAIRY-FREE
EGG-FREE
NUT-FREE

Butter Chicken
MEATBALLS

Yield: 18 meatballs **Prep Time:** 15 minutes **Cook Time:** 25 minutes

This fun spin on butter chicken is a wonderful hearty winter dish that packs a lot of flavor. The rich and creamy sauce is the star of the show, and the tender meatballs soak a lot of it up to make every bite saucy and delicious. Serve these meatballs with a side of cauliflower rice to ensure that you don't let a drop of sauce go to waste.

Meatballs

1¼ pounds ground chicken

⅓ cup blanched almond flour

1 medium egg

1 tablespoon finely chopped fresh ginger

1 tablespoon chopped fresh cilantro

2 cloves garlic, minced

1 teaspoon ground cumin

1 teaspoon ground coriander

½ teaspoon ground black pepper

¼ teaspoon salt

Sauce

1 tablespoon extra-virgin olive oil

1 medium yellow onion, diced

2 cloves garlic, minced

¾ cup canned full-fat coconut milk

½ cup chicken stock

½ cup tomato paste

2 teaspoons garam masala

2 teaspoons ground cumin

2 teaspoons ground coriander

½ teaspoon cayenne pepper

½ teaspoon ground ginger

1½ tablespoons unsalted butter or ghee

2 tablespoons chopped fresh cilantro, for garnish

1. Preheat the oven to 400°F. Line a sheet pan with parchment paper.

2. Place all of the ingredients for the meatballs in a large bowl and use your hands to mix everything together. Wet your hands and form the mixture into 18 meatballs, about 1½ inches in diameter. Place on the prepared sheet pan and bake for 18 to 20 minutes, until golden and cooked through.

3. While the meatballs are cooking, prepare the sauce: Heat the oil in a large skillet over medium-high heat. Add the onion and garlic and sauté for 4 to 5 minutes, until the onion is translucent. Stir in the coconut milk, chicken stock, tomato paste, and spices and allow the sauce to boil gently for about 6 minutes, until it has begun to thicken.

4. Stir in the butter. Once the meatballs are cooked, transfer them to the skillet with the sauce. Spoon the sauce over the meatballs to coat them and simmer for a minute or two. Garnish with the chopped cilantro before serving.

SUBSTITUTIONS: *Omit the onion and garlic for low-FODMAP and use 1 tablespoon of garlic-infused oil in place of the extra-virgin olive oil. For dairy-free, use coconut oil in place of the ghee or butter. Swap the almond flour for coconut flour to make the meatballs nut-free.*

STORAGE: *Leftovers will last in the fridge for up to 4 days or in the freezer for up to 2 months. To reheat, place the frozen meatballs in a pot on the stove with a splash of water.*

Ground Chicken

You can make your own ground chicken by cutting boneless, skinless chicken breasts and/or thighs into cubes and pulsing in a food processor until the meat is broken down into a minced texture.

SCD BASICS
Tomato Paste (page 35), **Chicken Stock** (page 53)

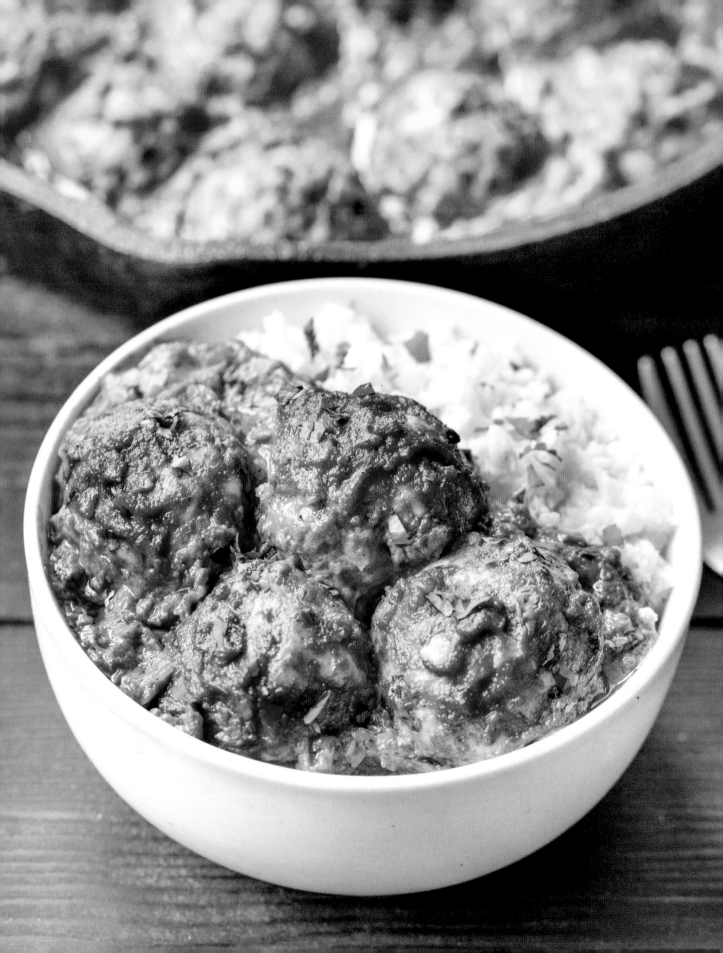

Creamy Chicken &
SPINACH CANNELLONI

Yield: 16 cannelloni   **Prep Time:** 15 minutes   **Cook Time:** 45 minutes

My nana used to make the most incredible creamy cannelloni. She didn't have a written recipe; she'd just describe measurements as "a good-sized amount of this" and "a little bit of that." Before she passed away, she took the time to write out the recipes for more than twenty of her dishes so that I would always have them. I wish that I could say that this was her recipe for cannelloni, but it turns out that there was not a single ingredient listed in the recipe that I could use in this book, so these SCD cannelloni are inspired by her. The filling is creamy and delicious, wrapped in thin strips of eggplant—a stand-in for the traditional pasta tubes that give the dish its name—and then topped with tomato sauce. It may not be quite as good as my nana's cannelloni, but it's close.

Tomato Sauce

2 tablespoons extra-virgin olive oil

½ medium yellow onion, diced

1 clove garlic, minced

1 teaspoon salt

½ teaspoon ground black pepper

1 (14-ounce) can diced tomatoes, or 1½ cups chunky tomato sauce

Cannelloni

1½ teaspoons extra-virgin olive oil

3 eggplants

Filling

⅔ cup raw cashews, soaked in boiling water for 10 minutes and drained

½ cup unsweetened almond milk

2 cloves garlic, peeled

1 tablespoon extra-virgin olive oil

1 medium yellow onion, diced

6 ounces ground chicken

3 cups spinach

Chopped fresh basil and/or grated Parmesan cheese, for garnish (optional)

SPECIAL EQUIPMENT
High-powered blender

1. Preheat the oven to 350°F.

2. To make the tomato sauce, heat the oil in a medium-sized saucepan over medium heat. Add the onion and garlic and cook for 5 minutes, until the onion begins to soften. Add the salt, pepper, and tomatoes and simmer for 25 minutes, stirring every 5 minutes, until the tomatoes have broken down and the sauce has reduced to a thick consistency.

3. While the sauce is cooking, make the cannelloni: Preheat a panini press or a grill pan over medium-high heat, then grease the press or pan with the oil. Cut the eggplants lengthwise into sixteen ¼-inch-thick slices. Place the slices on the greased panini press or grill pan and cook for 4 minutes, until the eggplant slices have softened and grill marks form. Transfer to a plate and set aside.

4. To make the filling, place the cashews, almond milk, and garlic in a high-powered blender and blend until completely smooth. Set the cashew cream aside while you prepare the rest of the filling ingredients.

5. Heat the oil in a large skillet over medium heat and add the onion. Cook for 5 minutes, until the onion begins to soften, then add the chicken. Use a wooden spoon to break the meat into crumbles and cook for 5 minutes, until the chicken is cooked through. Mix in the spinach and cashew cream and cook for 4 to 5 more minutes, until the spinach has wilted.

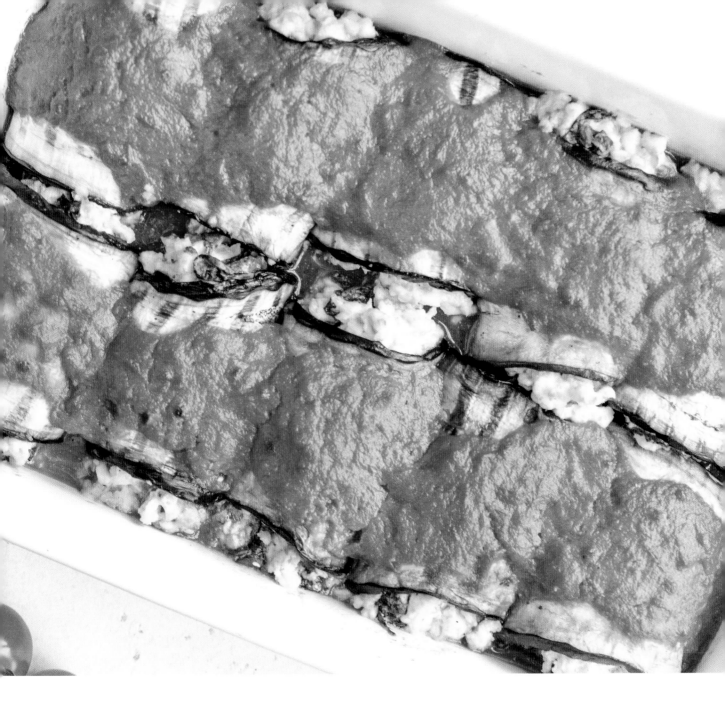

STORAGE: *Leftovers will last in the fridge for up to 3 days or in the freezer for up to 2 months.*

SCD BASICS
Tomato Sauce (page 36)

6. Spoon one-third of the tomato sauce into an 11 by 7-inch baking dish and evenly spread it on the bottom. Place 2 tablespoons of the filling at the base of a slice of eggplant and roll it tightly. Place the eggplant roll seam side down in the baking dish. Repeat with the remaining eggplant slices and filling, until the baking dish is full. Spoon the remaining sauce over the rolls and bake for 15 minutes, until the sauce is bubbling and the rolls are heated through.

7. Serve garnished with chopped basil and/or Parmesan cheese, if using.

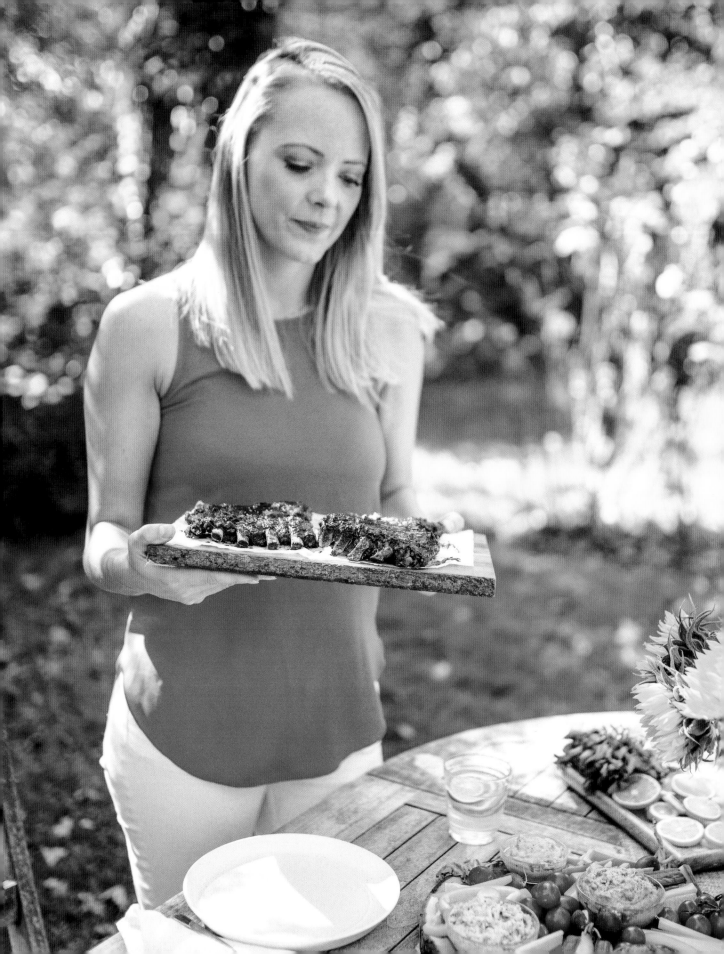

Meat

Grilled Skirt Steak
WITH ASIAN SALSA VERDE

Yield: 4 servings   **Prep Time:** 20 minutes, plus at least 1 hour to marinate   **Cook Time:** 5 minutes

Skirt steak is one of my favorite cuts of meat, but it's often overlooked because of its flat shape and tendency to become tough when overcooked. However, it's more affordable than the thicker cuts of beef and becomes flavorful and tender when marinated for a few hours and cooked quickly over high heat. If you can't find skirt steak, flank steak is a good second choice. Like skirt steak, it's a thin cut of meat that takes well to marinating. This dish is great for a crowd at a summer cookout and always gets 10/10 rave reviews.

⅓ cup coconut aminos

1 tablespoon honey, or 1 Medjool date, pitted, soaked for 10 minutes, and drained

1 (1-inch) piece fresh ginger, roughly chopped

3 cloves garlic, peeled

1 red chili pepper, such as Fresno

1 tablespoon toasted sesame oil

2 pounds skirt steak or flank steak

Asian Salsa Verde

¾ cup chopped fresh cilantro

⅔ cup chopped scallions

1 jalapeño pepper, minced

¼ cup apple cider vinegar

3 tablespoons extra-virgin olive oil

2 tablespoons toasted sesame oil

1 tablespoon white sesame seeds

1 tablespoon black sesame seeds

1 lime, halved (for garnish)

1. Put the coconut aminos, honey, ginger, garlic, chili pepper, and sesame oil in a blender and blend until smooth. Place the beef in a zip-top bag and pour the marinade over the top. Allow to marinate in the fridge for a minimum of 1 hour.

2. To make the Asian salsa verde, place all of the ingredients in a bowl and stir until well mixed. Set aside.

3. Heat a grill to high heat; alternatively, heat a grill pan over high heat. Once hot, grill the marinated beef for exactly 2½ minutes per side for medium-rare. Transfer the steak to a cutting board to rest for 5 minutes before slicing thinly across the grain. Serve with the Asian salsa verde spooned over the top and lime halves on the side.

SUBSTITUTIONS: *Omit the honey to make this dish keto.*

MAKE AHEAD/STORAGE: *The Asian salsa verde can be made and the steak left to marinate a day in advance. Leftovers will last in the fridge, with the grilled steak and salsa verde stored separately, for up to 3 days. A delicious use for the leftover steak is to cut it up and toss it into a salad and use the salsa verde as dressing.*

SCD BASICS
Coco-not Aminos (page 47)

Rest Time

Whether you're preparing chicken, steak, pork, or lamb, once the meat is done cooking, always allow it to rest before slicing. This will give the juices time to redistribute throughout the meat rather than letting them escape onto the cutting board. The result is more flavorful and juicy meat. As a general rule, leave the steak to rest for 5 minutes per inch of thickness.

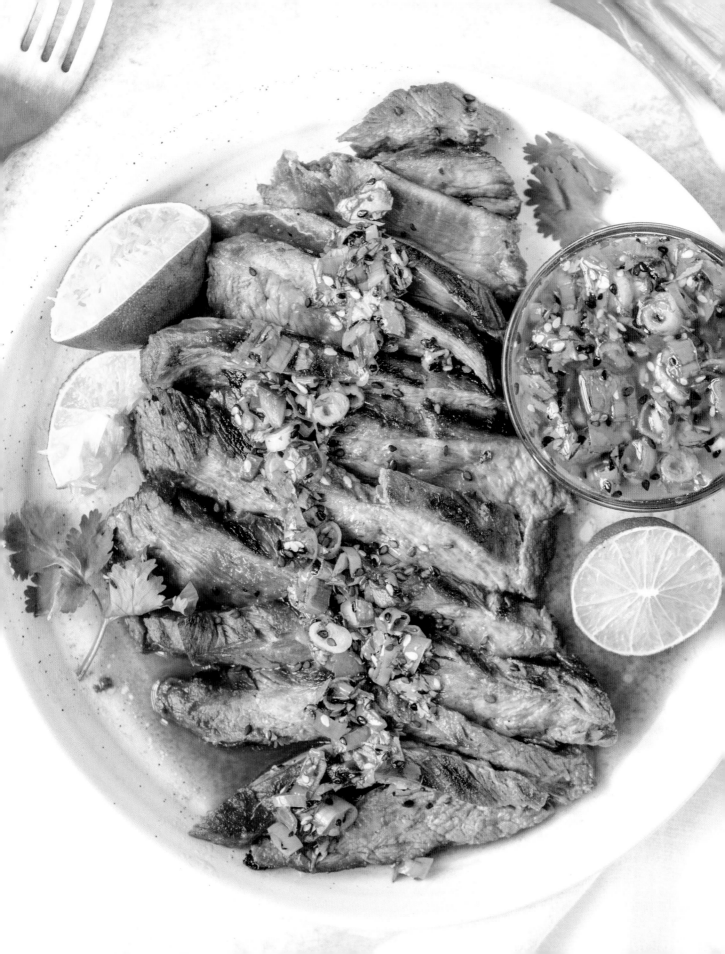

The Most Epic
GRAIN-FREE BEEF LASAGNA

Yield: 8 servings   **Prep Time:** 30 minutes   **Cook Time:** 1 hour 15 minutes

When it comes to comfort food, it's hard to beat lasagna, and this grain-free version is 100 percent satisfying. Thinly sliced butternut squash sheets make the perfect noodle replacement. If you can't find precut sheets in stores, it's not hard to slice them yourself (see the sidebar, opposite).

On my blog, this recipe receives rave reviews for just how much it tastes like traditional lasagna. Even my husband, SA, who grew up eating his Italian mom's incredible homemade lasagna, gives this healthier version two thumbs up. Although it takes a bit of time to make, it freezes really well, so double or triple the recipe and freeze small portions for those weeknights when you are in need of fast comfort food.

Meat Sauce

1 tablespoon extra-virgin olive oil

1 medium yellow onion, diced

2 cloves garlic, minced

1¼ pounds ground beef

1 pound ground pork

¼ teaspoon salt

3 cups chunky tomato sauce, or 1 (21-ounce) can diced tomatoes

2 tablespoons tomato paste

1 tablespoon fresh oregano leaves

1½ teaspoons red pepper flakes

Cashew "Cheese"

1 cup raw cashews, soaked in boiling water for 10 minutes and drained

⅔ cup unsweetened almond milk

2 cloves garlic, peeled

2 tablespoons roughly chopped fresh basil

10 to 12 butternut squash sheets (see sidebar)

Chopped fresh Italian parsley, for garnish

1. Preheat the oven to 375°F.

2. Heat the oil in a large pot over medium-high heat. Add the onion and minced garlic and sauté for 4 minutes, or until the onion begins to soften.

3. Add the ground beef and pork and season with the salt. Cook for about 10 minutes, until the meat is cooked through, using a wooden spoon to break the meat into a fine crumble.

4. Stir in the tomato sauce, tomato paste, oregano, and red pepper flakes. Simmer for 10 minutes.

5. While the meat sauce simmers, place the cashews, almond milk, and 2 cloves of garlic in a high-powered blender and blend until completely smooth; there should be no small bits. Transfer the mixture to a bowl and stir in the basil.

6. Spread about one-quarter of the meat sauce in an even layer on the bottom of an 11 by 7-inch baking dish. Place the butternut squash sheets on top of the sauce, followed by a layer of meat sauce, then a thin layer of the cashew "cheese." Create two more layers of squash, sauce, and "cheese."

7. Bake for 45 to 50 minutes, until a golden-brown crust has formed and the butternut squash sheets are tender when tested with a knife. If the lasagna browns too quickly while baking, loosely cover it with a sheet of aluminum foil. Sprinkle with fresh parsley before serving.

SPECIAL EQUIPMENT
High-powered blender

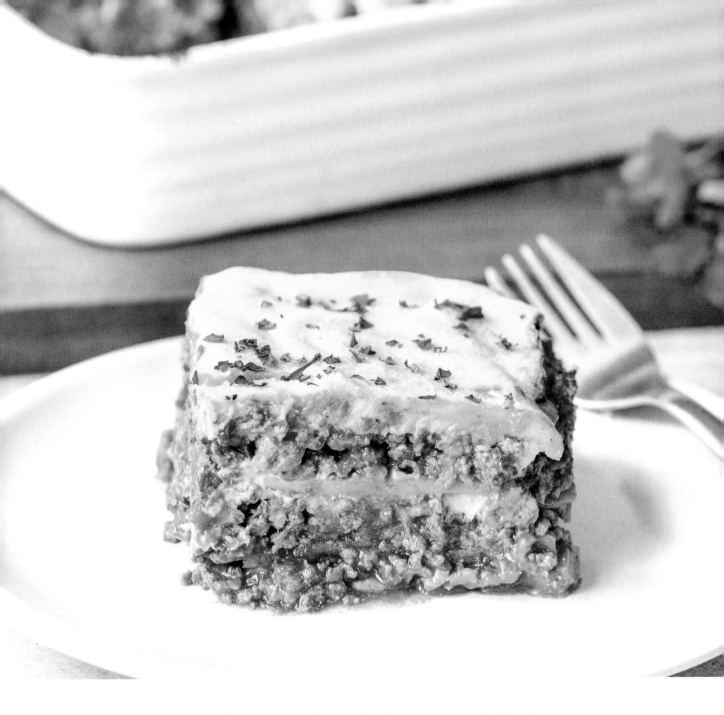

STORAGE: *Leftovers will last in the fridge for up to 3 days or in the freezer for up to 3 months. I recommend freezing it in small portions to speed the thaw time.*

SCD BASICS
Tomato Paste (page 35)
Tomato Sauce (page 36)

Making Butternut Squash Sheets

If you can't find butternut squash sheets in the grocery, buy a butternut squash with a large, thin neck. Follow these steps to make the sheets:

1. Cut the neck from the base of the squash and use a vegetable peeler to peel it.

2. Cut the neck in half lengthwise and use a mandoline to cut very thin slices.

If you don't have a mandoline, you can bake the squash halves in a preheated 400°F oven for 20 minutes to soften the squash, which makes it much easier to use a knife to cut thin slices without losing a finger.

KETO
LOW-FODMAP
PALEO
DAIRY-FREE
EGG-FREE
NUT-FREE

Shredded
BEEF RAGU

Yield: 8 servings   **Prep Time:** 15 minutes   **Cook Time:** 3 hours 20 minutes

If you check my freezer at any time, I guarantee you will find at least two containers of this ragu. It's my favorite thing to pull out on a cold day when I'm craving a hearty and comforting bowl of food. Unlike ragu made with ground meat, I find this shredded beef version to be a bit fancier and more impressive. I love serving it over a bowl of zucchini noodles, spaghetti squash, or sautéed cubes of eggplant and garnishing it with chopped parsley or Parmesan cheese.

3½ pounds boneless beef chuck roast or brisket, cut into 3-inch cubes

1 teaspoon salt

1 teaspoon ground black pepper

1 tablespoon extra-virgin olive oil

1 cup diced carrots (about 1 large carrot)

1 cup diced celery (about 2 medium stalks)

1 medium yellow onion, diced

4 cloves garlic, minced

1 teaspoon dried thyme leaves

1 teaspoon dried rosemary leaves

½ teaspoon red pepper flakes

2 (14-ounce) cans diced tomatoes, or 3⅓ cups chunky tomato sauce

2½ cups beef stock

3 tablespoons tomato paste

½ cup red wine, or ¼ cup red wine vinegar

2 bay leaves

1. Preheat the oven to 350°F.

2. Use a paper towel to pat the beef dry, then season on all sides with the salt and pepper.

3. Heat the oil in a large Dutch oven or ovenproof pot over high heat. Working in batches, sear the beef for about 2 minutes per side until browned. Use a slotted spoon to transfer the seared beef to a plate and set aside.

4. Lower the heat to medium and add the carrots, celery, onion, garlic, thyme, rosemary, and red pepper flakes to the pot. Cook for 8 minutes, until the carrots have begun to soften.

5. Add the tomatoes, stock, tomato paste, and red wine and bring to a gentle simmer, then return the seared beef to the pot. Add the bay leaves, cover with a lid, and place in the oven to cook for 3 hours, or until the beef is fall-apart tender.

6. Use a slotted spoon to transfer all of the pieces of beef from the pot to a cutting board. Place a potato masher into the pot of sauce and mash the vegetables to break down any larger pieces and thicken the sauce.

7. Use two forks to shred the beef, then return the shredded beef to the pot and stir to completely coat the meat in the sauce.

SUBSTITUTIONS: *Omit the garlic and onion and use 1 tablespoon of garlic-infused oil in place of the extra-virgin olive oil to make it low-FODMAP.*

STORAGE: *Leftovers will last in the fridge for up to 5 days or in the freezer for up to 4 months. To thaw the frozen ragu, place ½ inch of water and the frozen ragu in a pot on the stove over medium heat, stirring occasionally until warmed through.*

SCD BASICS
Tomato Paste (page 35)
Tomato Sauce (page 36)
Beef Stock (page 52)

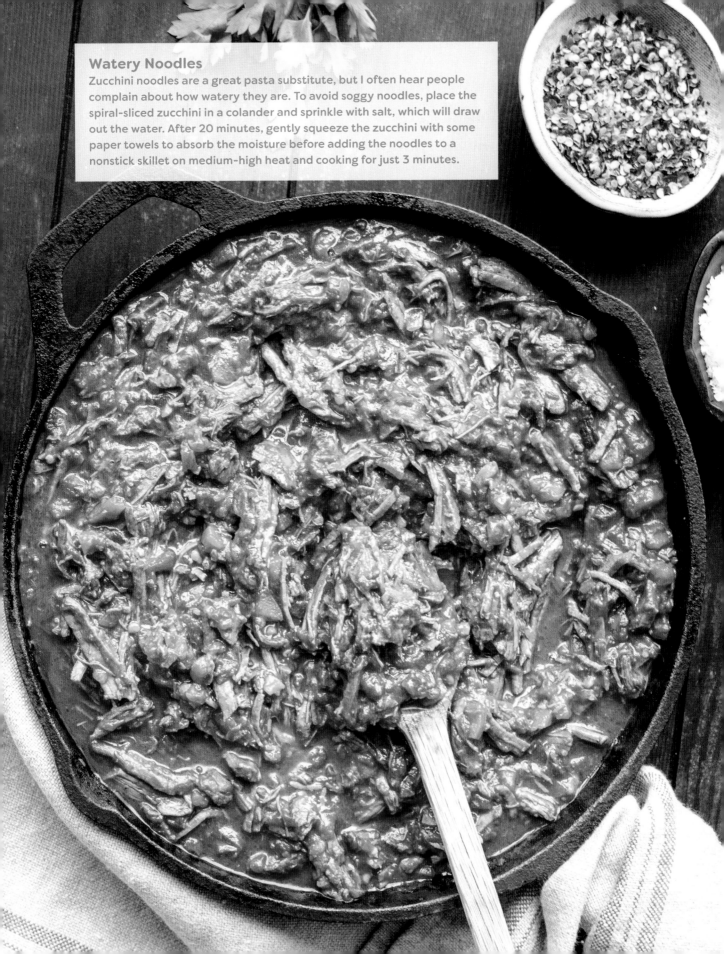

Watery Noodles

Zucchini noodles are a great pasta substitute, but I often hear people complain about how watery they are. To avoid soggy noodles, place the spiral-sliced zucchini in a colander and sprinkle with salt, which will draw out the water. After 20 minutes, gently squeeze the zucchini with some paper towels to absorb the moisture before adding the noodles to a nonstick skillet on medium-high heat and cooking for just 3 minutes.

Korean
BEEF TACOS

Yield: 8 tacos   **Prep Time:** 20 minutes, plus at least 2 hours to marinate   **Cook Time:** 10 minutes

These tacos filled with Korean beef (or *bulgogi*) are seriously epic. After two hours of marinating, the thinly sliced beef is incredibly tender and becomes slightly caramelized when seared. This meal quickly became a family favorite in my house; it's a great alternative to the usual Mexican-inspired tacos we eat. I like serving these tacos in warm grilled celery root tortillas, but lettuce cups would work just as well. I highly recommend making extra beef so that you can enjoy it with freshly made coleslaw the next day; it's a delicious use for leftovers that you shouldn't pass up.

Beef

1¼ pounds boneless sirloin, flank, or skirt steak

1 (1-inch) piece fresh ginger, roughly chopped

3 cloves garlic, peeled

2 tablespoons coconut aminos

2 tablespoons toasted sesame oil

1½ tablespoons honey

Spicy Mayonnaise

⅓ cup mayonnaise

1 red chili pepper, such as Fresno

1 tablespoon freshly squeezed lime juice

1 clove garlic, peeled

Coleslaw

2 cups shredded red cabbage

1 tablespoon toasted sesame oil

1½ teaspoons coconut aminos

1 teaspoon white sesame seeds

For Serving

8 Celery Root Tortillas (page 44)

¼ medium red onion, thinly sliced

¼ cup sliced scallions

1. Cut the beef very thinly against the grain (see tip) and place it in a bowl.

2. To make the marinade, place the ginger, garlic, coconut aminos, sesame oil, and honey in a blender and blend until smooth. Pour the marinade over the sliced beef, cover, and put in the fridge for a minimum of 2 hours (but ideally overnight). Rinse out the blender.

3. To make the spicy mayonnaise, put the mayo, chili pepper, lime juice, and garlic in a blender and blend until completely smooth. If the sauce is too thick, add a splash of water and blend to thin it out.

4. Place the cabbage, sesame oil, coconut aminos, and sesame seeds in a medium-sized bowl and toss until well coated. Set aside.

5. Heat a medium-sized nonstick skillet over high heat. Once the skillet is very hot, add the beef and any excess marinade and cook untouched for 3 to 4 minutes so that the meat browns on one side. Stir and cook the beef for another 2 to 3 minutes, until cooked through and the sauce has thickened and created a caramelized glaze on the beef.

6. To assemble, fill each tortilla with some shredded cabbage, a large spoonful of the beef, and slices of onion; drizzle with the spicy mayonnaise. Garnish with chopped scallions and serve.

SUBSTITUTIONS: *For keto, omit the honey.*

STORAGE: *The coleslaw is best made only a few hours before serving to prevent it from getting mushy. Leftover steak will last in the fridge for up to 3 days.*

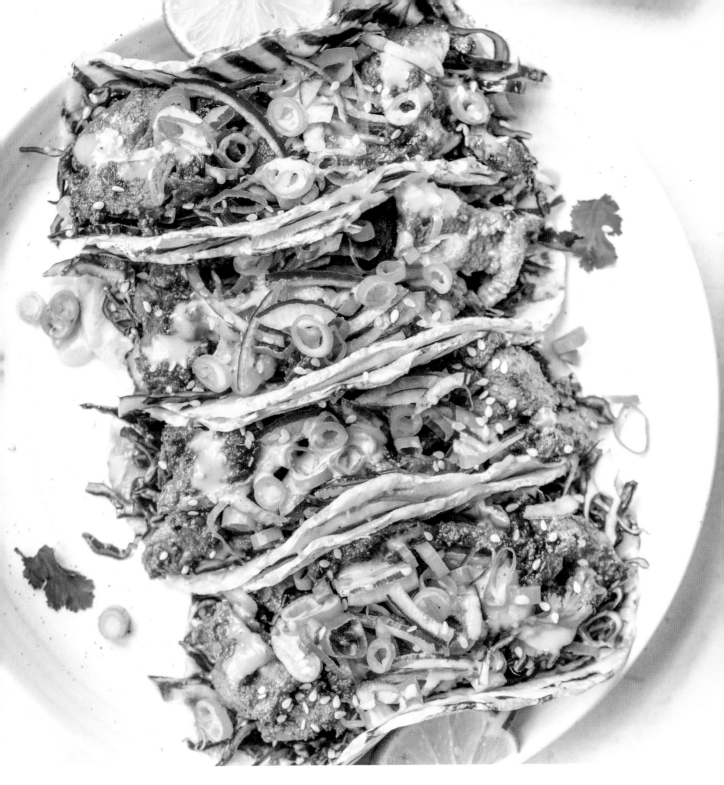

Against the Grain

To make cheap tough cuts of beef—such as flank steak, skirt steak, and brisket—easier to chew, always cut against the grain to break through the muscle fibers of the meat. The long fibers appear as lines in the meat and are easiest to identify when the meat is still raw. For more expensive but still lean cuts, such as filet and sirloin, the fibers are harder to identify; therefore, cutting against the grain isn't as important.

SCD BASICS

Easy 3-Minute Mayonnaise (page 42)

Coco-not Aminos (page 47)

every last bite   215

KETO
LOW-FODMAP
PALEO
DAIRY-FREE
EGG-FREE
NUT-FREE

Steak Fajita Skewers with
CILANTRO CHIMICHURRI

Yield: 8 skewers   **Prep Time:** 20 minutes, plus at least 10 minutes to marinate   **Cook Time:** 8 minutes

This is a fun spin on fajitas that's perfect for cookout season. The beef is marinated in a spicy sauce, quickly grilled, and then served with a cilantro chimichurri, which really packs a punch of flavor. There are many fun ways to serve these: on small skewers with chimichurri on the side as an appetizer, tossed into a salad, or with Celery Root Tortillas (page 44) as part of a build-your-own-fajita bar with all of the fixings.

Steak Skewers

3 tablespoons extra-virgin olive oil, plus more for the grill

1½ tablespoons ground cumin

2 teaspoons cayenne pepper

1 teaspoon paprika

1½ pounds boneless sirloin or rib-eye steak, cut into 1-inch cubes

1 green bell pepper, cut into 1-inch pieces

1 red bell pepper, cut into 1-inch pieces

2 medium white onions, cut into quarters

Cilantro Chimichurri

½ cup extra-virgin olive oil

½ cup fresh Italian parsley leaves

½ cup fresh cilantro leaves

⅓ cup chopped scallions

2 tablespoons red wine vinegar

1½ teaspoons freshly squeezed lime juice

2 cloves garlic, peeled

1 jalapeño pepper

1. In a bowl, whisk together the oil, cumin, cayenne pepper, and paprika. Add the steak and marinate for a minimum of 10 minutes (but ideally at least 1 hour).

2. To make the chimichurri, place all of the cilantro chimichurri ingredients in a food processor and blend until smooth. Refrigerate until ready to serve.

3. Preheat a grill to medium-high heat or a grill pan over medium-high heat.

4. Thread the marinated steak, green bell peppers, red bell peppers, and onions onto the skewers, alternating among each until the skewers are filled.

5. Lightly oil the grill or grill pan. Place the skewers onto the grill and brush with any leftover marinade. Grill for 8 minutes, turning every 2 minutes to ensure that they cook evenly.

6. Serve the skewers with the chimichurri sauce drizzled on top or on the side for dipping.

SUBSTITUTIONS: *For low-FODMAP, omit the garlic, scallions, and onion, and use garlic-infused oil in place of the extra-virgin olive oil.*

MAKE AHEAD/STORAGE: *The chimichurri can be made up to 3 days in advance and will last in the fridge for up to a week. Leftover cooked skewers will last in the fridge for up to 4 days. .*

Extra Chimichurri
You can use any extra chimichurri as a marinade for chicken or shrimp, serve it as a sauce on roasted veggies, or thin it out with olive oil and use it as a salad dressing.

SPECIAL EQUIPMENT
8 (10-inch) stainless steel or wooden skewers (see tip on page 184)

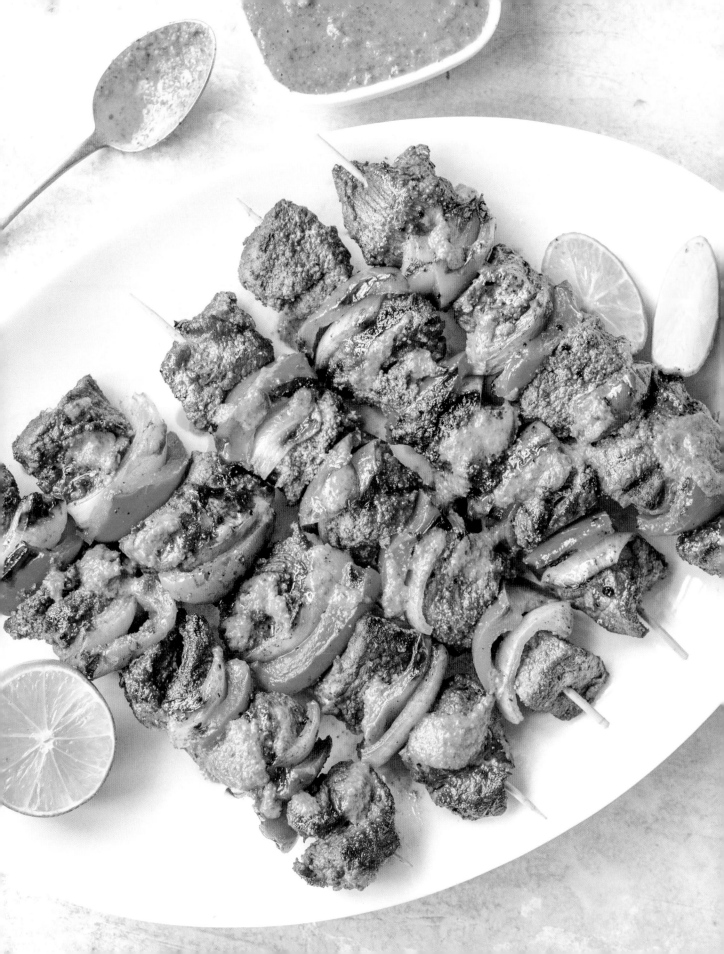

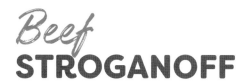
STROGANOFF

Yield: 4 servings **Prep Time:** 10 minutes **Cook Time:** 15 minutes

This beef stroganoff is hearty, richly flavored, and surprisingly quick to prepare, making it a great dish for a weeknight dinner during the colder winter months. I like using a mix of oyster, shiitake, and portobello mushrooms for an earthy flavor, but you can stick with just cremini or button mushrooms if that's what you have on hand. I recommend serving this saucy dish on a bed of spaghetti squash or cauliflower mash, such as the one on page 282. To make this dish more wallet-friendly, swap the beef for pork tenderloin.

1 tablespoon extra-virgin olive oil

1 pound boneless sirloin, beef tenderloin, or flank steak, cut into thin strips

12 ounces mushrooms, such as oyster, shiitake, cremini, and button, sliced

1 medium yellow onion, thinly sliced

3 cloves garlic, minced

1 cup beef stock

1½ tablespoons red wine vinegar

1 tablespoon Dijon mustard

⅔ cup coconut cream

½ teaspoon paprika

½ teaspoon salt

½ teaspoon ground black pepper

Chopped fresh Italian parsley, for garnish

1. Heat the oil in a large skillet over high heat. Add the beef strips and sear for about 2 minutes before flipping and cooking on the other side for another minute. Once the beef is browned, remove it from the skillet and set aside on a plate.

2. Lower the heat to medium, then add the mushrooms, onion, and garlic. Cook for 5 to 6 minutes, until the mushrooms and onion have softened, then stir in the beef stock, vinegar, and Dijon mustard. Use a wooden spoon to scrape the bits from the bottom of the skillet.

3. Stir in the coconut cream and paprika and let simmer for 5 minutes, until the mixture has thickened and reduced by half.

4. Season the sauce with the salt and pepper before returning the cooked beef and any juices on the plate to the skillet. Cook for another minute or two, until the meat has heated through, then serve garnished with chopped parsley.

STORAGE: *Leftovers will last in the fridge for up to 3 days or in the freezer for up to 2 months.*

SCD BASICS
Beef Stock (page 52)

Thin-Sliced Beef
To make it easier to cut thin slices of beef, place it in the freezer for 20 minutes before you need to slice it. The beef will become slightly firm and much easier to cut thinly.

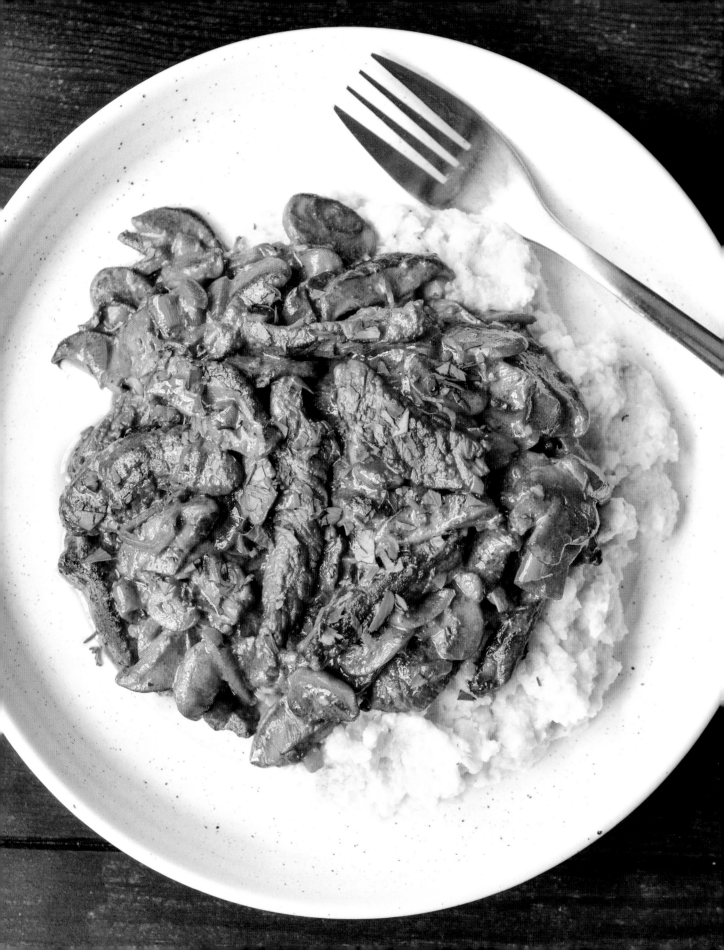

Short Rib Beef
BOURGUIGNONNE

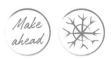

Yield: 6 servings   **Prep Time:** 25 minutes   **Cook Time:** 3 hours 15 minutes

Braised short ribs and beef bourguignonne are my two go-to dishes in the winter when I'm trying to impress, so I'm not sure why it has taken me so long to combine them into one. You get all of the rich flavors of the stew coupled with big tender pieces of short rib; it really is the best of both worlds. I find the flavors of the sauce are even better when this dish is made the day before and left to rest overnight in the fridge.

1 tablespoon extra-virgin olive oil

4 pounds boneless beef short ribs, cut into 2-inch pieces

½ teaspoon salt

½ teaspoon ground black pepper

7 ounces pancetta, roughly chopped

2 cups diced carrots (about 5 medium carrots)

1 medium yellow onion, diced

5 cloves garlic, minced

3 cups beef stock

2 cups red wine

2 tablespoons tomato paste

1½ cups pearl onions

2 bay leaves

1 teaspoon dried thyme leaves

1 tablespoon unsalted butter, ghee, or coconut oil

2 cups quartered cremini mushrooms (about 1 pound)

1 tablespoon chopped fresh Italian parsley, for garnish

1. Preheat the oven to 400°F.

2. Heat the oil in a Dutch oven or ovenproof pot over medium-high heat. Season the short ribs on all sides with the salt and pepper. Working in batches, sear the short ribs for about 2 minutes per side, until browned. Transfer the seared meat to a plate and set aside.

3. Lower the heat to medium and add the pancetta to the pot. Cook for 3 to 4 minutes, until it begins to crisp, then add the carrots, onion, and garlic and cook for another 3 minutes, until the onion begins to soften.

4. Drain the fat from the pot, then pour in the stock and red wine and use a wooden spoon to stir in the tomato paste. Make sure to scrape up any bits stuck to the bottom of the pot. Bring the liquid to a gentle simmer, then return the short ribs to the pot and stir in the pearl onions, bay leaves, and thyme. Transfer the pot to the oven and cook for 2½ to 3 hours, until the meat is fork-tender.

5. With 15 minutes left of cooking, melt the butter in a medium-sized skillet over medium-high heat. Add the mushrooms and sauté for 6 to 8 minutes, until the mushrooms have softened and developed a slightly golden color.

6. Once the beef is tender, remove the pot from the oven and stir in the mushrooms. At this point, you can allow the dish to cool before refrigerating overnight to develop the flavor, or you can garnish with the chopped parsley and serve it immediately.

SUBSTITUTIONS: *For keto, omit the carrots.*

MAKE AHEAD/STORAGE: *This is best made a day ahead and then reheated on the stove before serving. Leftovers will last in the fridge for up to 4 days or in the freezer for up to 3 months.*

SCD BASICS
Tomato Paste (page 35)
Beef Stock (page 52)

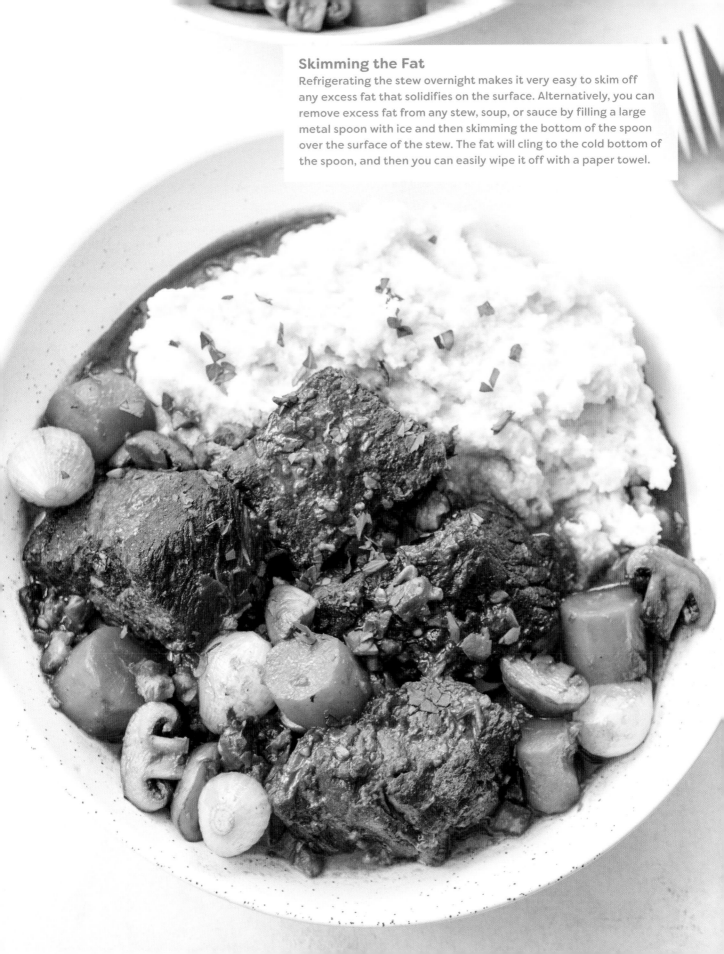

Skimming the Fat

Refrigerating the stew overnight makes it very easy to skim off any excess fat that solidifies on the surface. Alternatively, you can remove excess fat from any stew, soup, or sauce by filling a large metal spoon with ice and then skimming the bottom of the spoon over the surface of the stew. The fat will cling to the cold bottom of the spoon, and then you can easily wipe it off with a paper towel.

KETO
LOW-FODMAP
PALEO
DAIRY-FREE
EGG-FREE
NUT-FREE

Make ahead <30 min

Greek 7-Layer
LAMB DIP

Yield: 4 servings **Prep Time:** 18 minutes **Cook Time:** 12 minutes

This is a healthy spin on a dish from a restaurant in London that SA and I love. It can be served as either a main or an appetizer with lettuce cups on the side for scooping the seven layers (or you can use pita for anyone who's not a grain-free eater). The creamy tahini base and richly spiced ground lamb are the real stars of this dish, while the Greek salad adds a nice fresh flavor. You could also serve tzatziki (such as the one on page 98) on the side for an eighth layer.

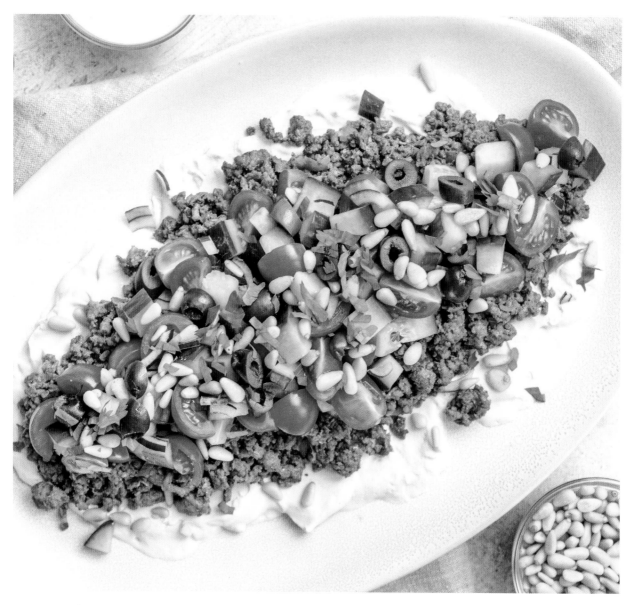

Tahini Sauce

½ cup tahini

⅓ cup water

2 tablespoons freshly squeezed lemon juice (see tip)

1½ tablespoons red wine vinegar

1 clove garlic, peeled

Greek Salad

1½ cups diced cucumber (about 1 medium cucumber)

1½ cups quartered cherry tomatoes (about 8 ounces)

⅓ cup sliced Kalamata olives

¼ cup crumbled feta cheese (optional)

2 tablespoons chopped red onions

1 tablespoon chopped fresh Italian parsley

1 tablespoon extra-virgin olive oil

1 teaspoon red wine vinegar

Lamb

1 tablespoon extra-virgin olive oil

1 medium yellow onion, diced

3 cloves garlic, minced

1 pound ground lamb

1 tablespoon grated lemon zest

1 tablespoon ground cumin

2 teaspoons ground coriander

1 teaspoon ground allspice

1 teaspoon turmeric powder

1 teaspoon paprika

½ teaspoon red pepper flakes

¼ teaspoon salt

2 tablespoons pine nuts, for garnish

1. Place the tahini sauce ingredients in a blender and blend until completely smooth and light in consistency. Set aside.

2. To make the Greek salad, place the cucumber, tomatoes, olives, feta (if using), red onions, and parsley in a bowl and mix together. Drizzle with the oil and vinegar and toss to coat. Set aside.

3. To make the lamb, place the oil, yellow onion, and garlic in a medium-sized skillet over medium heat and cook for 5 minutes, until the onion has softened.

4. Add the lamb to the skillet and use a wooden spoon to break up the meat into crumbles, making sure that there are no big chunks. Stir in the rest of the ingredients and continue to cook until the lamb is completely cooked through, about 7 minutes.

5. To assemble, spread the tahini sauce in a thin layer on a serving platter. Spoon the seasoned ground lamb over the sauce, ensuring that a border of tahini sauce is visible all around the meat. Spoon the Greek salad over the meat and garnish with the pine nuts. Serve immediately.

SUBSTITUTIONS: *For low-FODMAP, omit the onions and garlic, and use 1 tablespoon of garlic-infused oil in place of the extra-virgin olive oil. For Paleo or dairy-free or if you're new to SCD, omit the feta cheese from the Greek salad.*

MAKE AHEAD/STORAGE: *The seasoned meat and tahini sauce can be made a day in advance and stored separately, but the salad is best prepared right before serving. The meat freezes well and will last in the freezer for up to 2 months.*

Grating Zest

Any time you need both grated citrus zest and citrus juice, grate the zest before you juice the fruit. It's much easier to grate the zest from a whole, unjuiced fruit.

AIP
KETO
PALEO
DAIRY-FREE
EGG-FREE
NUT-FREE

Slow Cooker Honey
BALSAMIC RIBS

Yield: 6 servings **Prep Time:** 10 minutes **Cook Time:** 4 or 8 hours

In my opinion, a slow cooker is the easiest and most stress-free way to get fall-off-the-bone ribs (but see the oven instructions if you prefer that method). The rich honey balsamic sauce makes these ribs seem slightly more sophisticated than those served with barbecue sauce, but you still end up with a sticky glaze that you can't help but lick off your fingers.

2 racks baby back pork ribs

½ cup aged balsamic vinegar, divided

1 medium yellow onion, diced

⅓ cup beef stock

5 cloves garlic, minced

1 teaspoon dried thyme leaves

1 teaspoon dried rosemary leaves

½ teaspoon salt

2 tablespoons honey

SUBSTITUTIONS: *To make these ribs keto, omit the honey from the glaze.*

MAKE AHEAD/STORAGE: *The ribs can be cooked in the slow cooker up to 2 days in advance and then coated in the sauce and broiled before serving. These ribs freeze well; package any extra sauce separately in a zip-top bag so you can brush it over the top when you reheat the ribs.*

SCD BASICS
SCD Balsamic Vinegar (page 46)
Beef Stock (page 52)

1. Remove the membrane from the ribs: Put the ribs on a cutting board with the meaty side down and run a knife under the opaque layer of tissue to separate it from the meat and bones. Once you have begun to loosen the membrane, you should be able to use your fingers to peel it all up as one piece. Make sure to take time to do this step; it's the key to getting the tenderest fall-off-the-bone ribs.

2. Place ¼ cup of the vinegar, the onion, stock, garlic, thyme, rosemary, and salt in a 2-quart slow cooker and stir until well mixed. Arrange the pork ribs in the slow cooker and spoon the sauce over the top. Cover with the lid and cook for 8 hours on low or 4 hours on high. The ribs will be done when they are fork tender.

3. Preheat the oven to 400°F.

4. Transfer the ribs to an aluminum foil-lined sheet pan. Pour the liquid from the slow cooker into a saucepan over medium heat and add the remaining ¼ cup of the vinegar and the honey. Bring to a gentle simmer and cook for 10 minutes until the sauce is reduced and has thickened enough to coat the back of a spoon; remove it from the heat.

5. Brush the ribs on both sides with the sauce and broil them in the oven for 5 to 6 minutes, until the corners begin to char. Keep a close eye on the ribs to ensure that they don't burn. Serve the ribs with any remaining sauce on the side for dipping.

Oven Instructions

If you prefer to cook the ribs in the oven, preheat the oven to 250°F. Line the bottom and sides of a 9 by 13-inch baking dish with aluminum foil, and fold the foil over the sides of the dish to secure it. Add the balsamic vinegar (¼ cup), onion, beef stock, garlic, herbs, and salt to the baking dish and then place the ribs in the dish with the meat side down. Cover with aluminum foil so that the ribs are tightly enclosed and bake in the oven for 4 hours. Continue with Steps 3 and 4.

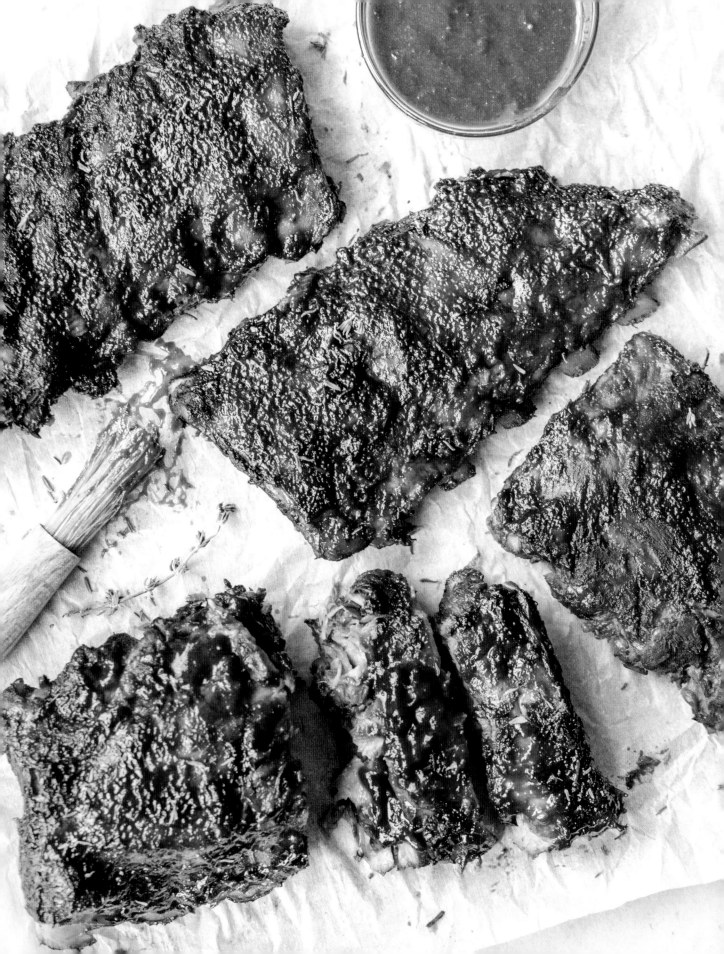

KETO
LOW-FODMAP
PALEO
DAIRY-FREE
EGG-FREE
NUT-FREE

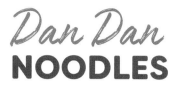

Dan Dan NOODLES

Yield: 2 servings   **Prep Time:** 10 minutes   **Cook Time:** 20 minutes

This lip-tinglingly spicy, slightly sweet and salty bowl of noodles packs a seriously flavorful punch. The chili oil really makes the dish. Cucumber noodles might seem like a weird base for the hot Dan Dan sauce, but the cold noodles add a much-needed freshness to each bite. If you don't eat pork, use ground chicken, turkey, or beef.

Dan Dan Sauce

⅓ cup chicken stock

2 tablespoons unsweetened almond butter

2 tablespoons coconut aminos

4 cloves garlic, peeled

1 (2-inch) piece fresh ginger, roughly chopped

1 tablespoon apple cider vinegar

½ teaspoon Chinese five-spice powder

2 Medjool dates, pitted, soaked for 10 minutes, and drained, or 2 tablespoons honey

1½ teaspoons toasted sesame oil

1 pound ground pork

For Serving

2 large cucumbers, spiral-sliced into long thin noodles

3 tablespoons chili oil (from below)

¼ cup sliced scallions

2 tablespoons chopped roasted cashews

Chili Oil

⅓ cup avocado oil

1 stick cinnamon

1 tablespoon Sichuan peppercorns

1 star anise

2 tablespoons red pepper flakes

½ teaspoon Chinese five-spice powder

1. Place all of the chili oil ingredients in a small saucepan over high heat and stir. Put a candy thermometer in the oil and heat it to 325°F, about 5 minutes. Then remove the pan from the heat and let cool to room temperature.

2. Place the stock, almond butter, coconut aminos, garlic, ginger, vinegar, Chinese five-spice powder, and dates in a blender and blend until completely smooth. Set aside.

3. Heat the sesame oil in a large skillet over medium heat. Add the ground pork and use a wooden spoon to break up the meat into crumbles. Continue cooking until the meat is no longer pink, about 5 minutes, then pour the sauce from the blender over the top and stir until it's well mixed.

4. To serve, divide the noodles between two bowls, top the noodles with equal portions of the Dan Dan sauce, and spoon 1½ tablespoons of the chili oil over each serving. Garnish with the chopped scallions and cashews.

SUBSTITUTIONS: *For keto, omit the Medjool dates or honey. For low-FODMAP, omit the garlic and scallions and use peanuts in place of cashews. For nut-free, swap the almond butter for sunflower seed butter and skip the cashews.*

STORAGE: *The sauce can be stored in the fridge for up to 4 days or in the freezer for up to 4 months. I recommend storing the sauce and cucumbers separately in the fridge until ready to serve.*

Chili Oil

This recipe makes more chili oil than is required for the noodles; don't let it go to waste! The chili oil will last in the fridge for up to 4 weeks, and it's fantastic drizzled over stir-fries, soups, or salads.

SCD BASICS
Coco-not Aminos (page 47), **Chicken Stock** (page 53)

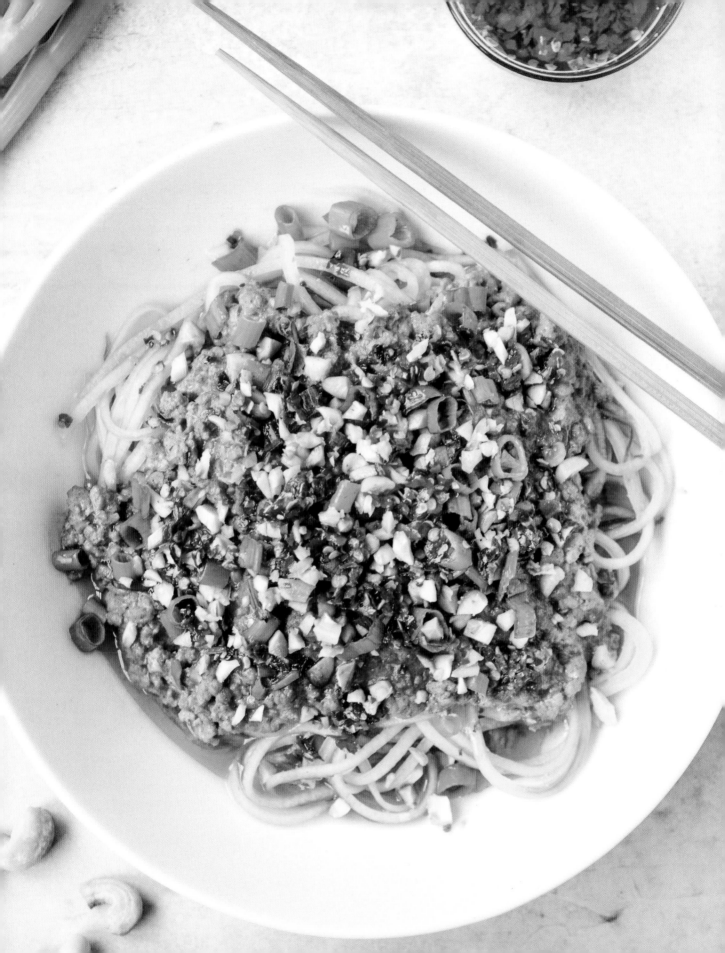

Make ahead

BBQ Pulled Pork & COLESLAW BOWL

Yield: 4 servings   **Prep Time:** 20 minutes   **Cook Time:** 5 or 8 hours

This recipe gives you all of the deliciousness of a pulled-pork sandwich without restricting yourself to the small amount of filling that fits between two buns. You can pack these bowls sky-high with the saucy BBQ shredded pork, creamy coleslaw, tender oven-roasted cubes of butternut squash, and pickles. This is a real crowd-pleasing dish that doesn't require a lot of time if you prepare the pork in advance. I like making extra pork to freeze for last-minute game day spreads.

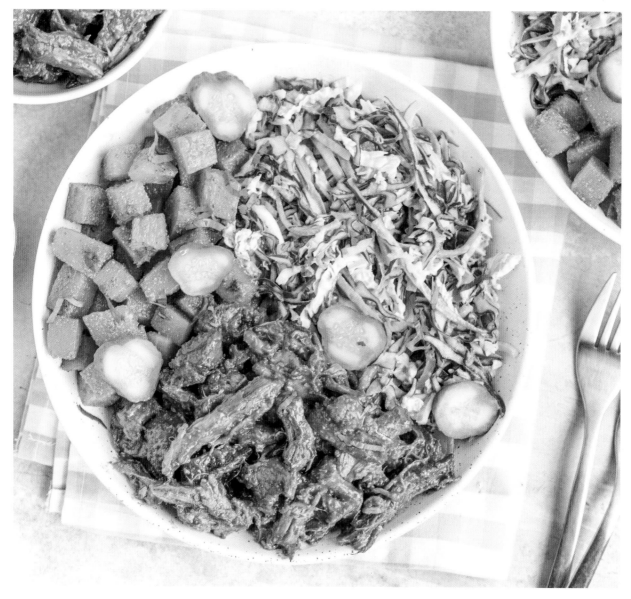

Shredded Pork

1 tablespoon extra-virgin olive oil

Salt and pepper

4 pounds boneless pork shoulder, fat trimmed

2 cups chopped tomatoes (about 4 medium tomatoes)

1 large yellow onion, diced

1⅓ cups beef stock

3 tablespoons apple cider vinegar

3 cloves garlic, minced

1 tablespoon chipotle paste, or 1½ teaspoons chipotle chili powder

1 teaspoon paprika

1 tablespoon ground coriander

1 tablespoon ground cumin

Butternut Squash

1 medium butternut squash

1 tablespoon extra-virgin olive oil

2 teaspoons ground cumin

1 teaspoon paprika

½ teaspoon salt

Coleslaw

½ cup mayonnaise

2 tablespoons apple cider vinegar

½ teaspoon ground black pepper

¼ teaspoon salt

1 teaspoon Dijon mustard

4 cups shredded green, red, or mixed cabbage

1 cup shredded carrots (about 1 large carrot)

½ medium red onion, diced

2 pickles, thinly sliced, for garnish

2 tablespoons chopped fresh Italian parsley, for garnish

1. Heat the oil in a large skillet over high heat. Season the pork on all sides with salt and pepper, and then sear it in the skillet on all sides, about 3 minutes per side.

2. Place the tomatoes, yellow onion, stock, vinegar, garlic, chipotle paste, and spices in a 4-quart slow cooker and stir to mix. Place the seared pork shoulder in the slow cooker and spoon the tomato mixture over the top. Cover with the lid and cook for 5 hours on high or 8 hours on low. The pork is done when you can easily pull it apart with a fork. Alternatively, you can cook the pork in the oven at 300°F for 3 hours.

3. With 30 minutes left of cooking, prepare the rest of the bowl. Preheat the oven to 425°F. Peel the butternut squash and cut it into 1-inch cubes. Place the butternut squash cubes on a sheet pan, toss with the oil, cumin, paprika, and salt and roast for 20 minutes, until tender.

4. To prepare the coleslaw, whisk together the mayonnaise, apple cider vinegar, pepper, salt, and Dijon mustard in a small bowl. Place the cabbage, carrots, and red onion in a salad bowl, pour the dressing over the veggies, and toss until the veggies are well coated.

5. Transfer the pork to a cutting board and shred using two forks. Pour the sauce from the slow cooker into a blender and blend until smooth (or use an immersion blender). Pour the sauce over the shredded pork and toss until well coated.

6. To serve, divide the shredded pork, coleslaw, and butternut squash among 4 bowls. Garnish with the pickles and parsley and serve with any extra sauce on the side.

SUBSTITUTIONS: *For keto, omit the carrots from the coleslaw and skip the butternut squash cubes. For low-FODMAP, skip the garlic, onions, and pickles.*

MAKE AHEAD/STORAGE: *The pulled pork can be made up to 2 days in advance. The coleslaw and dressing can be made a day in advance but should be stored in separate containers in the fridge. The pork will last in the fridge for up to 4 days or in the freezer for up to 3 months.*

Home Fries
Make extra roasted butternut squash and reheat for breakfast to enjoy as home fries with eggs.

SCD BASICS
Chipotle Paste (page 34), **Easy 3-Minute Mayonnaise** (page 42), **Quick Pickled Veggies** (page 48), **Beef Stock** (page 52)

Pork Belly, Applesauce &
PICKLED ONION LETTUCE CUPS

Yield: 12 to 15 lettuce cups   **Prep Time:** 20 minutes   **Cook Time:** 1 hour

I had a version of these lettuce cups at a Vancouver restaurant and still think about them ten years later...a clear sign that I needed to figure out how to re-create them. Although it may seem like a random combination, the sweet applesauce, crunchy pork belly, and acidic pickled onions are a wonderful contrast of flavors that make these lettuce cups both rich and fresh tasting.

2 medium apples

1 pound pork belly

1 tablespoon chopped fresh rosemary

1 tablespoon chopped fresh thyme

1 tablespoon salt

1 cup 100% pure, no-sugar-added apple juice or apple cider

½ medium red onion, thinly sliced

½ cup apple cider vinegar

2 small heads of gem or butter lettuce, cleaned and separated into leaves

MAKE AHEAD/STORAGE: *The onions can be pickled up to 4 days in advance. Unfortunately, the crackling on the pork belly loses its crunchiness when reheated and is best cooked right before serving.*

Pickled Onions

Make extra pickled onions; they will last in the fridge for 2 to 3 weeks, although they're best within 4 days of being made, and are a flavorful addition to salads.

1. Preheat the oven to 350°F.

2. Core the apples and cut them into eighths. Place the apple slices in a roasting pan.

3. Using a sharp paring knife, score the skin of the pork belly. Rub both sides of the pork belly with the rosemary, thyme, and salt and place the pork on top of the apples. Pour the apple juice into the roasting pan and bake for 40 minutes.

4. While the pork is roasting, place the red onion slices in a mason jar and cover the onion with the apple cider vinegar. They should be completely submerged. Set aside.

5. After the pork belly has roasted for 40 minutes, remove it from the oven and increase the temperature to 425°F. Spoon the apples and any excess apple juice from the roasting pan into a small saucepan.

6. Return the pork belly to the oven and roast for another 20 minutes. After 20 minutes, the skin on the pork belly should be golden brown and crispy.

7. Meanwhile, heat the apples and liquid in the saucepan over medium heat for 5 minutes or until the apple slices are very soft. Remove from the heat and use a potato masher to mash the apples into a chunky purée. Set the applesauce aside to cool to room temperature.

8. Remove the roasting pan from the oven and allow the pork belly to rest for 5 minutes before transferring it to a cutting board and slicing into ½-inch-thick pieces.

9. To assemble the lettuce cups, place 12 to 15 lettuce leaves on a serving tray. Place a slice of pork belly on each of the leaves; top with a spoonful of the applesauce and 2 or 3 slices of the pickled red onion.

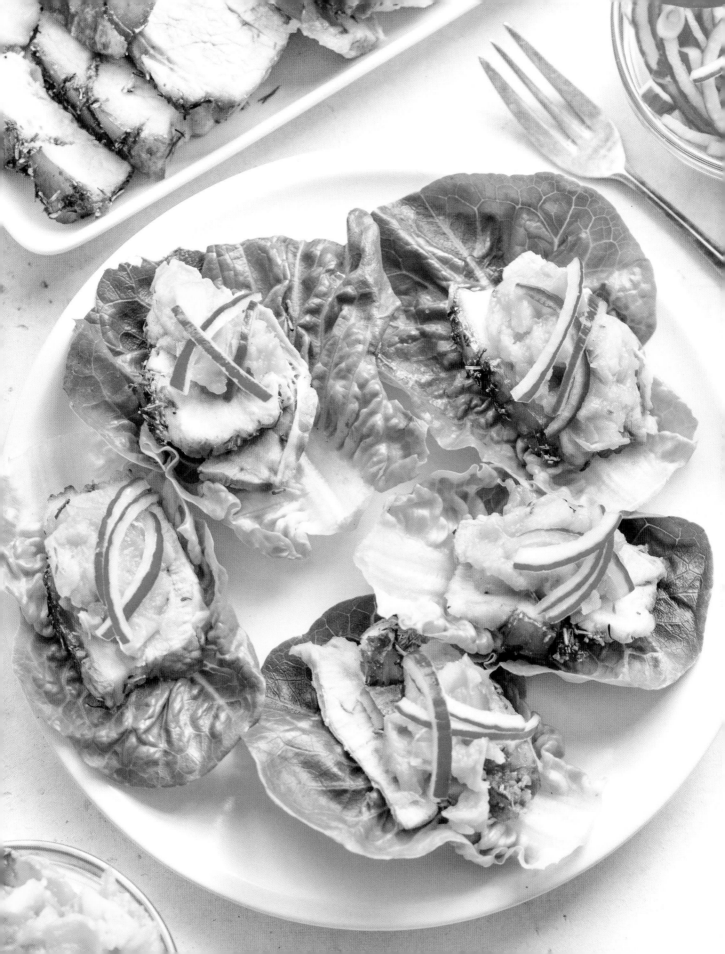

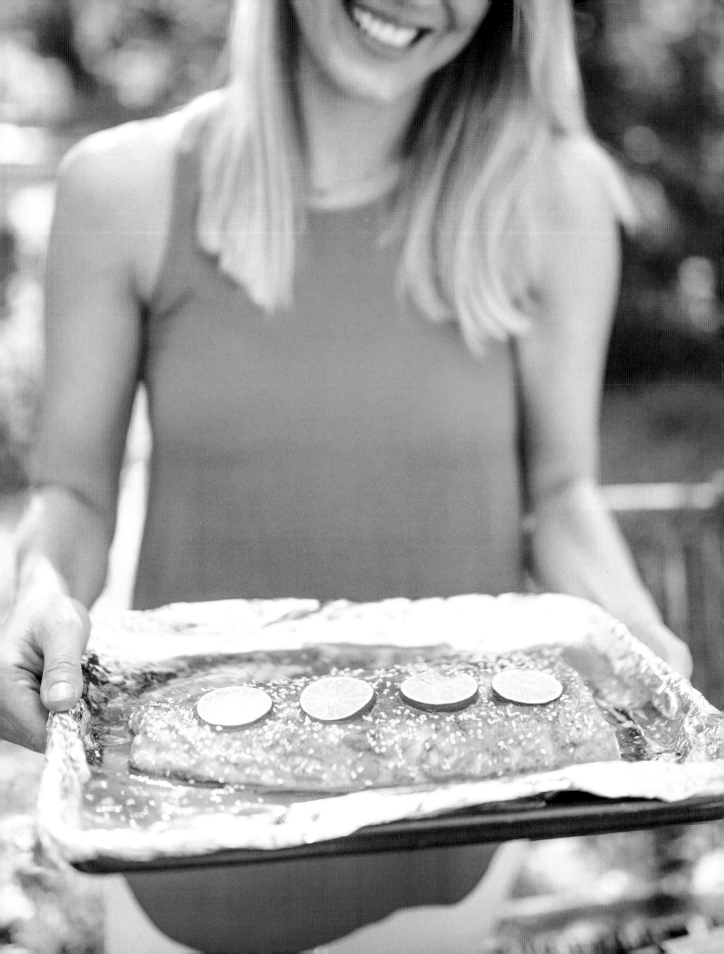

Seafood

Sweet Chili
SALMON

Yield: 4 servings **Prep Time:** 8 minutes **Cook Time:** 22 minutes

An oven-baked side of salmon is one of my favorite main dishes to serve guests because it's so easy and quick to prepare, and it always looks impressive. This salmon is topped with a deliciously sticky Asian sauce that you can make in minutes in a blender. Halve the sauce and you can top a few fillets of salmon with it for a weeknight dinner for two.

1 side skin-on salmon, deboned (about 2 pounds)

¼ teaspoon salt

¼ teaspoon ground black pepper

¼ cup honey

3 cloves garlic, minced

1 tablespoon apple cider vinegar

1 tablespoon coconut aminos

1 tablespoon toasted sesame oil

1 (1-inch) piece fresh ginger, roughly chopped

½ red chili pepper, such as Fresno

½ lime, thinly sliced

1 tablespoon sliced scallions, for garnish

1 teaspoon white sesame seeds, for garnish

1. Preheat the oven to 400°F and place a large piece of aluminum foil on a sheet pan.

2. Place the salmon on the prepared pan and season it with the salt and pepper. Fold the sides of the foil around the salmon so that it's surrounded by a tight border.

3. Place the honey, garlic, vinegar, coconut aminos, sesame oil, ginger, and chili pepper in a blender and blend into a smooth sauce. Pour the sauce into a small saucepan over medium-high heat and bring to a simmer. Let the sauce simmer for 8 to 10 minutes, until it has begun to thicken and has reduced by about one-third.

4. Spoon the sauce over the salmon and arrange 3 or 4 slices of lime on top. Place the sheet pan in the oven and bake for 12 to 15 minutes, until the thickest part of the salmon easily flakes with a fork.

5. Remove from the oven and spoon any of the sauce that's collected around the sides of the salmon back onto the salmon. Garnish with the scallions and sesame seeds before serving.

STORAGE: *The salmon is best prepared right before serving. Leftovers will last in the fridge for up to 3 days and are delicious eaten cold.*

SCD BASICS
Coco-not Aminos (page 47)

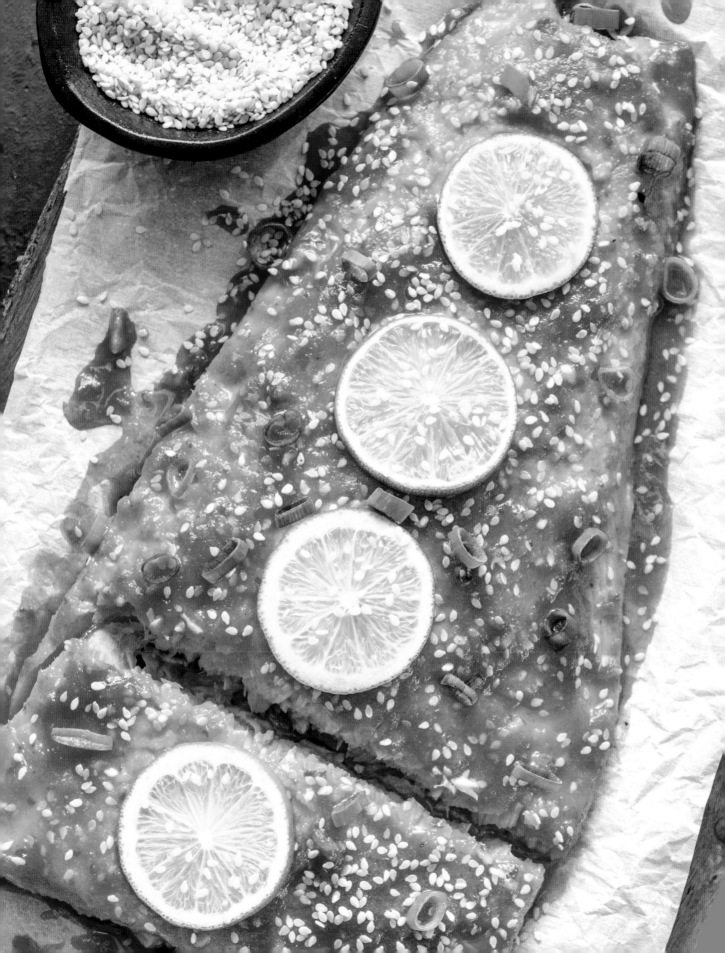

Creamy Honey Mustard
BAKED SALMON

Yield: 4 servings   **Prep Time:** 5 minutes   **Cook Time:** 7 minutes

This salmon is one of my go-to dishes when I'm in need of a fast and easy weeknight dinner. Start to finish, it takes just 12 minutes. I'm a girl from the west coast of Canada, where salmon is practically its own food group, so I know a thing or two about how to cook salmon (and what a dry disaster it can become when overcooked!). This super easy high-temperature, short-cook-time method ensures you get flaky, moist salmon every time. Not a fan of salmon? The sauce would be delicious served on cod, halibut, or oven-baked shrimp!

4 (4-ounce) skinless salmon fillets

½ teaspoon ground black pepper

¼ teaspoon salt

⅓ cup mayonnaise

2 tablespoons Dijon mustard

1 tablespoon honey

2 cloves garlic, minced

1 teaspoon chopped fresh dill, plus more for garnish

Lemon slices, for garnish

1. Preheat the oven to 450°F.

2. Arrange the salmon fillets evenly in a baking dish and season with the pepper and salt.

3. Place the mayonnaise, Dijon mustard, honey, garlic, and dill in a bowl and stir until well mixed. Spoon the sauce onto each of the salmon fillets and spread it evenly into a thin layer over the top and sides.

4. Bake for 7 minutes, until the salmon is opaque and flakes with a fork. Garnish with a few sprigs of fresh dill and slices of lemon before serving.

SUBSTITUTIONS: *To make this dish keto, skip the honey.*

STORAGE: *Leftovers will last in the fridge for up to 3 days. I prefer to enjoy leftover salmon cold, but if you like it warm, I recommend reheating it in a preheated 250°F oven for 15 minutes.*

SCD BASICS
Easy 3-Minute Mayonnaise
(page 42)

Seasoning Fish

I recommend seasoning fish with salt and pepper rather than adding the seasoning to the sauce or glaze. That way, you can ensure that each fillet or piece is seasoned evenly. Season the fish with salt just a minute or two before cooking; any longer and the salt will begin to draw moisture out of the fish.

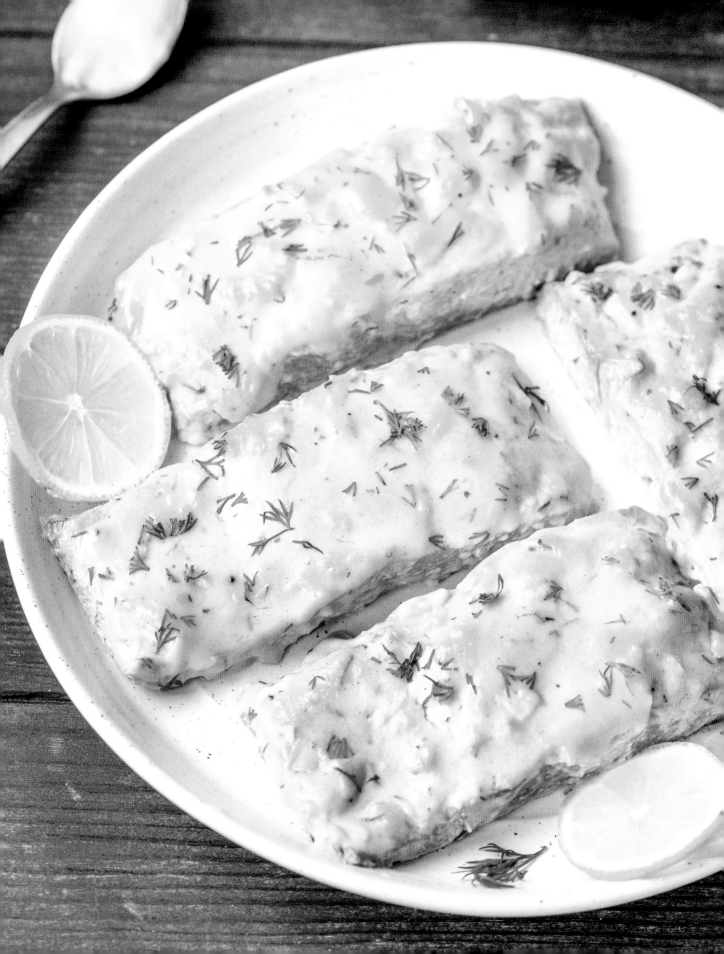

Easy Canned TUNA CAKES

Yield: 6 servings **Prep Time:** 10 minutes **Cook Time:** 8 minutes

I first created the recipe for these tuna cakes during a there's-no-food-in-the-house, what-should-I-make-for-dinner moment. I grabbed the few random things I could find in the fridge and pantry and mixed them up in a bowl to create these simple yet really flavorful tuna cakes. They quickly became a big hit on my blog; people loved how fast and easy they are to make with just a few ingredients that are often already in the pantry and fridge. I like serving them with tartar sauce (such as the one on page 42) and a simple salad for dinner, and then reheating leftovers for lunch the next day or topping them with a poached egg for breakfast.

Tuna Cakes

2 (5-ounce) cans tuna, packed in water

½ cup blanched almond flour

¼ cup chopped scallions

1 medium egg

2 tablespoons chopped fresh Italian parsley

2 tablespoons grated red onions

1 teaspoon grated lemon zest

1 tablespoon freshly squeezed lemon juice

1½ teaspoons Dijon mustard

½ teaspoon ground black pepper

¼ teaspoon salt

1 tablespoon extra-virgin olive oil, for frying

Lemon wedges, for serving

Tartar sauce, for serving

1. Drain the liquid from the cans of tuna, reserving 1 tablespoon of the liquid from the cans. Place the tuna and the reserved liquid in a medium-sized bowl and use a fork to break up the tuna.

2. Add all of the remaining ingredients to the bowl and stir until well mixed. Taste and adjust the seasoning as desired. Form the mixture into 6 patties.

3. Heat the oil in a large skillet over medium heat. Once hot, add the patties and cook for about 4 minutes, until a golden crust forms. Flip and cook on the other side for another 3 to 4 minutes.

4. Serve the patties with lemon wedges and tartar sauce.

SUBSTITUTIONS: *For AIP, use coconut flour in place of the almond flour and omit the mustard and pepper. For low-FODMAP, omit the scallions and red onions.*

STORAGE: *Leftovers will last in the fridge for up to 3 days. I recommend reheating them in a nonstick skillet for 2 to 3 minutes per side.*

Canned Tuna on SCD

Canned tuna is allowed on the Specific Carbohydrate Diet as long as it's packed in water or its own juices.

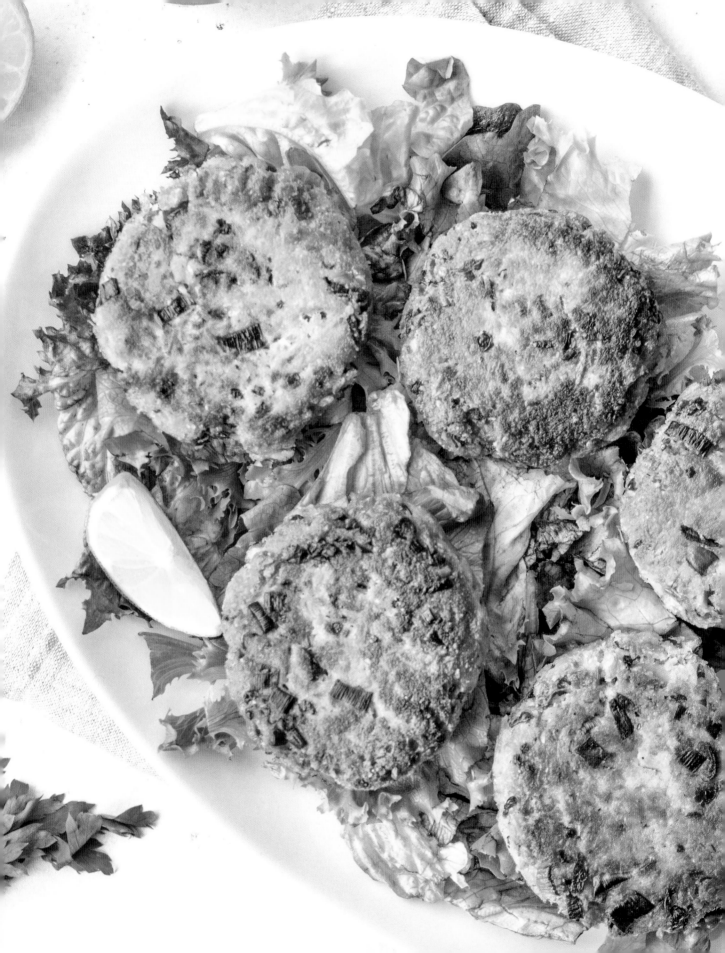

Spicy
FISH TACOS

Yield: 4 servings   **Prep Time:** 20 minutes   **Cook Time:** 8 minutes

Because they have a few different components, these tacos may seem like a lot of work, but the whole recipe (including cutting and grilling the celery root tortillas) can be done in less than 30 minutes. This is a great dish to double and serve to a big group of friends: lay everything out, including both celery root tortillas and regular tortillas for the non–grain-free folks, and let everyone assemble their own.

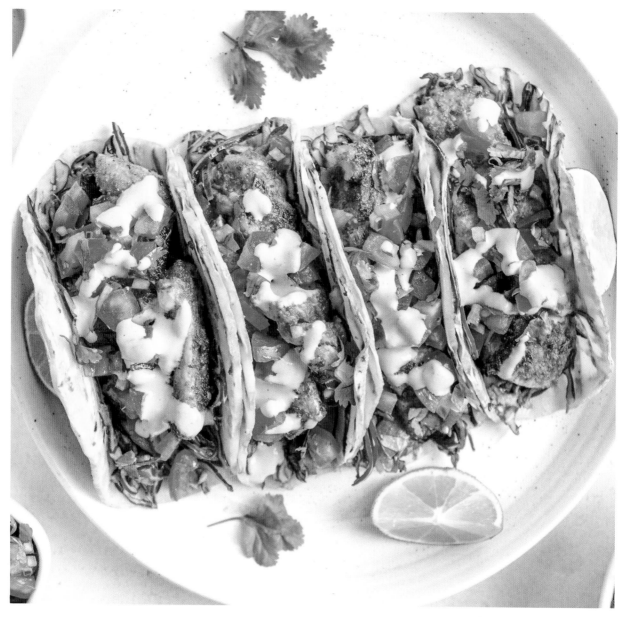

Pico de Gallo

1 cup diced tomatoes (about 2 medium tomatoes)

½ cup chopped fresh cilantro

¼ cup chopped red onions

1 jalapeño pepper, thinly sliced, plus more if needed

1 tablespoon freshly squeezed lime juice, plus more if needed

½ teaspoon salt

Coleslaw

3 cups shredded red or green cabbage (about 1 small head)

⅓ cup plus ¼ cup chopped scallions, divided

½ cup mayonnaise

⅓ cup chopped fresh cilantro

2 cloves garlic, peeled

2 tablespoons freshly squeezed lime juice

Pinch of salt

Spicy Fish

2 teaspoons ground cumin

1 teaspoon smoked paprika

1 teaspoon dried oregano leaves

½ teaspoon cayenne pepper

¼ teaspoon ground black pepper

¼ teaspoon salt

1 pound skinless white fish fillets, such as halibut, mahi mahi, tilapia, or cod

1 tablespoon light olive oil or avocado oil, for frying

2 to 3 lime wedges

8 Celery Root Tortillas (page 44), warmed, for serving

Chopped fresh cilantro, for garnish

SCD BASICS
Easy 3-Minute Mayonnaise
(page 42)

1. Place all of the pico de gallo ingredients in a bowl and stir to combine. Taste and add more lime juice, jalapeño, or salt as desired. Refrigerate until ready to serve.

2. To make the coleslaw, place the shredded cabbage and ¼ cup of the scallions in a bowl. Put the mayonnaise, cilantro, garlic, lime juice, salt, and the remaining ⅓ cup of scallions in a blender and blend until smooth. Pour about half of this cilantro lime sauce over the cabbage and toss until well coated. Set aside.

3. On a plate, stir together the spices and salt for the spicy fish. Cut the fish into 8 strips, about 1½ inches in thickness. Place the fish pieces in the spice mixture and pat the spices all over the fish so that each piece is well coated on all sides.

4. Heat the oil in a large skillet over medium-high heat. Add the pieces of seasoned fish and cook for 3 to 4 minutes per side, until golden and easily flaked with a fork. Once the fish pieces are done cooking, squeeze the lime juice over the top.

5. To assemble the tacos, fill each tortilla with some coleslaw and two pieces of fish. Spoon the pico de gallo over the fish and drizzle with the reserved cilantro lime sauce. Garnish with chopped cilantro.

STORAGE: *Leftovers will last in the fridge for up to 2 days. Everything is best stored separately in the fridge and can be eaten in reheated celery root tortillas or as a salad.*

KETO
LOW-FODMAP
PALEO
DAIRY-FREE
EGG-FREE
NUT-FREE

Sheet Pan Roasted Cod with Fennel, Olives, RED ONION & TOMATOES

Yield: 4 servings **Prep Time:** 5 minutes **Cook Time:** 35 minutes

This is an easy all-in-one dish that you can throw together, put in the oven, and leave alone. When fennel is roasted, it loses its sharp licoricey flavor and becomes deliciously soft and buttery. The combination of roasted fennel, salty olives, cherry tomatoes, and red onion is a great pairing with cod. You can swap the code with another type of white fish, such as halibut, hake, or sole.

2 fennel bulbs

1 large red onion, cut into eighths

1 cup cherry tomatoes (about 7 ounces)

¼ cup extra-virgin olive oil

1 tablespoon freshly squeezed lemon juice (see tip, page 223)

2 cloves garlic, minced

1 teaspoon dried thyme leaves

¾ teaspoon ground black pepper, divided, plus more for garnish

½ teaspoon salt, divided

4 (5-ounce) skinless cod fillets

1½ teaspoons grated lemon zest

½ teaspoon paprika

½ cup pitted Kalamata olives

Fresh thyme sprigs, for garnish

1. Preheat the oven to 350°F.

2. Remove any tough outer layers from the fennel and cut each bulb into wedges.

3. Place the fennel, onion, and tomatoes in a large baking dish or on a sheet pan. Try to lay everything in a single layer.

4. In a bowl, whisk together the oil, lemon juice, garlic, thyme, ½ teaspoon of the pepper, and ¼ teaspoon of the salt and drizzle over the veggies. Roast for 20 minutes.

5. Season the cod fillets with the lemon zest, paprika, the remaining ¼ teaspoon of pepper, and remaining ¼ teaspoon of salt.

6. After 20 minutes, remove the veggies from the oven and scatter the olives around the baking dish. Arrange the seasoned cod fillets among the vegetables, then spoon some of the liquid from the dish over each fillet. Return to the oven to bake for 15 minutes, until the fish is opaque and easily flakes with a fork.

7. Garnish with pepper and sprigs of thyme before serving.

SUBSTITUTIONS: *For low-FODMAP, omit the garlic and red onion and use ¼ cup of garlic-infused oil in place of the extra-virgin olive oil.*

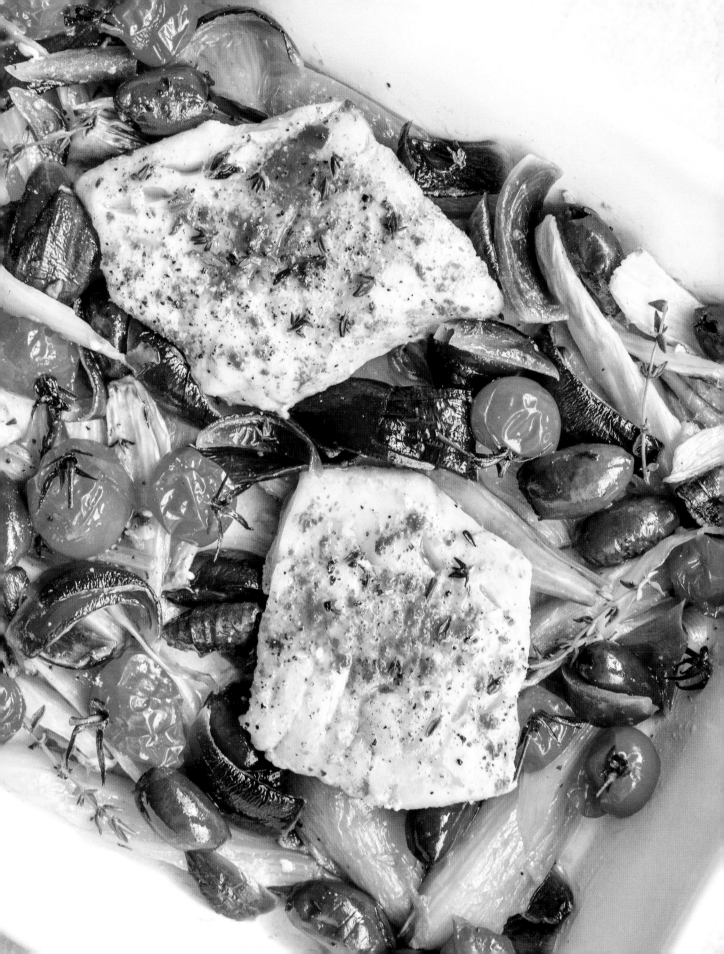

Chili Mayo Shrimp
LETTUCE CUPS

Yield: 4 lettuce cups **Prep Time:** 10 minutes **Cook Time:** 6 minutes

This is a great 20-minute dish that might not look like much, but boy are these lettuce cups tasty! The quickly seared shrimp are tossed in the most delicious creamy, spicy, and slightly tangy sauce and then served in crisp lettuce cups. Coating the shrimp in coconut flour helps the sauce stick to them, but you can skip the coating if you prefer; they'll still be delicious.

Sauce

⅓ cup mayonnaise

2 cloves garlic, peeled

1 tablespoon tomato paste

1 tablespoon apple cider vinegar

1 teaspoon coconut aminos

1 teaspoon finely chopped red chili peppers, such as Fresno

2 teaspoons fish sauce

Shrimp

¼ cup coconut flour

½ teaspoon salt

½ teaspoon ground black pepper

1 pound large shrimp, peeled and deveined

2 tablespoons avocado oil

For Serving

4 large butter lettuce leaves, cleaned

2 tablespoons sliced scallions

1 tablespoon white sesame seeds

½ lime, cut into 4 wedges

1. Place all of the sauce ingredients in a blender and blend until the sauce is completely smooth; there should be no small bits. Set aside.

2. In a bowl, stir together the coconut flour, salt, and pepper. Add the shrimp and toss so that they are lightly dusted with the seasoned coconut flour.

3. Heat the oil in a large skillet over medium-high heat. Add the shrimp to the skillet and cook for about 3 minutes per side, until golden. Pour the sauce into the skillet and gently stir to coat the shrimp.

4. To assemble the lettuce cups, place 4 lettuce leaves on a serving platter. Evenly divide the shrimp among the lettuce leaves and evenly garnish each cup with the sesame seeds and chopped scallions. Serve with a lime wedge on the side.

SUBSTITUTIONS: *For low-FODMAP, omit the scallions. Skip the coconut flour if you have an allergy.*

SCD BASICS
Tomato Paste (page 35)
Easy 3-Minute Mayonnaise (page 42)
Coco-not Aminos (page 47)

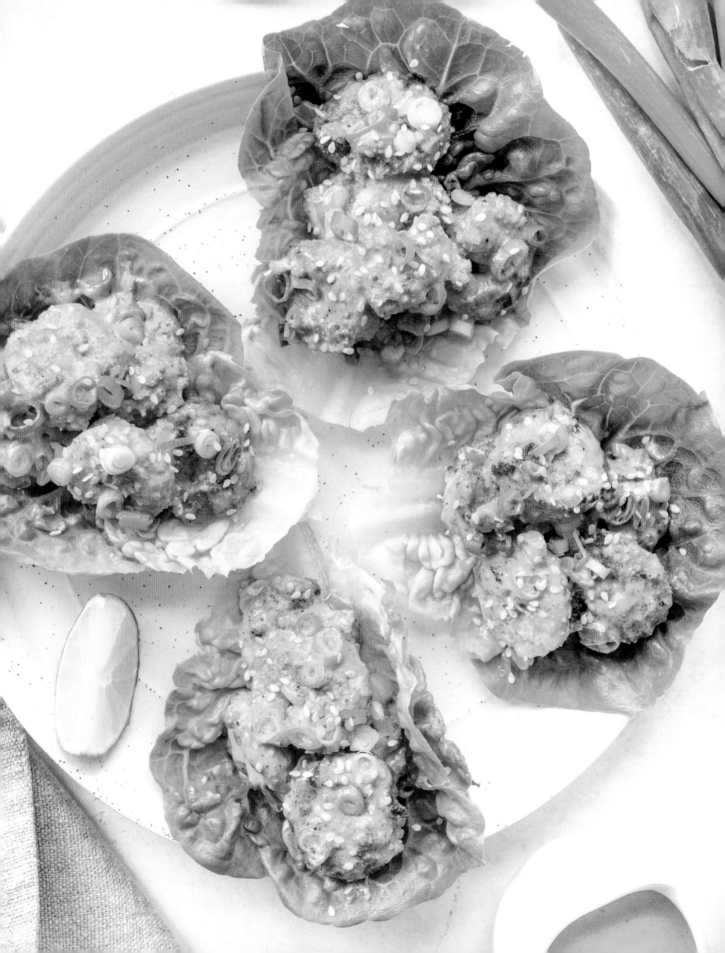

AIP
KETO
PALEO
DAIRY-FREE
EGG-FREE
NUT-FREE

Ginger & Black Pepper
SHRIMP STIR-FRY

< 30 min

Yield: 4 servings **Prep Time:** 15 minutes **Cook Time:** 15 minutes

This is a great weeknight dinner that comes together quickly, is packed with flavor, and gives you a big dose of your daily vegetables. Serve this stir-fry with Coconut Cauliflower Rice (page 272) to soak up the extra sauce.

Sauce

½ cup beef stock

3 tablespoons coconut aminos

2 tablespoons apple cider vinegar

1 tablespoon honey

1 teaspoon fish sauce

2 tablespoons toasted sesame oil, divided

2 tablespoons finely chopped fresh ginger

1 clove garlic, chopped

¾ pound medium shrimp, peeled and deveined

1 medium yellow onion, thinly sliced

1 red bell pepper, thinly sliced

5 ounces broccolini, long stems cut into 3-inch pieces

4 ounces shiitake mushrooms, thinly sliced

1 head bok choy, thinly sliced, whites and leafy greens separated

3 scallions, sliced into ½-inch pieces

2 teaspoons ground black pepper

1 tablespoon white sesame seeds, for garnish

1. Stir together all of the sauce ingredients in a small saucepan over medium heat and bring to a simmer. Simmer for 5 minutes, or until it has reduced by a third, then remove the pan from the heat.

2. Heat 1 tablespoon of the sesame oil in a large skillet or wok over medium-high heat. Add the ginger and garlic and cook for 1 minute until they become fragrant, then add the shrimp. Cook the shrimp for 3 minutes, until they turn pink. (Don't overcook them.) Then transfer them from the skillet to a plate.

3. Heat the remaining 1 tablespoon of the sesame oil in the skillet over medium-high heat. Once hot, add the onion, bell pepper, broccolini, mushrooms, and the whites of the bok choy and cook for 5 minutes, until the broccolini is tender.

4. Pour the sauce into the skillet and stir to coat the veggies before adding the scallions, greens of the boy choy, black pepper, and the cooked shrimp. Cook for another minute until the bok choy greens have wilted. Garnish with the sesame seeds before serving.

SUBSTITUTIONS: *For AIP, omit the sesame seeds, black pepper, and bell pepper and use light olive oil in place of the sesame oil. For keto, omit the honey.*

STORAGE: *Leftovers will last in the fridge for up to 2 days.*

SCD BASICS
Coco-not Aminos (page 47)
Beef Stock (page 52)

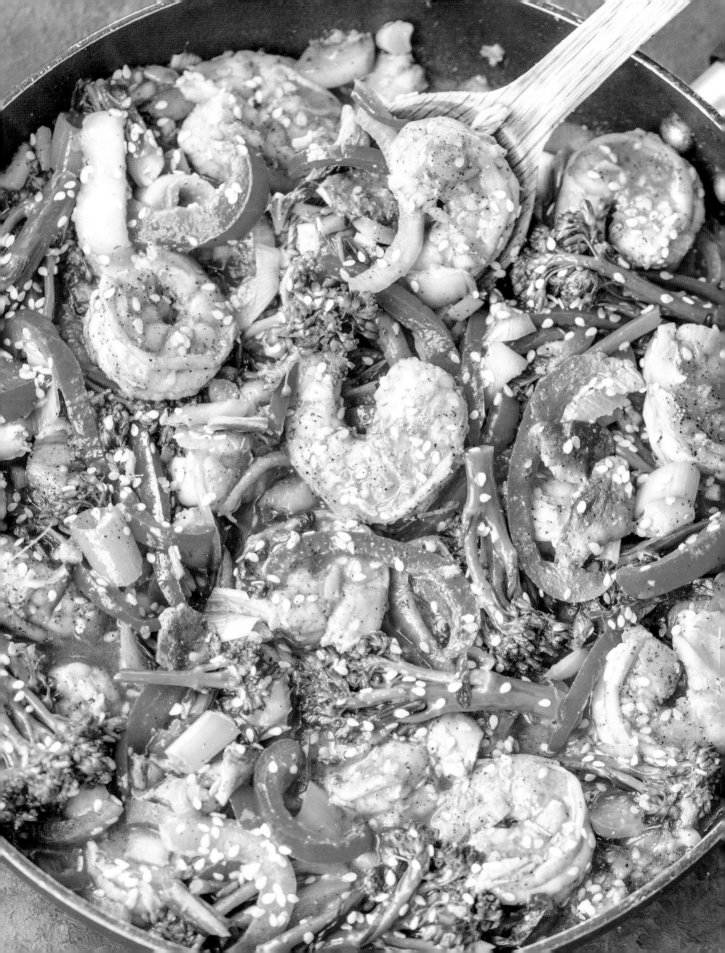

Creamy Lemon
DILL SHRIMP

Yield: 4 servings **Prep Time:** 15 minutes **Cook Time:** 12 minutes

Lemon and garlic cream sauce is one of my favorite pairings with seafood. Although this sauce is really creamy, fresh herbs and lemon help lighten it up. With a start-to-finish cook time of less than 15 minutes, this is a great weeknight dish that you can serve over cauliflower mash, spaghetti squash, zucchini noodles, or even steamed broccoli.

⅓ cup raw cashews, soaked in boiling water for 10 minutes and drained

⅓ cup unsweetened almond milk

1 clove garlic, peeled

3 tablespoons freshly squeezed lemon juice (see tip, page 223)

1 tablespoon unsalted butter or ghee

1 pound medium shrimp, peeled and deveined

¾ cup chicken or vegetable stock

2 tablespoons chopped fresh dill, plus more for garnish

1 teaspoon grated lemon zest

¼ teaspoon salt

¼ teaspoon ground black pepper plus more for garnish

5 to 6 lemon slices (see tip)

SPECIAL EQUIPMENT
High-powered blender

SCD BASICS
Chicken or Vegetable Stock
(page 53)

1. Place the cashews, almond milk, garlic, and lemon juice in a high-powered blender and blend until completely smooth. Set aside.

2. Heat the butter in a large skillet over medium-high heat. Once hot, add the shrimp and cook for 3 minutes until the shrimp are pink on both sides. Transfer to a plate and set aside.

3. Lower the heat to medium and pour the cashew cream mixture into the skillet. Add the stock and whisk to combine. Simmer for 4 to 5 minutes, until the mixture has thickened and reduced by about one-third (or more depending on how thick you'd like the sauce to be).

4. Stir the dill, salt, pepper, and lemon zest into the sauce, then add the cooked shrimp and the lemon slices. Cook for 1 to 2 minutes, until the shrimp are warmed, then remove from the heat. Garnish with extra dill and pepper before serving.

SUBSTITUTIONS: *For keto, use macadamia nuts in place of the cashews. For dairy-free, use coconut oil in place of butter or ghee.*

STORAGE: *Leftovers will last in the fridge for up to 3 days.*

TIPS: *This lemon dill sauce is great to have in your repertoire for serving over pan-seared salmon, chicken, or even pork chops.*

For an extra bit of fanciness, heat a grill pan over medium-high heat and grill the lemon slices for 4 minutes or until nice grill marks have developed. Garnish the dish with the grilled lemon slices.

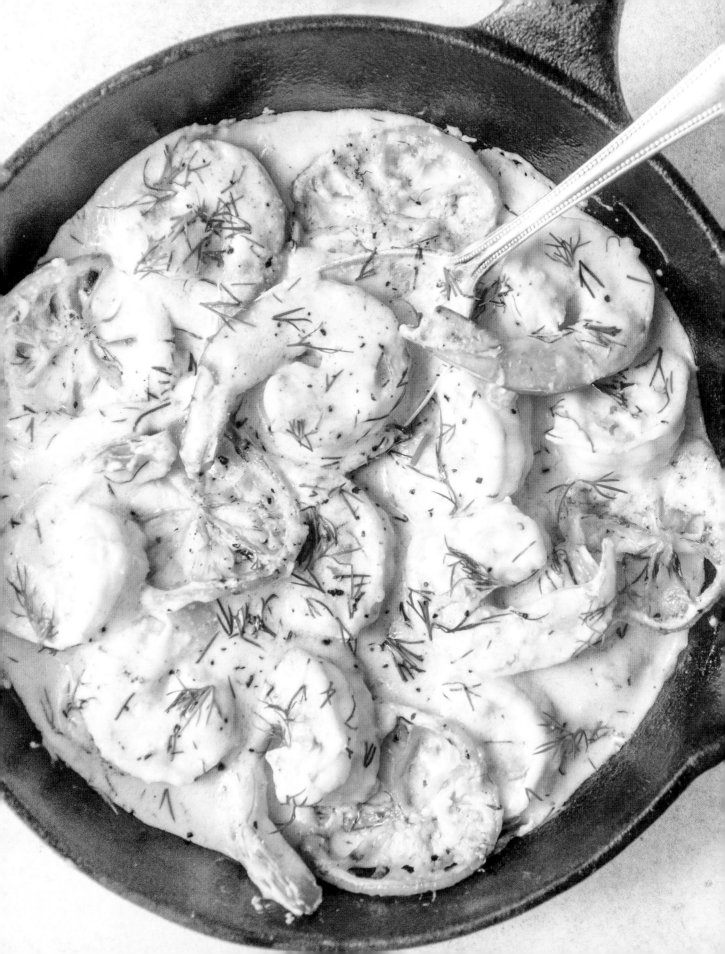

KETO
LOW-FODMAP
PALEO
DAIRY-FREE
EGG-FREE
NUT-FREE

Bacon & Garlic Herb
BUTTER SEARED SCALLOPS

Yield: 4 servings **Prep Time:** 15 minutes **Cook Time:** 15 minutes

Scallops are a great quick dinner to make when you are trying to impress. I've found that the majority of people who don't like scallops attribute their dislike to the texture, which becomes chewy when the scallops are overcooked. A perfectly cooked scallop should have a slightly caramelized crust and a tender, almost buttery center. I recommend serving these scallops with a side of cauliflower mash to absorb some of the delicious buttery sauce.

12 large sea scallops (about 12 ounces)

5 strips bacon

½ teaspoon ground black pepper

¼ teaspoon salt

1 tablespoon unsalted butter or ghee

2 cloves garlic, minced

½ cup chicken stock

1 tablespoon coconut cream

2 teaspoons apple cider vinegar

2 tablespoons chopped fresh Italian parsley, for garnish

SUBSTITUTIONS: *Omit the garlic for low-FODMAP. For dairy-free, use coconut oil in place of the butter or ghee. For pescatarians, skip the bacon and use vegetable stock in place of chicken.*

STORAGE: *Scallops should be eaten immediately after cooking; they do not reheat or freeze well once cooked.*

1. Take the scallops out of the fridge 10 minutes before cooking to allow them to come to room temperature.

2. Heat a large skillet on medium-high heat and cook the bacon until crisp, 5 to 6 minutes. Transfer the bacon to a paper towel, leaving the bacon grease in the skillet.

3. Prep the scallops by removing the muscle if it's attached, then pat the scallops dry with a paper towel. Increase the heat to high and season the scallops with the pepper and salt. Once the skillet is very hot, add the scallops, making sure there is space around each one, and cook without moving them for 1½ minutes, until a golden crust forms. Flip the scallops and cook for another 1½ minutes, then transfer to a plate.

4. Reduce the heat to medium-high and add the butter and garlic to the skillet and cook for 1 minute. Add the stock and stir with a wooden spoon. scraping any browned bits from the bottom of the skillet. Add the coconut cream and vinegar and simmer for 4 to 5 minutes, until the liquid begins to reduce.

5. While the sauce is cooking, chop the cooked bacon into small crumbly bits. Add the chopped bacon and the cooked scallops to the skillet, then garnish with the chopped parsley. Serve immediately.

Tips for the Perfect Golden Sear

Use these tips for achieving a golden crust when searing scallops—or for searing fish, chicken, steak, lamb, or pork!

- Pat the scallops dry with a paper towel before seasoning with salt and pepper.
- Make sure the skillet is very, very hot before adding the scallops.
- Don't overcrowd the pan; it's better to work in batches than add too many at once.
- Don't move the scallops after you've put them in the skillet; leave them untouched while a crust forms, then flip.

SCD BASICS
Chicken Stock (page 53)

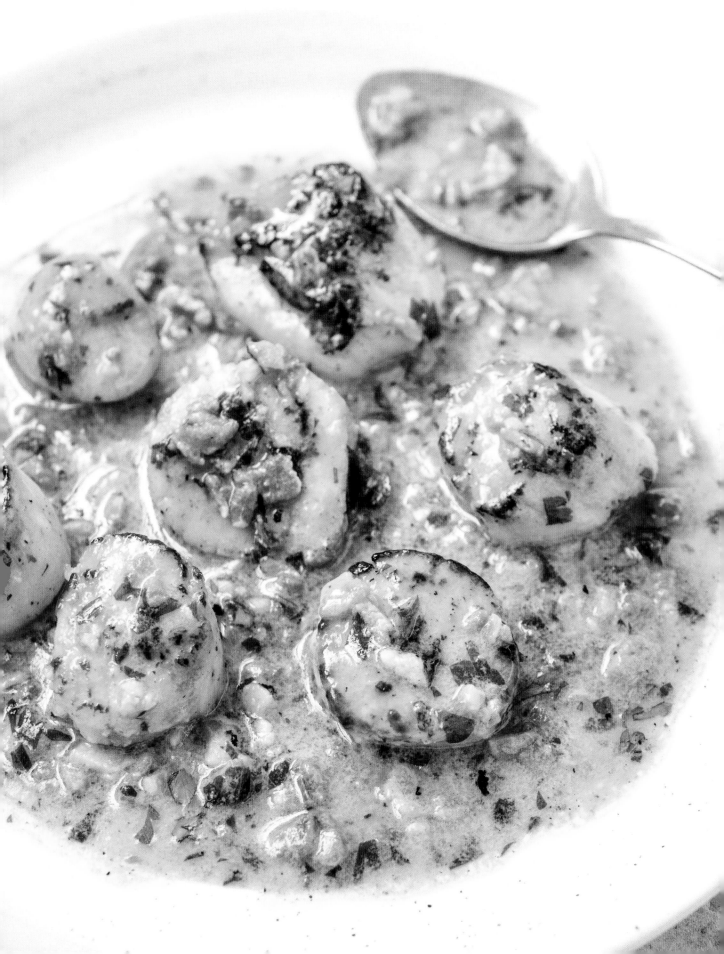

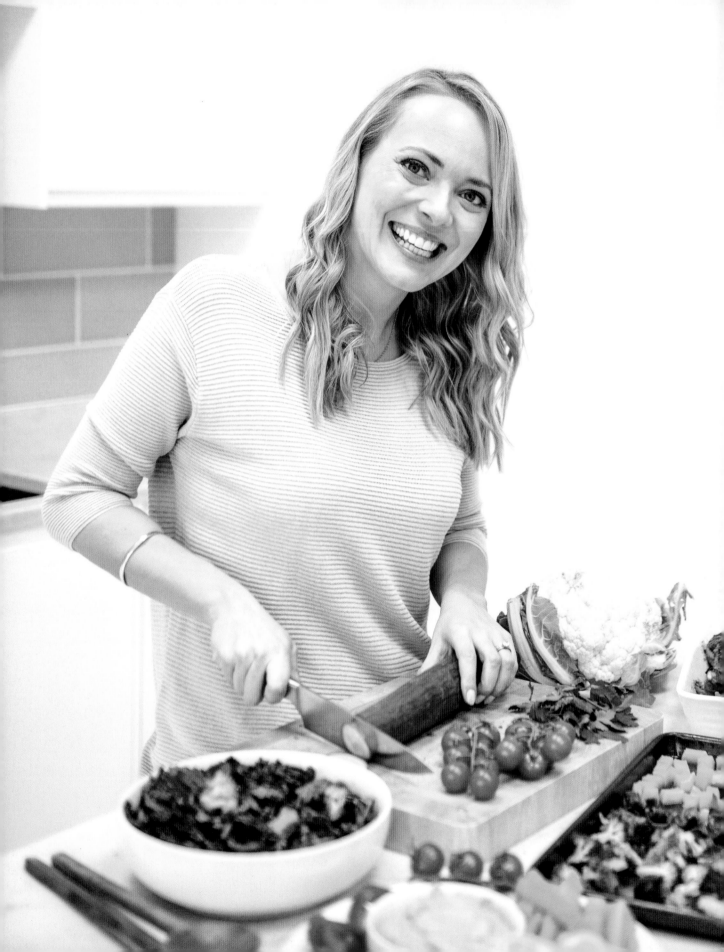

Vegetarian

Cashew e PEPE

Yield: 2 servings   **Prep Time:** 15 minutes   **Cook Time:** 12 minutes

If I had to choose my last meal, it would without question be cacio e pepe—one of the simplest yet most comforting of dishes. This version of the classic Italian pasta dish uses a cashew sauce to replicate the creaminess of the original, which is traditionally made with lots and lots of cheese and starchy pasta water. The creamy cashew sauce coats each noodle, while the flecks of black pepper add a sharp spiciness to each bite to make this one heck of a comforting meal.

1¼ pounds butternut squash noodles

1 tablespoon extra-virgin olive oil

⅓ cup raw cashews, soaked in boiling water for 10 minutes and drained

1 cup unsweetened almond milk, divided

2 tablespoons unsalted butter, ghee, or coconut oil

2 teaspoons freshly cracked black pepper, plus more for garnish

⅓ cup grated Parmesan cheese

¼ teaspoon salt

Chopped fresh Italian parsley, for garnish (optional)

SPECIAL EQUIPMENT
High-powered blender

1. Preheat the oven to 400°F.

2. Lay the butternut squash noodles out evenly on a sheet pan and drizzle with the oil. Bake for 10 minutes, until tender.

3. Place the cashews and ½ cup of the almond milk in a high-powered blender and blend until completely smooth; there should be no small bits.

4. Melt the butter in a medium-sized skillet over medium heat. Add the pepper and toast for 1 minute, then pour in the cashew sauce. Whisk in the remaining ½ cup of almond milk, Parmesan cheese, and salt and reduce the heat to low before adding the roasted butternut squash noodles. Gently toss the noodles so that they are evenly coated in the sauce.

5. Serve garnished with a sprinkle of chopped parsley, if desired, and freshly cracked black pepper.

SUBSTITUTIONS: *Use 2 tablespoons of nutritional yeast in place of the Parmesan cheese for Paleo, vegan, dairy-free. Use olive oil in place of butter and nutritional yeast in place of the Parmesan cheese to make it vegan. You can swap out the butternut squash noodles for sweet potato noodles (although this will not be SCD legal).*

STORAGE: *Leftovers will last in the fridge for up to 4 days. Before reheating, stir in a splash of unsweetened almond milk to prevent the sauce from being too thick.*

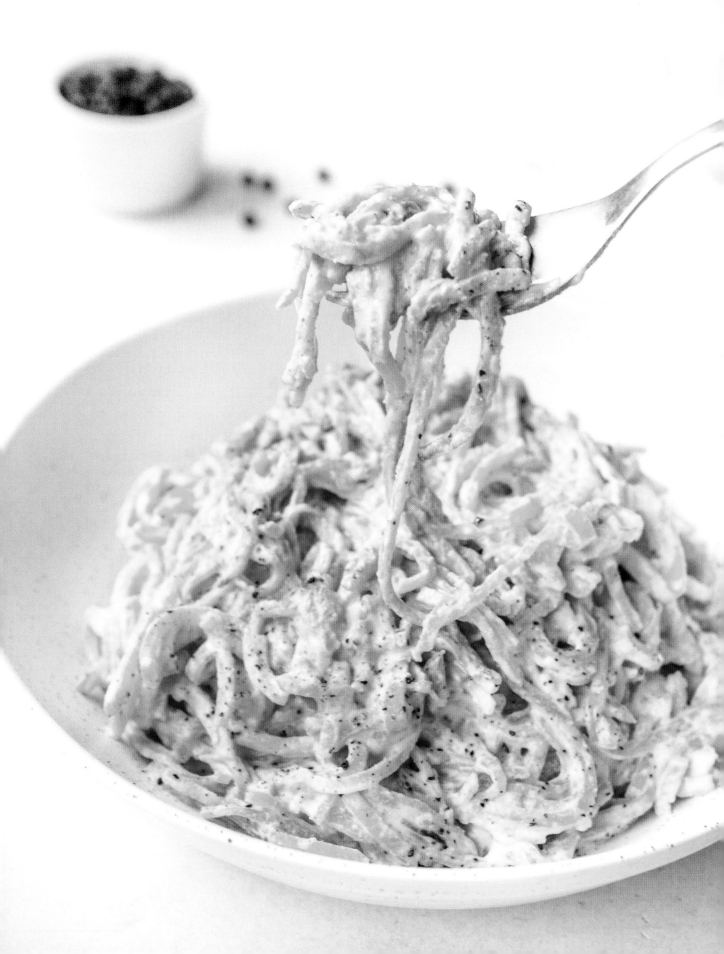

PALEO
VEGAN
VEGETARIAN
DAIRY-FREE
EGG-FREE
NUT-FREE

Creamy Spring
RISOTTO

Yield: 4 servings   **Prep Time:** 10 minutes   **Cook Time:** 16 minutes

My dad has always considered himself to be quite the risotto aficionado, and he regularly declares to absolutely anyone who will listen that he makes the BEST risotto in the world. In fairness, it is pretty good, but that likely comes down to the amount of butter, grated Parmesan cheese, and mascarpone that he secretly stirs in. Over the years, I've tried seeking his approval with cauliflower risotto—to no avail. It was my discovery of the wonders of celery root risotto that enabled me to finally get his stamp of approval. When cooked correctly, celery root rice becomes deliciously creamy, but it still holds its shape and doesn't turn into mush, making truly the BEST grain-free risotto around. Add more protein to this dish by including chicken, flaked salmon, shrimp, or seared scallops.

1 large celery root (about 2 pounds)

1 tablespoon extra-virgin olive oil

1 large yellow onion, diced

1 leek, diced

2 cloves garlic, minced

¼ teaspoon salt

1 cup unsweetened almond milk

1 cup chicken or vegetable stock

½ cup frozen peas, thawed

6 spears asparagus, cooked and cut into 1-inch pieces

½ cup grated zucchini

⅓ cup grated Parmesan cheese

1 tablespoon freshly squeezed lemon juice

¼ cup finely chopped fresh chives

1. Peel the celery root and cut it into chunks. Place the chunks into a food processor and pulse. The key is not to overprocess; you want the celery root to break down into small pieces about the size of rice. You should have about 4 cups of celery root rice.

2. Heat the oil in a large skillet over medium heat. Add the onion, leek, and garlic and season with the salt. Sauté until the onion has softened, about 3 minutes.

3. Stir in the celery root rice, almond milk, and stock and cook for about 10 minutes, until a lot of the liquid has evaporated and the rice is tender.

4. Stir in the peas, asparagus, zucchini, Parmesan cheese, and lemon juice. Cook for another 3 minutes, until all of the liquid has evaporated, then stir in the chives before serving.

SUBSTITUTIONS: *For Paleo, vegan, or dairy-free, omit the Parmesan cheese. Use coconut milk in place of almond milk to make it nut-free.*

STORAGE: *Leftovers will last in the fridge for up to 4 days. If the risotto has dried out in the fridge, stir in a splash of almond milk before reheating.*

SCD BASICS

Chicken or Vegetable Stock
(page 53)

Shelf Life

Celery root is in season during the winter months, but you can find it year-round in most large grocery stores. It has a long shelf life, so buy a few extra because you can store them in your fridge for 4 to 6 weeks.

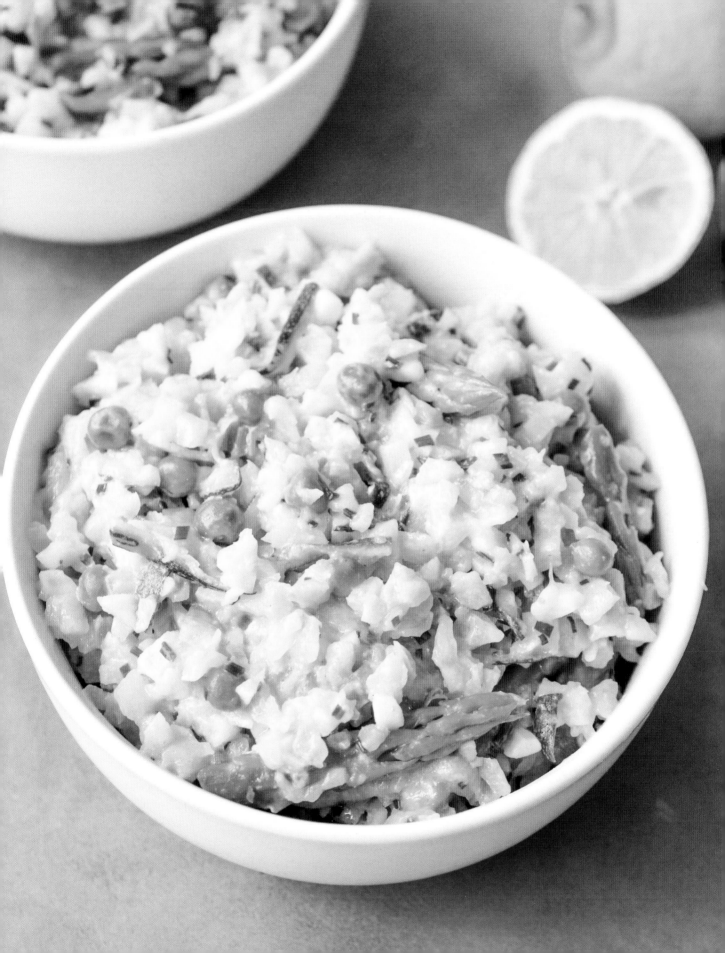

KETO
LOW-FODMAP
PALEO
VEGAN
VEGETARIAN
DAIRY-FREE
EGG-FREE

Butternut Squash Ravioli
WITH KALE PESTO

Make ahead

Yield: 10 ravioli   **Prep Time:** 20 minutes   **Cook Time:** 55 minutes

A lot of my blog readers who thought their days of ravioli were long gone love this healthy spin on the pasta dish. The butternut squash filling is deliciously rich and creamy and holds together well when wrapped with strips of zucchini. Use long and thin zucchini for this recipe because they're the easiest to cut with a vegetable peeler and result in the best strips for wrapping.

Ravioli Filling and "Pasta"

1 medium butternut squash, peeled and cubed (about 3 cups)

2 teaspoons extra-virgin olive oil

¼ teaspoon salt

⅓ cup grated Parmesan cheese

½ teaspoon ground dried sage

¼ teaspoon freshly grated nutmeg

¼ teaspoon ground black pepper

2 large thin zucchini

Kale Pesto

2 cups shredded Tuscan ("dino") kale

½ cup raw almonds

2 cloves garlic, peeled

1½ teaspoons freshly squeezed lemon juice

½ teaspoon salt

½ cup extra-virgin olive oil

1 tablespoon pine nuts, for garnish

SUBSTITUTIONS: *Omit the garlic for low-FODMAP and replace the extra-virgin olive oil with an equal amount of garlic-infused oil. Use ¼ cup of nutritional yeast instead of Parmesan cheese for Paleo, vegan and dairy-free.*

1. Preheat the oven to 400°F.

2. Place the butternut squash cubes on a sheet pan. Drizzle with the oil and sprinkle with the salt. Roast for 20 to 25 minutes, until the squash is tender and lightly browned.

3. Remove from the oven and transfer the cooked butternut squash to a blender or food processor. Add the Parmesan cheese, sage, nutmeg, and pepper and blend to a thick puree. Make sure that no chunks of squash remain in the puree. Put the puree in the fridge to cool while you prep the zucchini slices.

4. Cut the ends off of both zucchini, then cut each in half lengthwise. Using a vegetable peeler, cut 30 very thin strips of zucchini. (You can also use a knife for this task, but make sure the strips are very thin.)

5. Line a sheet pan with parchment paper. On a cutting board, lay out 3 zucchini strips so they overlap in the center to form a star (see diagram). Place about 1½ tablespoons of the butternut squash filling in the center of the strips where they overlap, then fold each strip of the zucchini over the top to cover. Place the ravioli on the prepared sheet pan so that the loose ends are on the bottom. Repeat with the remaining zucchini strips to form a total of 10 ravioli.

6. Bake the ravioli for 20 to 25 minutes, until the zucchini wrappings become tender.

7. While the ravioli are baking, make the pesto: Place the shredded kale, almonds, garlic, lemon juice, salt, and oil in a food processor and blend until a paste forms. Transfer the pesto to a medium-sized bowl.

8. Once the ravioli is finished baking, quickly microwave the pesto (or heat on the stove) until it's warm, then serve on top of the ravioli and garnish with the pine nuts before serving.

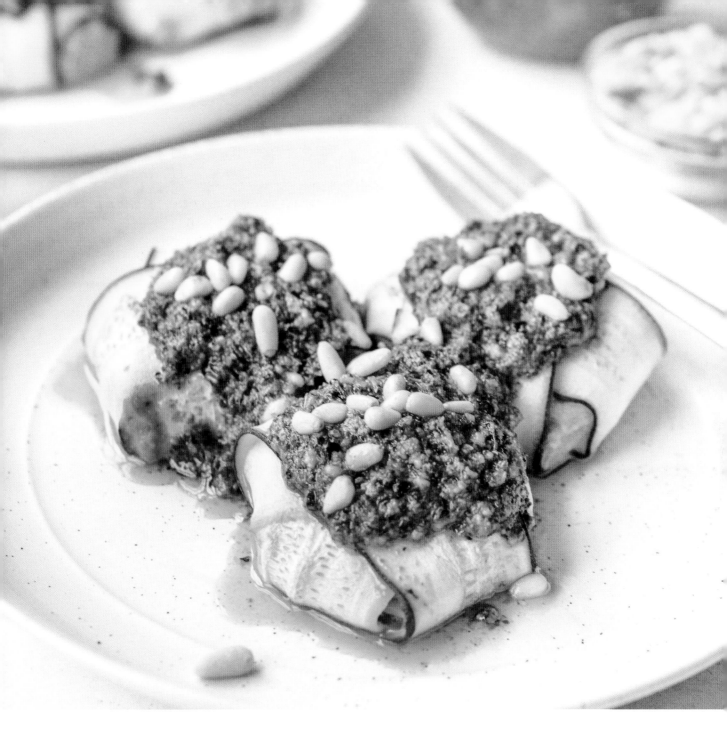

How to Make Zucchini Ravioli

MAKE AHEAD/STORAGE: *You can make the pesto and filling 2 days in advance and then assemble the ravioli just before baking. Leftovers will last in the fridge for up to 3 days and are best reheated in a preheated 350°F oven for 10 minutes.*

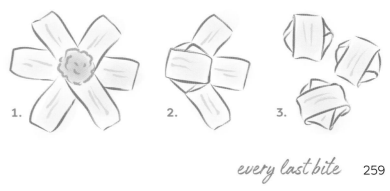

1.   2.   3.

KETO
LOW-FODMAP
PALEO
VEGAN
VEGETARIAN
DAIRY-FREE
EGG-FREE
NUT-FREE

Eggplant RAGU

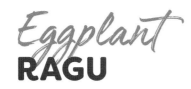

Yield: 4 servings **Prep Time:** 10 minutes **Cook Time:** 55 minutes

Slow-cooked chunks of eggplant make a wonderful hearty replacement for meat in this vegetarian ragu. This is an incredibly versatile dish; use it as a sauce for veggie noodles, try it as a sauce for fish or chicken, or even serve it as a side dish.

1 tablespoon extra-virgin olive oil

1 medium yellow onion, diced

4 cloves garlic, minced

1 teaspoon finely chopped capers

2 medium eggplants, cubed (about 4 cups)

3 tablespoons red wine vinegar

1 tablespoon tomato paste

1 teaspoon dried oregano leaves

½ teaspoon salt

3 cups chopped tomatoes (about 2 pounds tomatoes)

2 cups chicken or vegetable stock

Chopped fresh Italian parsley, for garnish

1. Heat the oil in a large skillet on medium heat. Add the onion, garlic, and capers and cook for 2 to 3 minutes, until the onion begins to soften.

2. Add the cubed eggplants, vinegar, tomato paste, oregano, and salt and stir to ensure the eggplant is well coated.

3. Stir in the tomatoes and stock and simmer for 45 to 50 minutes, stirring every 10 minutes, until the eggplant is very tender and the sauce has thickened into a ragulike consistency.

4. Serve the ragu garnished with a sprinkle of fresh parsley.

SUBSTITUTIONS: *For low-FODMAP, omit the garlic and onions and replace the extra-virgin olive oil with an equal amount of garlic-infused oil.*

STORAGE: *Leftovers will last in the fridge for up to 4 days or in the freezer for up to 4 months.*

SCD BASICS

Tomato Paste (page 35)

Chicken or Vegetable Stock (page 53)

Storing Tomatoes

For the best flavor, store unripened tomatoes stem side down on the countertop. Once they have fully ripened, transfer the tomatoes to the fridge to delay overripening and spoiling. Storing unripened tomatoes in the fridge will result in less flavorful, pale-colored tomatoes.

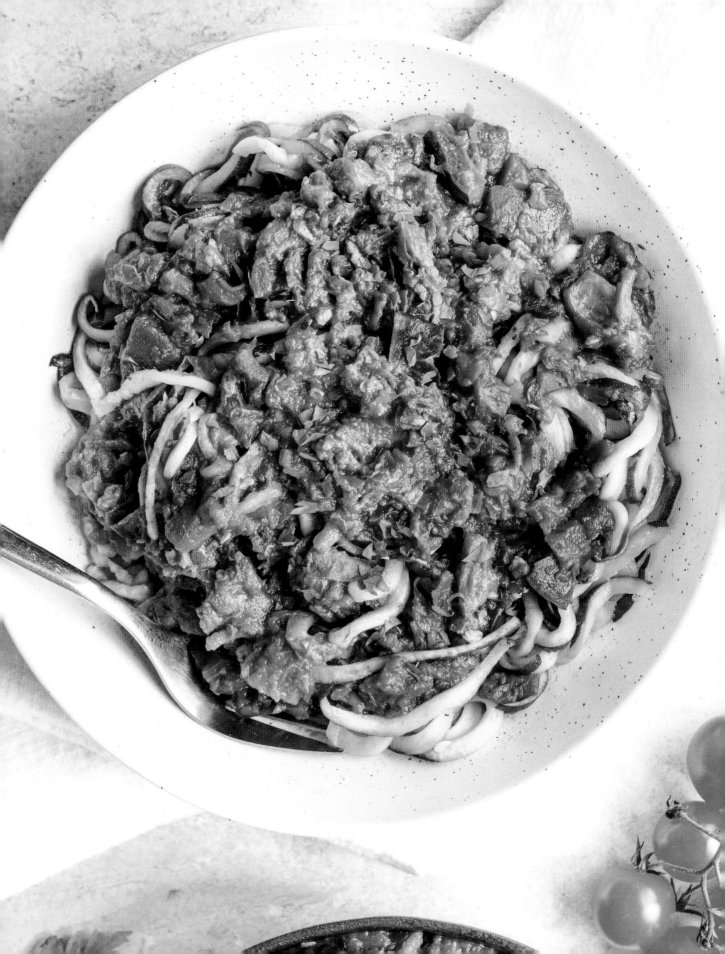

Eggplant Meatless MEATBALLS

Yield: 20 meatballs **Prep Time:** 15 minutes **Cook Time:** 1 hour 10 minutes

These little balls of deliciousness, which get rave reviews on my blog from both vegetarians and meat lovers, are a cross between meatballs and eggplant parmigiana. They are firm on the outside and soft in the center and will quickly have any carnivore forgetting that they're meat-free. Eggplant gives each ball a meatlike density, while the basil and garlic add delicious flavor. Eat them smothered in tomato sauce on a bed of veggie noodles with a garnish of Parmesan cheese and chopped basil for a hearty, satisfying meal.

Meatless Meatballs

1 tablespoon extra-virgin olive oil

2 medium eggplants, diced (about 3¾ cups)

1 medium yellow onion, diced

2 cloves garlic, minced

⅔ cup chicken or vegetable stock

¼ teaspoon salt

¼ teaspoon pepper

1¾ cups blanched almond flour

⅓ cup chopped fresh basil

⅓ cup grated Parmesan cheese

1 medium egg white, lightly beaten

Sauce

2 pounds tomatoes

1 tablespoon extra-virgin olive oil

½ medium yellow onion, chopped

1 clove garlic, minced

1 (14-ounce) can diced tomatoes, or 1⅔ cups chunky tomato sauce

¼ cup chopped fresh basil, plus more for garnish

1½ teaspoons red pepper flakes

1 teaspoon dried oregano leaves

½ teaspoon salt

½ teaspoon pepper

1. Preheat the oven to 350°F. Line a sheet pan with parchment paper, then spray it with cooking spray until well greased.

2. Heat the oil in a large skillet over medium heat. Add the diced eggplants, onion, garlic, and stock and season with salt and pepper. Cook for 15 to 20 minutes, until all of the eggplant has become soft and the liquid has been absorbed.

3. Transfer the eggplant mixture to a food processor or blender and pulse once or twice but no more. You want the larger pieces to break down, but you do not want the entire mixture to turn into a smooth puree. It should remain chunky.

4. Place the eggplant mixture, almond flour, basil, Parmesan cheese, and egg white in a bowl and mix with a wooden spoon until well combined.

5. Scoop heaping tablespoons of the mixture into your hands and roll into balls the size of a golf ball. Place on the prepared sheet pan about 1 inch apart. You should have a total of 20 balls.

6. Bake for 35 to 45 minutes, flipping the balls halfway through. Keep an eye on them to make sure they don't burn. They're done when they become firm to the touch.

7. While the meatballs are cooking, make the sauce: Chop the tomatoes into small pieces and place in a medium-sized pot over medium-low heat. Add the oil, onion, and garlic. Cook for 15 to 20 minutes, until the onion has softened.

8. Add the canned chopped tomatoes to the pot, lower the heat, and simmer for 45 minutes to 1 hour, stirring periodically to prevent burning.

9. Stir in the basil, red pepper flakes, and oregano. Season with the salt and pepper and serve topped with the cooked meatballs and more fresh basil.

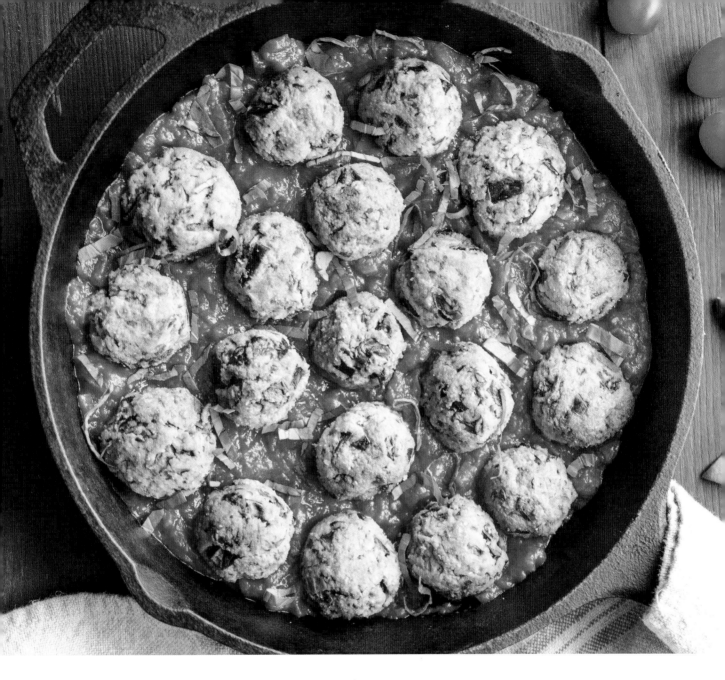

Garlic Potency

When cut and exposed to oxygen, garlic releases a sulfur compound, which creates a potent garlicky taste. The finer garlic is chopped, the more oxygen it's exposed to, and therefore the stronger its flavor, so minced garlic has a much stronger taste than roughly chopped garlic. An easy way to control the garlic flavor of a dish is to cut the cloves into smaller or larger pieces depending on your preference.

SUBSTITUTIONS: *For low-FODMAP, omit the garlic and onion and replace the extra-virgin olive oil with garlic-infused oil. Use 2 tablespoons of nutritional yeast in place of the Parmesan for Paleo or dairy-free.*

STORAGE: *Leftovers will last in the fridge for up to 4 days or in the freezer for up to 3 months; store the meatless meatballs separately from the sauce so they do not become mushy. To reheat, put the meatballs in a preheated 350°F oven for 15 minutes, or until warmed through; heat the sauce in a saucepan over medium-low heat.*

SCD BASICS
Tomato Sauce (page 36), **Chicken or Vegetable Stock** (page 53)

Tandoori Grilled
CAULIFLOWER STEAKS

Yield: 2 servings   **Prep Time:** 15 minutes   **Cook Time:** 10 minutes

Grilled cauliflower steaks are a great meat-free option to serve at a summer cookout. Although I love the texture of grilled cauliflower, I find that it needs some help in the flavor department to become outstanding. In this recipe, the cauliflower steaks are coated in a spicy tandoori sauce before being grilled until tender. The steaks are then garnished with a tahini mint sauce and fresh herbs to create one seriously flavorful dish that will satisfy carnivores and vegans alike.

1 medium head cauliflower

Tandoori Sauce

½ cup canned full-fat coconut milk

1 tablespoon freshly squeezed lemon juice

3 cloves garlic, peeled

1 (1-inch) piece fresh ginger, peeled

2 teaspoons garam marsala

1 teaspoon ground coriander

1 teaspoon paprika

1 teaspoon turmeric powder

1 teaspoon ground cumin

1 small red chili pepper, such as Fresno (optional)

Tahini Mint Sauce

¼ cup raw cashews, soaked in boiling water for 10 minutes and drained

¼ cup water

2 tablespoons freshly squeezed lemon juice

2 tablespoons canned full-fat coconut milk

1 tablespoon tahini

¼ teaspoon salt

3 tablespoons fresh mint leaves

¼ cup pomegranate seeds, for garnish

2 tablespoons shredded fresh mint, for garnish

1. Remove the leaves from the head of cauliflower and cut the head into 4 (½-inch-thick) steaks, being sure each slice includes a portion of the core so the steaks will hold together.

2. To make the tandoori sauce, place the coconut milk, lemon juice, garlic, ginger, spices, and red chili (if desired) in a high-powered blender. Blend until smooth.

3. Pour the sauce into a baking dish or sheet pan large enough to fit the steaks. Place the steaks in the dish and spoon the sauce over them so that they are well coated. Set aside. Rinse out the blender jar.

4. To make the tahini mint sauce, place the cashews in the blender. Add the water, lemon juice, coconut milk, tahini, and salt and blend until completely smooth. Add the fresh mint and pulse for 2 to 3 seconds just to break it into small pieces.

5. Heat a grill or panini press to medium-high heat; alternatively, heat a grill pan over medium-high heat. Lightly oil the grill, place the cauliflower steaks on the grill and cook for about 5 minutes or until grill marks form; flip and cook for 5 minutes on the other side, until the stem of the cauliflower is tender and can be pierced with a fork. If you're cooking the cauliflower steaks in batches, keep the cooked steaks warm in a warm oven.

6. Serve the cauliflower steaks drizzled with the tahini mint sauce and garnished with pomegranate seeds and shredded mint.

MAKE AHEAD/STORAGE: *You can cut the cauliflower steaks and let them marinate overnight in the tandoori sauce (Steps 1 through 3) before grilling. Once grilled, the cauliflower steaks will last in the fridge for up to 3 days. The tahini mint sauce can be made up to 3 days in advance and stored in the fridge until ready to serve.*

SPECIAL EQUIPMENT: High-powered blender

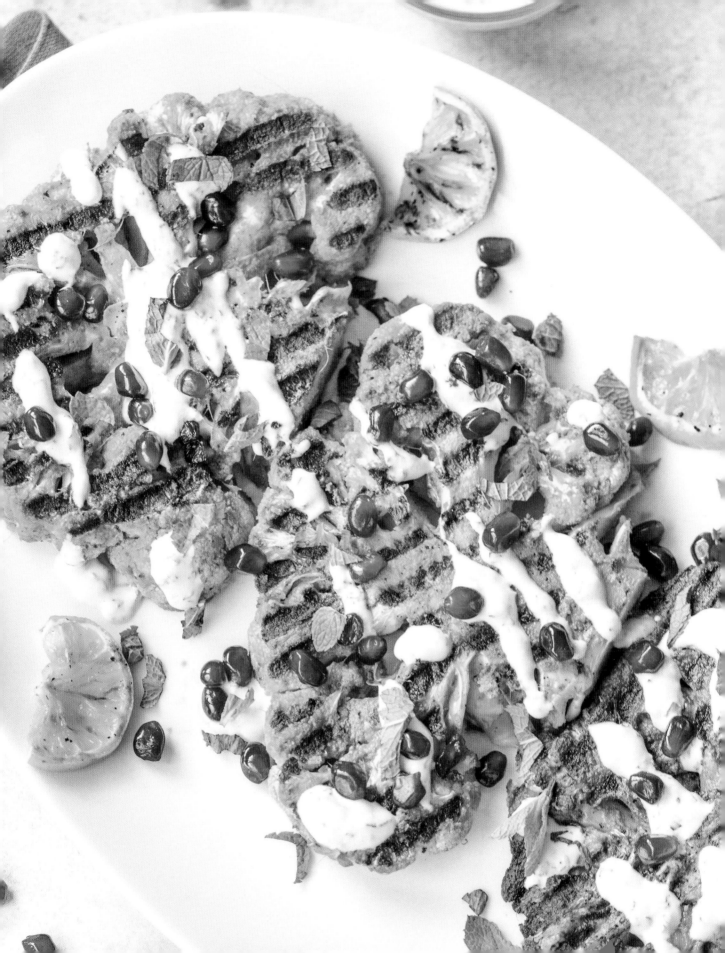

KETO
PALEO
VEGAN
VEGETARIAN
DAIRY-FREE
EGG-FREE
NUT-FREE

Mushroom & Onion
RISOTTO

Yield: 4 servings **Prep Time:** 15 minutes **Cook Time:** 30 minutes

Although I prefer using celery root to make risotto (as in the Creamy Spring Risotto on page 256), if you struggle to find it in stores you will find this recipe that uses cauliflower rice to be a great alternative. Dried porcini mushrooms are in the herb section of most grocery stores and add a wonderful earthiness to the dish. Sometimes, for extra fanciness, I add a drizzle of truffle oil before serving and top the dish with small sections of fresh thyme sprigs.

1 ounce dried porcini mushrooms

½ cup boiling water

2 tablespoons ghee or unsalted butter, divided

1 medium yellow onion, thinly sliced

2 cloves garlic, minced

½ teaspoon salt

5 ounces shiitake, button, or oyster mushrooms, thinly sliced

1 teaspoon dried thyme leaves

6 cups fresh riced cauliflower

1½ cups unsweetened almond milk

¼ cup chicken or vegetable stock

1 tablespoon white wine vinegar

¼ cup grated Parmesan cheese

1 tablespoon coconut cream

½ teaspoon salt

½ teaspoon pepper

1. Place the dried porcini mushrooms in a bowl with the boiling water and soak for 15 minutes. After 15 minutes of soaking, remove the porcini from the bowl, reserving the soaking water. Roughly chop the porcini and set aside.

2. Heat 1 tablespoon of the ghee in a large skillet over medium heat. Add the onion and garlic, sprinkle with the salt, and cook for 3 minutes or until the onion is translucent.

3. Stir in the rehydrated porcini, sliced mushrooms, and thyme. Cook for 6 to 8 minutes, until the mushrooms have softened, then transfer to a plate and set aside.

4. Place the remaining 1 tablespoon of ghee in the skillet. Once melted, add the riced cauliflower. Cook for 6 to 7 minutes, until the cauliflower begins to turn golden.

5. Add the almond milk, the reserved porcini soaking water, stock, vinegar, and sautéed mushroom mixture and cook for 10 minutes or until there is no liquid in the bottom of the skillet.

6. Stir in the Parmesan cheese and coconut cream, season with the salt and pepper, and serve.

SUBSTITUTIONS: *Omit the Parmesan cheese for Paleo. Use coconut oil instead of butter or ghee and omit the Parmesan cheese to make this risotto vegan and dairy-free. Use coconut milk in place of almond milk to make it nut-free.*

STORAGE: *Leftovers will last in the fridge for up to 3 days and are best reheated in the microwave for 2 minutes or in a skillet over medium heat for 5 minutes or until warmed through. If the risotto appears dry as you reheat it, stir in a splash of almond milk before serving.*

SCD BASICS

Chicken or Vegetable Stock
(page 53)

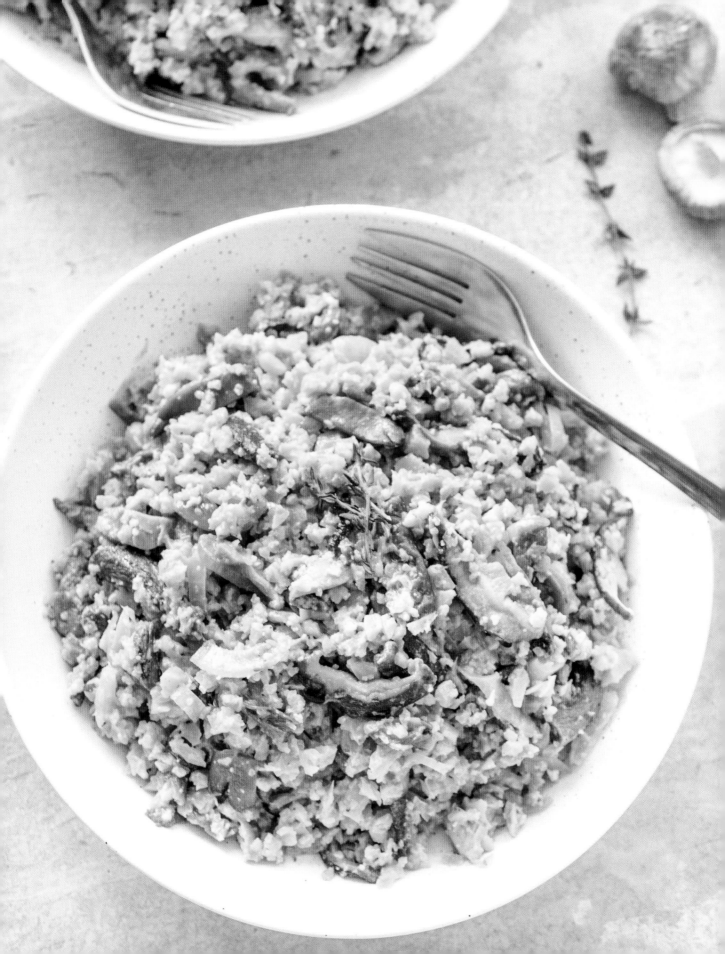

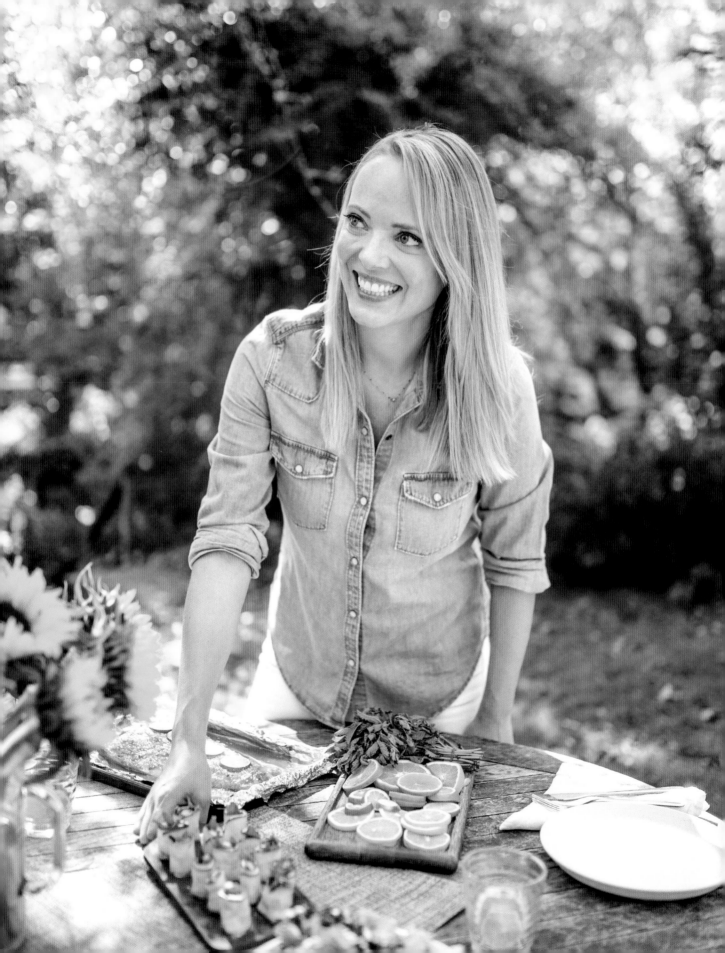

Side Dishes

KETO
PALEO
VEGAN
VEGETARIAN
DAIRY-FREE
EGG-FREE
NUT-FREE

Make ahead

Grilled Veggie Platter
WITH GREEN GODDESS SAUCE

Yield: 6 servings   **Prep Time:** 20 minutes   **Cook Time:** 15 minutes

This is a gorgeous side dish for summer cookouts. People seem to gravitate toward it because of its vibrant colors. It's fantastic served warm or cold, and it's also a great meal prep dish: grill the veggies on a Sunday and then toss them into salads for meals throughout the week. You also can add the leftover grilled veggies to a frittata like the one on page 70.

Green Goddess Sauce

1 medium avocado

¾ cup fresh basil leaves

½ cup chopped scallions

¼ cup extra-virgin olive oil

¼ cup fresh tarragon leaves

1 jalapeño pepper

2 tablespoons apple cider vinegar

1 tablespoon freshly squeezed lemon juice

1 clove garlic, peeled

½ teaspoon salt

2 to 3 tablespoons water

½ cup extra-virgin olive oil

¼ cup chopped fresh Italian parsley

2 cloves garlic, minced

½ teaspoon salt

½ teaspoon ground black pepper

2 red onions, cut into wedges

8 to 10 asparagus spears, trimmed

1 red bell pepper, stem and seeds removed and cut into quarters

1 large eggplant, cut into ½-inch slices

3 portobello mushrooms

1 large yellow squash, cut into ½-inch slices

1 bunch broccolini

1. To make the Green Goddess sauce, place all of the sauce ingredients except the water in a blender and blend until smooth. Add 2 tablespoons of water and blend again; add more water as needed to thin the sauce until it reaches your desired consistency. Transfer to a small bowl and refrigerate until ready to serve.

2. Preheat the grill to medium-high heat; alternatively, place a grill pan over medium-high heat.

3. In a large bowl, whisk together the oil, parsley, garlic, salt, and pepper. Working in batches, add the veggies and toss with your hands until they are well coated in the oil mixture. If there is any remaining oil mixture, reserve for serving. Place the vegetables on the grill and cook for 10 to 12 minutes, turning occasionally, until lightly charred.

4. Transfer the cooked veggies to a large platter and slice the mushrooms. Brush the vegetables with any of the remaining oil mixture and serve with the sauce on the side; alternatively, you can drizzle the sauce over the veggies.

SUBSTITUTIONS: *I've included my favorite vegetables for grilling, but feel free to include other veggies that you have on hand, such as scallions, carrots, zucchini, or radicchio.*

MAKE AHEAD/STORAGE: *You can cut and grill everything a day in advance and quickly brush with extra oil and herbs before serving. Leftover grilled veggies and green goddess sauce should be stored separately and will last in the fridge for up to 4 days.*

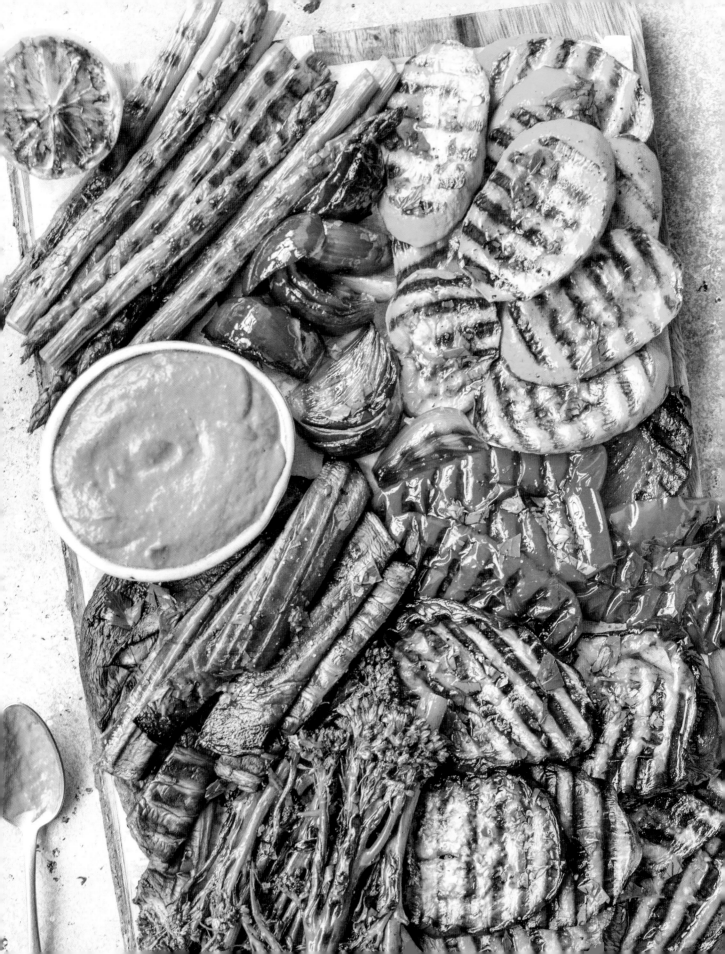

AIP
KETO
PALEO
VEGAN
VEGETARIAN
DAIRY-FREE
EGG-FREE
NUT-FREE

Coconut
CAULIFLOWER RICE

Yield: 4 servings **Prep Time:** 10 minutes **Cook Time:** 15 minutes

This rice isn't revolutionary or knock-your-socks-off flavorful; it's just an easy-to-prepare side dish to have in your repertoire. With its subtle flavors, it's a great dish to serve alongside saucy mains such as Kung Pao Chicken (page 180), Butter Chicken Meatballs (page 202), or Sweet Chili Salmon (page 234).

1 medium head cauliflower, or 4 cups fresh or frozen riced cauliflower

1 tablespoon coconut oil

½ teaspoon salt

½ cup full-fat canned coconut milk (see tip)

1½ teaspoons freshly squeezed lime juice

1. Cut the cauliflower into small florets. Place the florets in a food processor and pulse for 5 or 6 seconds, until broken down into rice-sized pieces.

2. Melt the coconut oil in a large skillet over medium-high heat. Add the riced cauliflower, season with salt, and cook for 3 to 4 minutes, until the rice begins to turn slightly golden.

3. Stir in the coconut milk and lime juice and cook for 8 minutes, stirring occasionally to ensure it doesn't burn. The cauliflower rice is done when it's tender and all of the coconut milk has evaporated.

STORAGE: *Leftovers will last in the fridge for up to 3 days.*

TIP: *If using frozen riced cauliflower, I recommend reducing the amount of coconut milk to ⅓ cup.*

Coconut Milk Versus Coconut Cream

Coconut milk is a blend of coconut flesh and water that has a consistency similar to cow's milk. When you chill a can of coconut milk overnight in the fridge, it separates, and the thick coconut cream rises to the top. Keep some cans of coconut milk in the cupboard; quickly shake the can to mix it well before adding it to recipes calling for coconut milk. Keep additional cans of coconut milk in the fridge so you can easily scoop off the thick cream for any recipes requiring coconut cream. Reserve the leftover water from the can to add to smoothies.

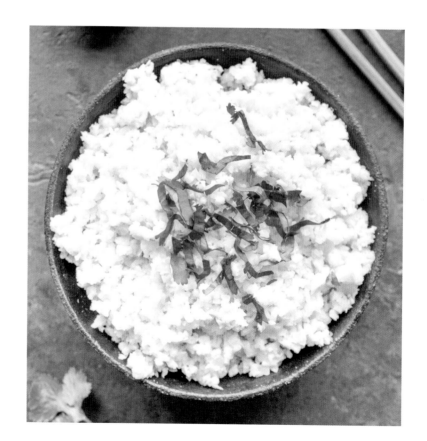

KETO
PALEO
VEGAN
VEGETARIAN
DAIRY-FREE
EGG-FREE
NUT-FREE

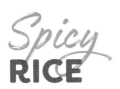

Spicy RICE

Yield: 4 servings   **Prep Time:** 5 minutes   **Cook Time:** 15 minutes

If you are new to the world of cauliflower rice, this is a great recipe to start with because it's packed with bold flavor. It's a quick-and-easy side dish to round out a meal of grilled chicken or fish.

1 medium head cauliflower, or 4 cups fresh or frozen riced cauliflower

1½ teaspoons extra-virgin olive oil

½ red bell pepper, diced

½ green bell pepper, diced

½ medium red onion, diced

2 teaspoons turmeric powder

2 teaspoons paprika

1 teaspoon ground cumin

½ teaspoon cayenne pepper

½ cup frozen peas

½ cup chicken or vegetable stock

1. Cut the cauliflower into small florets and place them in a food processor. Pulse for 5 or 6 seconds, until broken down into rice-sized pieces.

2. Heat the oil in a large skillet over medium-high heat. Once hot, add the bell peppers, onion, turmeric, paprika, cumin, and cayenne pepper. Cook for 5 to 6 minutes, until the vegetables begin to brown.

3. Lower the heat to medium and stir in the riced cauliflower and peas, making sure everything is well combined and then pour in the chicken stock. Cook for 5 minutes, until all of the liquid has been absorbed and the cauliflower rice is tender.

SUBSTITUTIONS: *Skip the frozen peas to make this dish keto.*

STORAGE: *Leftovers will last in the fridge for up to 2 days. Reheat in the microwave or in a skillet on low heat with a splash of chicken stock.*

TIP: *When making cauliflower rice, I find it's best to pulse the florets in the food processor in small batches so that the pieces are all evenly sized. Filling the food processor too full often results in larger chunks getting stuck while smaller pieces break down into a fine powder.*

SCD BASICS
Chicken of Vegetable Stock
(page 53)

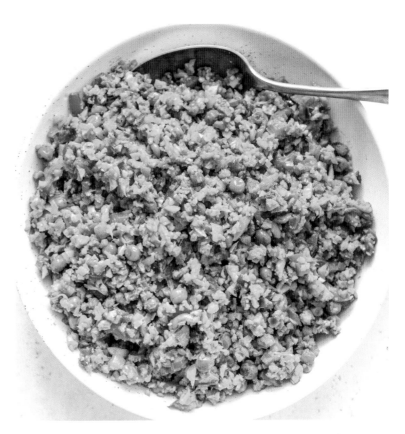

AIP
KETO
LOW-FODMAP
PALEO
VEGAN
VEGETARIAN
DAIRY-FREE
EGG-FREE
NUT-FREE

Make ahead

Patty's Melt-in-Your-Mouth
FENNEL & LEEKS

Yield: 4 servings **Prep Time:** 5 minutes **Cook Time:** 45 minutes

This is a dish that my mother-in-law, Patty, taught me to make. Over the past 10 years of watching her cook, I have learned that the secret to many of her comforting and richly flavored dishes is patience. Whether you're making a soup, a sauce, or a caramelized vegetable, letting things simmer low and slow for 30 minutes or more always results in a more flavorful dish. Which brings me to this fennel and leek dish: Although this recipe contains just a handful of ingredients, the extended cooking time results in the most buttery, melt-in-your-mouth, and tender vegetables. Even fennel haters will swoon over how deliciously soft and delicious it becomes when cooked this way.

1 large leek

3 bulbs fennel

1 tablespoon extra-virgin olive oil

2 tablespoons unsalted butter or ghee

2 cloves garlic, minced

⅓ cup chicken or vegetable stock, plus more as needed

3 tablespoons chopped fresh Italian parsley

1 teaspoon salt

½ teaspoon ground black pepper

1. Cut the leek in half lengthwise, then thinly slice it. Place the leek slices in a bowl of water and leave them submerged for 5 minutes to loosen any dirt from between the leaves. Use a slotted spoon to transfer the leek slices to a paper towel–lined plate to drain.

2. Trim the stems from the top of the fennel, cut each bulb in half, and then cut into ¼-inch-thick slices.

3. Heat the oil and butter in a large pot over medium-high heat. Cook the garlic for 30 seconds until fragrant. Add the fennel and leeks and cook for 5 minutes, until the fennel begins to soften slightly.

4. Stir in the stock and lower the heat to medium-low. Cook for 40 minutes, stirring every 8 to 10 minutes to ensure that it doesn't burn. (If it does, add a splash more stock.) After 40 minutes, the fennel should be very soft.

5. Stir in the parsley, salt, and pepper and serve.

SUBSTITUTIONS: *For AIP, use olive oil in place of the butter and omit the pepper. Skip the garlic to make it low-FODMAP. Omit the butter or ghee and use an additional 2 tablespoons of olive oil to make this dish vegan or dairy-free.*

MAKE AHEAD/STORAGE: *This dish can be made up to 2 days in advance and then reheated in a skillet over medium-high heat for 10 minutes or until warmed through. Leftovers will last in the fridge for up to 4 days.*

SCD BASICS
Chicken or Vegetable Stock
(page 53)

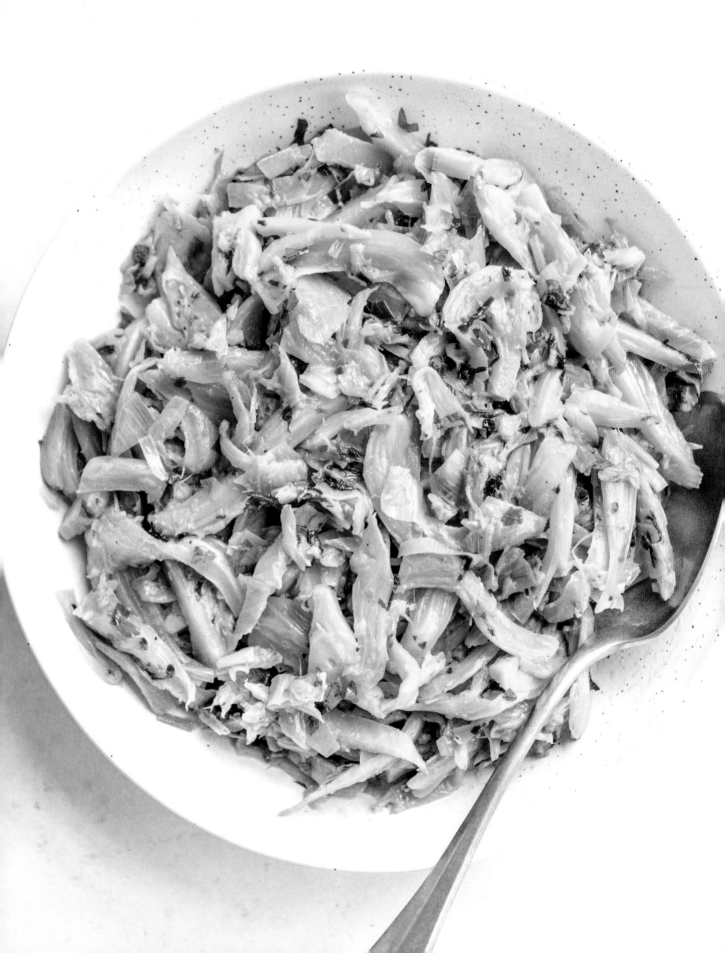

AIP
KETO
PALEO
VEGAN
VEGETARIAN
DAIRY-FREE
EGG-FREE
NUT-FREE

Lemon & Garlic
ROASTED ASPARAGUS

< 30 min

Yield: 4 servings   **Prep Time:** 5 minutes   **Cook Time:** 12 minutes

I love oven-roasted asparagus; the tips get slightly charred and the spears become much more flavorful than when they've been steamed. This is a really simple side dish that you can quickly toss in the oven while you work on preparing the rest of the meal. Lemon gives this dish a fresh flavor, making it a wonderful accompaniment to fish or grilled meat.

1 small shallot, minced

2 cloves garlic, minced

½ teaspoon grated lemon zest

1 tablespoon freshly squeezed lemon juice

1 tablespoon extra-virgin olive oil

1 teaspoon honey

½ teaspoon dried thyme leaves

1 pound asparagus, woody ends trimmed off

2 slices lemon, cut in half

½ teaspoon salt

½ teaspoon ground black pepper

2 tablespoons toasted sliced almonds

1. Preheat the oven to 400°F.

2. In a bowl, whisk together the shallot, garlic, lemon zest, lemon juice, oil, honey, and thyme. Lay the asparagus evenly in a baking dish and drizzle the sauce over the top. Toss the asparagus gently so that the spears are evenly coated in the sauce. Place the lemon slices on top of the spears.

3. Bake for 12 minutes, until the asparagus spears are tender. Sprinkle with the salt, pepper, and almonds before serving immediately.

SUBSTITUTIONS: *For AIP, omit the almonds and pepper. Skip the honey to make this dish keto. Swap the honey for maple syrup to make it vegan. Use raw hulled sunflower seeds in place of sliced almonds to make it nut-free.*

Keeping Asparagus Fresh
Asparagus stays fresh longer when stored in the fridge in a jar or glass filled with 2 inches of water.

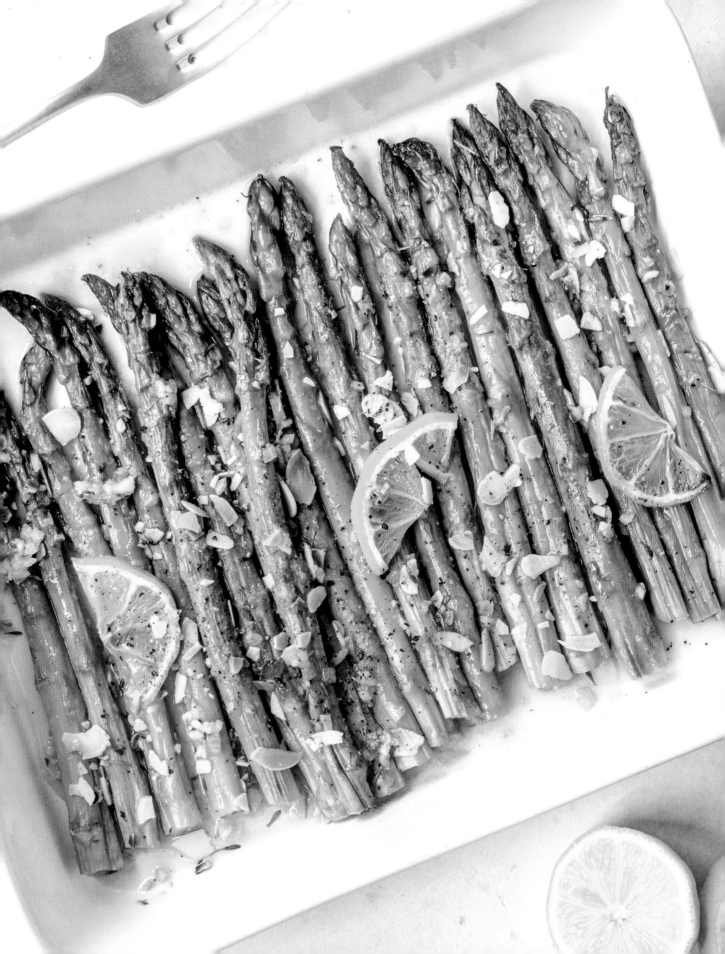

Green Beans with Hazelnuts & TAHINI LEMON SAUCE

Yield: 4 servings **Prep Time:** 10 minutes **Cook Time:** 4 minutes

Creamy tahini lemon sauce is a great way to bring green beans to life. The red onion adds a sharp kick of flavor, and the toasted hazelnuts add crunch. You can enjoy this dish warm or cold as a side dish or simple salad.

¼ cup water

2 tablespoons tahini

2 teaspoons red wine vinegar

1½ teaspoons grated lemon zest, for garnish

1 tablespoon freshly squeezed lemon juice

1 clove garlic, minced

1 teaspoon salt

1 pound green beans, ends trimmed

¼ medium red onion, very thinly sliced

¼ cup toasted hazelnuts, roughly chopped

1 teaspoon black sesame seeds, for garnish

1. In a small bowl, whisk together the water, tahini, vinegar, lemon juice, garlic, and salt until smooth. Set aside.

2. Bring a large pot of water to a boil. Add the green beans and cook for 4 minutes, until tender but not mushy. Transfer the green beans to a colander to drain them; rinse the beans with cold water to stop them from continuing to cook.

3. Place the green beans in a serving bowl along with the onion and hazelnuts. Drizzle the tahini sauce over the top and toss until well coated. Serve garnished with the lemon zest and sesame seeds.

SUBSTITUTIONS: *Skip the hazelnuts to make this dish nut-free.*

MAKE AHEAD/STORAGE: *This dish can be made a day ahead, and leftovers will last in the fridge for up to 4 days.*

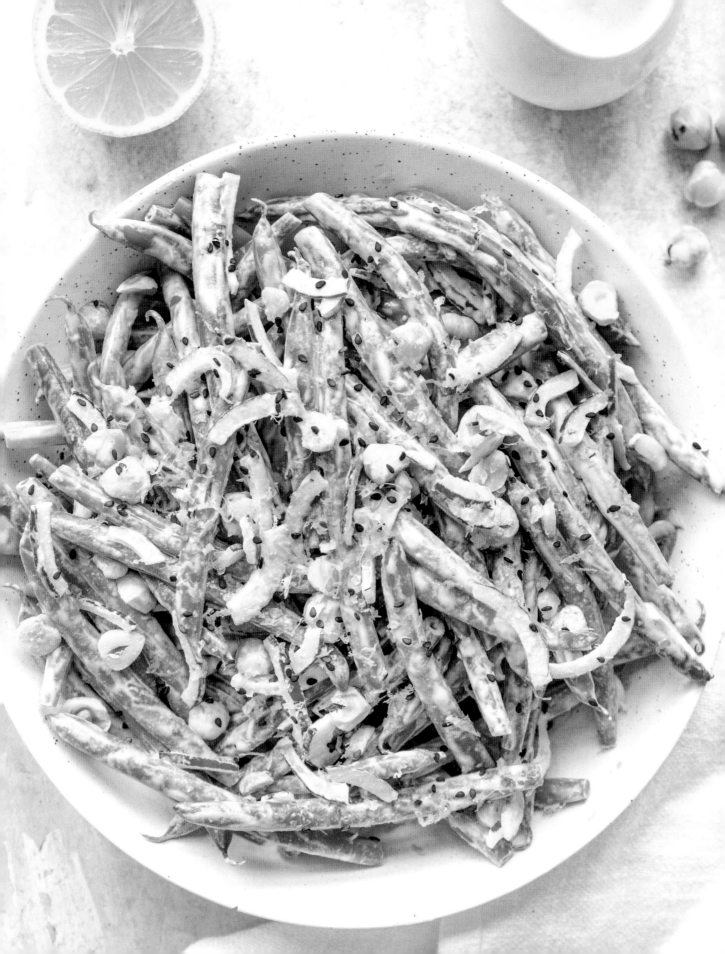

AIP
KETO
PALEO
VEGAN
VEGETARIAN
DAIRY-FREE
EGG-FREE
NUT-FREE

Garlic Roasted
MUSHROOMS

Make ahead *<30 min*

Yield: 4 servings   **Prep Time:** 5 minutes   **Cook Time:** 20 minutes

This is the ideal recipe to convert mushroom haters because, let's be honest, it's impossible to dislike something cooked in this much butter and garlic. This is the perfect low-maintenance side dish to serve with steak or chicken. Alternatively, use big portobello mushrooms and enjoy it as a main with a side of mash to sop up the sauce.

1 pound cremini or button mushrooms

3 tablespoons unsalted butter or ghee, melted

1 tablespoon extra-virgin olive oil

4 cloves garlic, minced

1 tablespoon aged balsamic vinegar, or 1 teaspoon red wine vinegar

½ teaspoon salt

½ teaspoon ground black pepper

¼ cup chopped fresh Italian parsley

1. Preheat the oven to 350°F.

2. Cut the mushrooms into quarters or halves, depending on the size, so that they are equally sized. Place the mushrooms in an 8-inch square baking dish.

3. In a bowl, whisk together the melted butter, oil, garlic, vinegar, salt, and pepper, then pour over the mushrooms. Toss until the mushrooms are well coated in the butter mixture.

4. Bake for 20 minutes, until the mushrooms are tender and golden. Stir in the parsley before serving.

SUBSTITUTIONS: *For AIP, use olive oil and omit the pepper. Use 2 additional tablespoons of olive oil in place of the butter or ghee to make this dish vegan and dairy-free.*

MAKE AHEAD/STORAGE: *You can prepare these mushrooms (without the parsley) a day in advance; reheat in a preheated 350°F oven for 10 minutes and top with the parsley before serving. Leftovers will last in the fridge for up to 3 days.*

Cleaning Mushrooms
Don't wash mushrooms! They're like sponges and will absorb excess moisture, which will be released when you cook them. The result is a watery dish. Instead, wipe mushrooms with a damp paper towel to remove any dirt.

SCD BASICS
SCD Balsamic Vinegar (page 46)

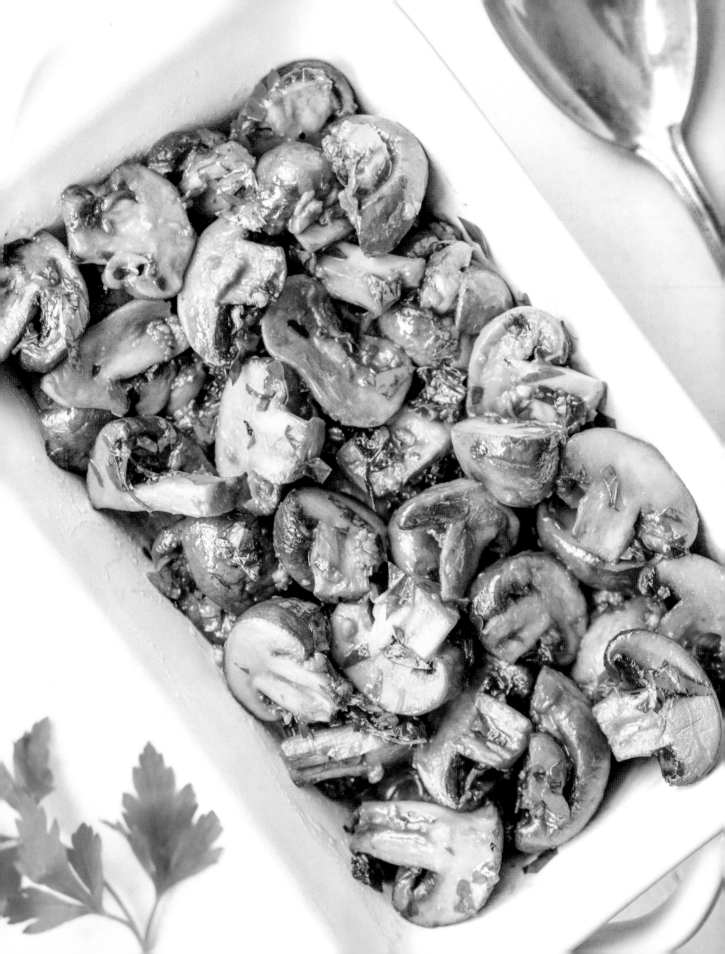

KETO
PALEO
VEGAN
VEGETARIAN
DAIRY-FREE
EGG-FREE
NUT-FREE

< 30 min

The BEST
CAULIFLOWER MASH

Yield: 2 servings   **Prep Time:** 5 minutes   **Cook Time:** 20 minutes

I know it's a bold statement, but this truly is the BEST and only cauliflower mash recipe that you will ever need. With just three ingredients and a bit of salt, it all comes down to two simple steps that really elevate this mash to the next level in both flavor and creaminess. This is my go-to side dish for anything saucy—such as the Balsamic Chicken & Grapes (page 188), Beef Stroganoff (page 218), and Short Rib Beef Bourguignonne (page 220)—and is guaranteed to win over even the most avid mashed potato fans. This recipe receives rave reviews on my blog for its delicious creaminess.

1 medium head cauliflower, or 4 cups fresh or frozen riced cauliflower

2 tablespoons unsalted butter, ghee, or coconut oil

¼ teaspoon salt

1¾ cups unsweetened almond milk

For Garnish

Chopped fresh Italian parsley

Fresh cracked black pepper

Olive oil (optional)

1. Cut the cauliflower into chunks, place in a food processor and pulse for 5 or 6 seconds, until the cauliflower is broken into small pieces. Alternatively, you can chop up the cauliflower by hand. (Don't stress about the sizes of the cauliflower pieces; they don't need to be completely even.)

2. Melt the butter in a large skillet over medium-high heat. Add the cauliflower and sprinkle with the salt. Cook for 6 to 7 minutes, until the cauliflower begins to turn golden.

3. Stir in the almond milk and let the cauliflower cook for about 10 minutes, until there is no liquid in the bottom of the skillet; it should all be absorbed into the cauliflower. Don't rush this step because leaving too much milk in the cauliflower before blending will result in a liquidy mash.

4. Transfer the mixture to a food processor and blend until completely smooth. Serve warm garnished with chopped parsley, cracked black pepper, and olive oil, if desired.

SUBSTITUTIONS: *Canned full-fat coconut milk can be used in place of the almond milk to make this dish nut-free.*

STORAGE: *Leftover cauliflower mash will last in the fridge for up to 3 days. Alternatively, you can freeze it in single-serving portions in a silicone muffin pan for up to 1 month.*

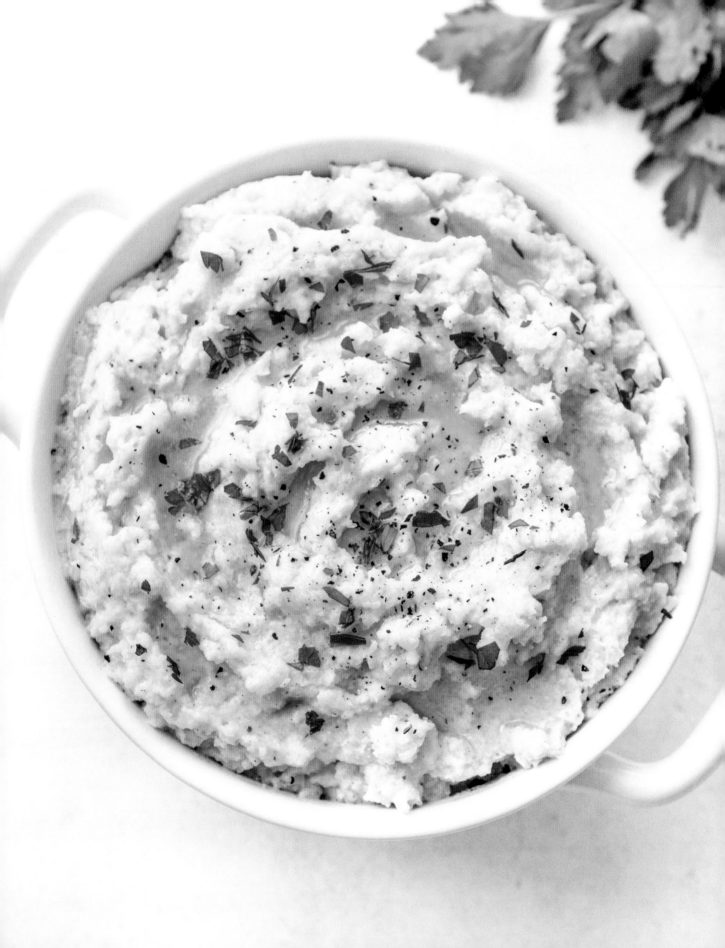

AIP
KETO
PALEO
VEGAN
VEGETARIAN
DAIRY-FREE
EGG-FREE
NUT-FREE

Make ahead

Roasted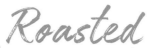
BRUSSELS SPROUTS & BACON

Yield: 4 servings   **Prep Time:** 10 minutes   **Cook Time:** 30 minutes

Everyone needs a Brussels sprouts recipe in their repertoire to make for Thanksgiving or Christmas with the knowledge that it will be a hit rather than pushed to the side of everyone's plate. In this recipe, Brussels sprouts and bacon (my favorite food tag team) are tossed in a honey, mustard, and balsamic sauce and then roasted until slightly charred and tender. It's a flavor-packed combination that's guaranteed to be a hit with even kids and Brussels sprouts–hating adults.

1 pound Brussels sprouts, halved

5 strips bacon, cut into small pieces

2 tablespoons aged balsamic vinegar, or 1 tablespoon red wine vinegar

1 tablespoon extra-virgin olive oil

1½ teaspoons Dijon mustard

1½ teaspoons honey

½ teaspoon ground black pepper

¼ teaspoon salt

1. Preheat the oven to 425°F.

2. Place the Brussels sprouts and bacon on a large sheet pan or in a large baking dish, ensuring they are in an even single layer.

3. In a small bowl, whisk together the remaining ingredients. Pour the mixture over the Brussels sprouts and bacon and toss with your hands to coat evenly.

4. Roast for 25 to 30 minutes, until the Brussels sprouts are tender and golden brown, and the bacon is crisp.

SUBSTITUTIONS: *Omit the mustard and pepper to make it AIP. For keto, omit the honey. Swap the bacon for thinly sliced red onions and use maple syrup in place of the honey to make this dish vegan or vegetarian.*

MAKE AHEAD/STORAGE: *The Brussels sprouts and bacon can be tossed in the sauce mixture a day before baking. Leftovers will last in the fridge for up to 3 days and are delicious tossed into a salad.*

SCD BASICS
SCD Balsamic Vinegar (page 46)

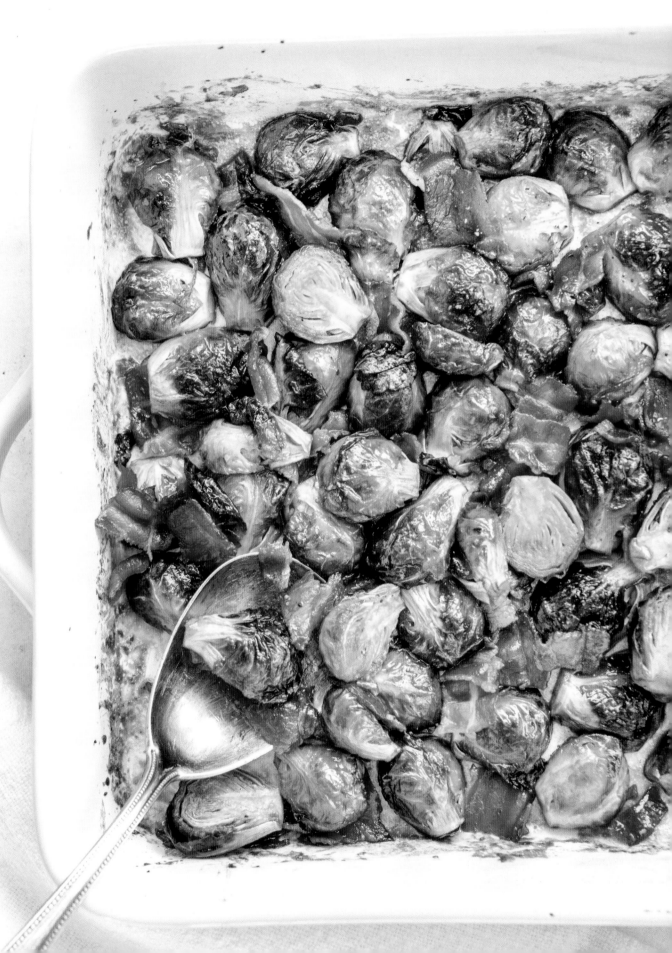

KETO
PALEO
VEGAN
VEGETARIAN
DAIRY-FREE
EGG-FREE

Make ahead

Loaded Cauliflower
CASSEROLE

Yield: 10 servings **Prep Time:** 20 minutes **Cook Time:** 25 minutes

This is a great casserole to feed to a crowd. It's packed with tender cauliflower florets coated in a deliciously cheesy sauce (which tastes cheesy even if you opt for the dairy-free version!) and mixed with flavorful pieces of bacon and chopped scallions.

2 small heads or 1 large head cauliflower, cut into bite-sized florets

1½ cups unsweetened almond milk

1 cup cashews, soaked in boiling water for 10 minutes and drained

2 tablespoons Dijon mustard

3 cloves garlic, peeled

1½ cups chicken or vegetable stock

½ cup shredded cheddar cheese

1 teaspoon paprika

½ teaspoon cayenne pepper

½ cup diced scallions, plus more for garnish

6 strips bacon, cooked and roughly chopped

SPECIAL EQUIPMENT
High-powered blender

1. Preheat the oven to 375°F.

2. Bring a large pot with 1 inch of water to a gentle simmer over medium-high heat. Add the cauliflower florets, cover with a lid, and cook for about 5 minutes, until the florets are just tender. Alternatively, you can cook the cauliflower florets in a steamer basket. Transfer the cooked florets to a colander to drain any excess water.

3. While the cauliflower is cooking, place the almond milk, cashews, Dijon mustard, and garlic in a high-powered blender and blend until completely smooth and creamy. Transfer the mixture to the empty pot along with the stock, cheese, paprika, and cayenne pepper and bring to a gentle simmer over medium-low heat. Whisk until the cheese has melted and the sauce is smooth; remove from the heat.

4. Add the cauliflower florets to the pot along with the scallions and bacon and gently toss until everything is well coated in the sauce. Pour everything into an 11 by 7-inch baking dish.

5. Bake 20 minutes until hot and bubbly. Garnish with additional scallions before serving.

SUBSTITUTIONS: *For keto, use macadamia nuts in place of the cashews to reduce the carbs. For Paleo, replace the cheese with ¼ cup of nutritional yeast. For vegan or vegetarian, use ¼ cup of nutritional yeast in place of the cheese and skip the bacon.*

MAKE AHEAD/STORAGE: *This casserole can be prepped a day in advance and baked just before serving. Leftovers will last in the fridge for up to 3 days.*

SCD BASICS
Chicken or Vegetable Stock
(page 53)

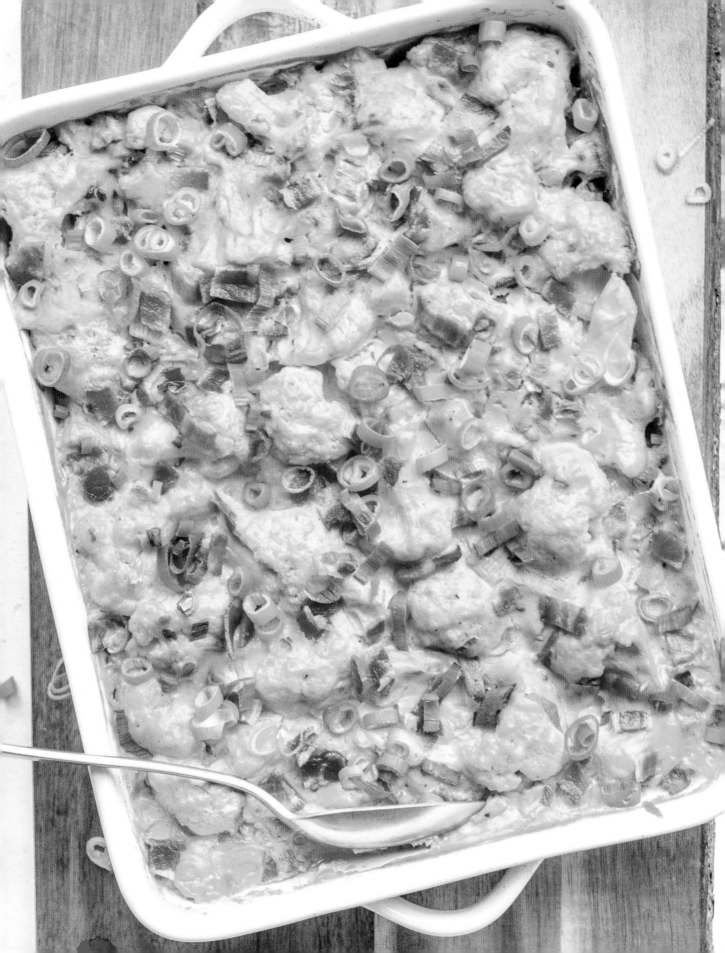

KETO
PALEO
VEGAN
VEGETARIAN
DAIRY-FREE
EGG-FREE

Creamed
SPINACH & KALE

Yield: 6 servings   **Prep Time:** 20 minutes   **Cook Time:** 10 minutes

Creamed spinach has always been one of my favorite side dishes, but it often contains just as much dairy as spinach. This version has all of the same delicious creaminess, and no one will suspect it's because of cashews—not dairy! I like using a combination of kale and spinach to give the dish a bit more texture; just be sure to cook the kale longer so that it doesn't come out chewy.

8 ounces curly kale, destemmed

8 ounces fresh spinach

⅔ cup cashews, soaked in boiling water for 10 minutes and drained

⅔ cup unsweetened almond milk

1 teaspoon freshly squeezed lemon juice

Pinch of ground nutmeg

1 tablespoon unsalted butter, ghee, or coconut oil

1 medium yellow onion, minced

4 cloves garlic, minced

½ teaspoon salt

SPECIAL EQUIPMENT
High-powered blender

1. Bring a pot with 3 inches of water to a boil over high heat. Place the kale in the pot and cook for 3 minutes, until tender, then use a slotted spoon to remove it from the water and transfer to a colander. Run cold water over the kale to cool it. Next, return the pot of water to the stove and bring it to a boil before placing the spinach in the pot to cook for 2 minutes. Remove the spinach from the water and place it in the colander with the kale to cool.

2. Place the cashews, almond milk, lemon juice, and nutmeg in a high-powered blender and blend until completely smooth.

3. Once the kale and spinach have cooled enough to handle, use your hands to squeeze out as much liquid as possible and then roughly chop the greens.

4. Melt the butter in a large skillet over medium-high heat. Add the onion, garlic, and salt and sauté for 4 to 5 minutes, until the onion is translucent. Add the chopped kale and spinach to the skillet; stir in the cashew cream mixture until the greens are well coated in the cream. Remove from the heat and serve immediately.

Delicious Dip

This is so deliciously creamy you can eat it as a hot dip! Add ¼ cup grated Parmesan cheese (or 2 tablespoons nutritional yeast for dairy-free or vegan) and bake in a preheated 350°F oven for 15 minutes. Serve the creamed spinach and kale hot and bubbly in a bowl with Seeded Crackers (page 292) for dipping.

SUBSTITUTIONS: *For keto, use macadamia nuts in place of the cashews to reduce the carbs. Use coconut oil to make this dish vegan and dairy-free.*

MAKE AHEAD/STORAGE: *This can be made a day in advance and reheated in a preheated 350°F oven for 10 to 15 minutes, or until warmed through. Leftovers can be stored in the fridge for up to 3 days.*

SCD BASICS
Chicken Stock (page 53)

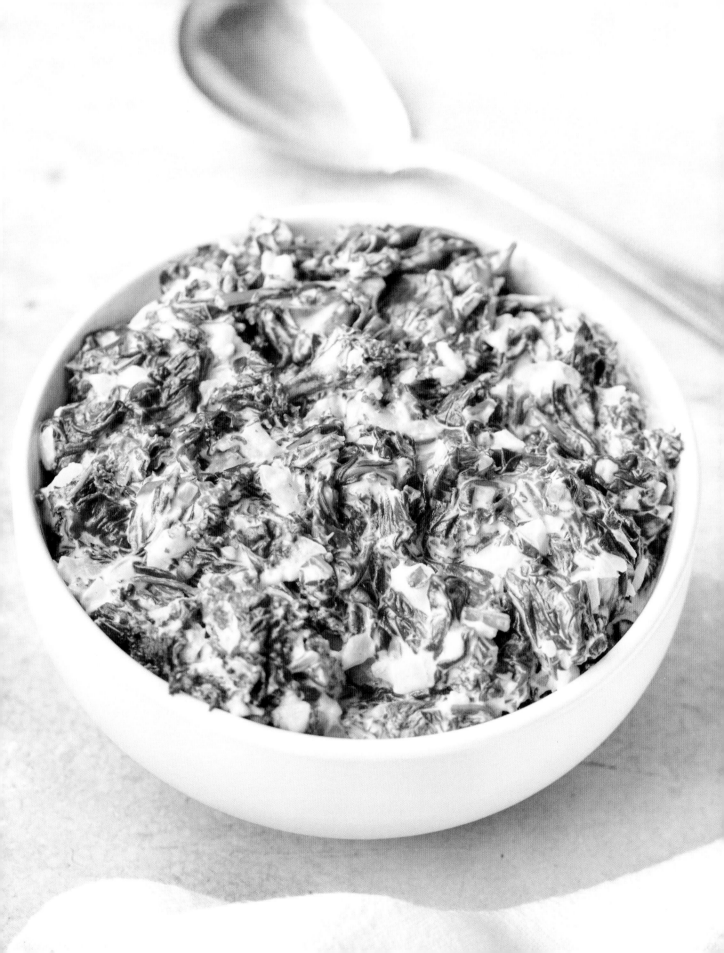

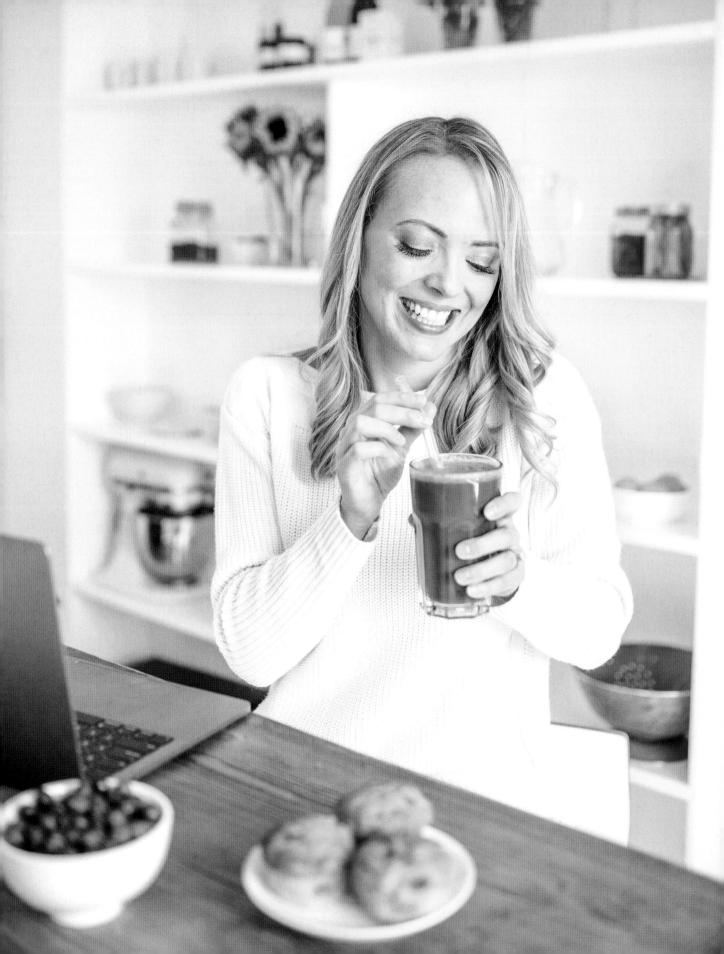

Snacks

< 30 min

Seeded CRACKERS

Yield: 40 crackers   **Prep Time:** 15 minutes   **Cook Time:** 15 minutes

Because I'm a major snacker, it didn't take me long after starting the Specific Carbohydrate Diet to realize that I needed a reliable cracker recipe in my repertoire. These crackers are crispy, salty, and perfect for topping with cheese or hummus, and they're even delicious on their own. I love the combination of seeds in this recipe, but feel free to switch things up by adding chopped herbs, chopped oil-packed sun-dried tomatoes, or spices like cayenne pepper or paprika.

Crackers

1½ cups blanched almond flour

1 medium egg

1½ teaspoons poppy seeds

1½ teaspoons white sesame seeds

1½ teaspoons black sesame seeds

1 clove garlic, minced

½ teaspoon salt

½ teaspoon ground black pepper

Egg Wash

1 medium egg

1½ teaspoons water

Seeds and SCD

Seeds are considered a more advanced food on SCD, and you should eat them only after you're symptom free. Replace the seeds in these crackers with chopped fresh rosemary and thyme if you are new to the diet and not yet in remission.

1. Preheat the oven to 350°F.

2. Place the ingredients for the crackers in a medium-sized bowl and stir for 2 minutes until the mixture is well combined and has formed into a loose dough.

3. Place the dough on the counter between two large sheets of parchment paper and use a rolling pin to roll the dough into a rectangle that's approximately 12 by 9 inches. The dough should be almost paper thin (the thinner the dough, the crispier the crackers).

4. Using the edges of the parchment paper, transfer the dough to a sheet pan. Remove the top parchment sheet and use a paring knife to cut a grid in the dough to form 1½-inch squares. This will make it easier to break the crackers into a uniform size after baking.

5. In a small bowl, whisk together the egg and water until frothy, then brush the dough with the egg wash.

6. Bake for 15 minutes, until the crackers are golden brown. Keep an eye on them while baking to make sure they don't burn. You may need to rotate the sheet pan halfway through to ensure even baking.

7. Allow the crackers to cool on the sheet pan for 5 minutes before breaking them into squares.

SUBSTITUTIONS: *Skip the garlic to make these crackers low-FODMAP.*

STORAGE: *The crackers will last in an airtight container in the fridge for up to 4 weeks.*

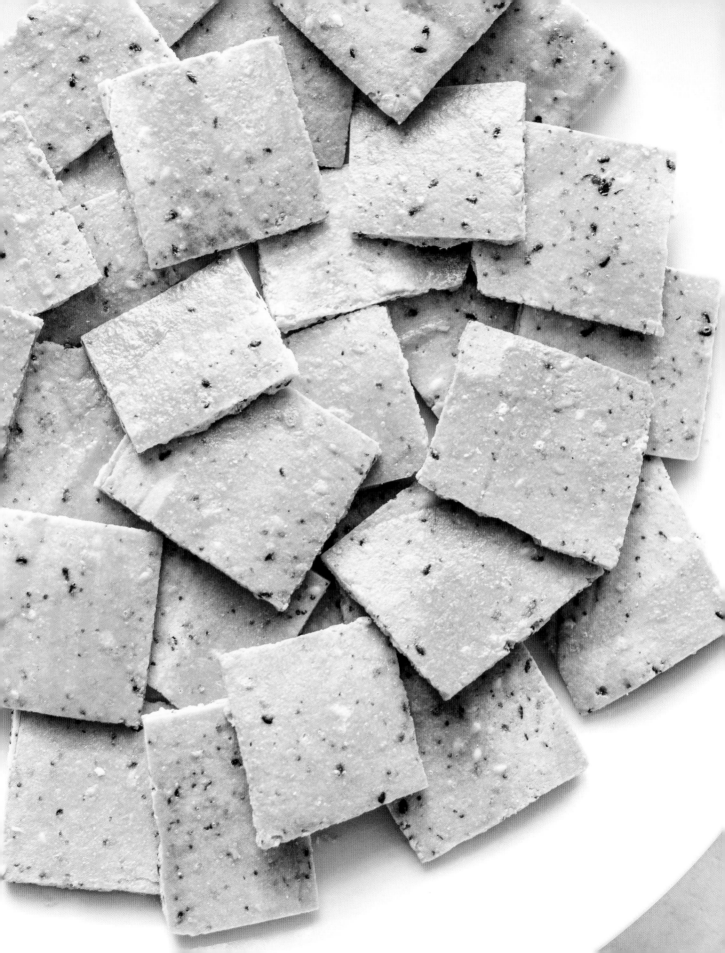

Jalapeño, Bacon & CAULIFLOWER MUFFINS

Yield: 16 mini muffins **Prep Time:** 10 minutes **Cook Time:** 20 minutes

These mini muffins have a secret ingredient that makes them light and moist: cauliflower! An entire head of cauliflower is hidden in a batch of these muffins, but you will never be able to tell. They're a great bite-sized snack to add to a packed lunch or bring with you on long car rides. You also can form the batter into small mounds on a sheet pan to make small buns.

1 small head cauliflower

1½ cups blanched almond flour

2 tablespoons coconut flour

2 medium eggs

2 tablespoons melted coconut oil

1 teaspoon Dijon mustard

1 teaspoon freshly squeezed lemon juice

1 teaspoon baking soda

½ teaspoon salt

1 teaspoon ground black pepper

½ teaspoon paprika

¼ teaspoon cayenne pepper

¼ cup chopped cooked bacon

¼ cup chopped jalapeño peppers plus 16 thin slices jalapeño pepper (about 3 jalapeños)

SPECIAL EQUIPMENT
1 (24-well) mini muffin pan

1. Preheat the oven to 350°F and grease 16 wells of a mini muffin pan with coconut oil or use 16 mini muffin liners.

2. Cut the cauliflower into small chunks and place in a food processor. Pulse until the cauliflower is broken into a fine meal-like texture (finer than rice). You should have 2 cups of powdered cauliflower.

3. Transfer the cauliflower meal to a large bowl, then add the almond flour, coconut flour, eggs, coconut oil, mustard, lemon juice, baking soda, salt, and spices and stir until well combined.

4. Add the bacon and chopped jalapeños and stir until they are evenly distributed throughout the batter.

5. Spoon the batter into the greased muffin cups or muffin liners, ensuring that you fill each to the top. (These muffins will not rise when they bake.)

6. Bake for 15 minutes, then remove from the oven and top each muffin with a slice of jalapeño. Return to the oven to bake for another 5 minutes, until the muffins are golden and a toothpick inserted in the center comes out clean.

SUBSTITUTIONS: *To make this recipe vegetarian, omit the bacon.*

STORAGE: *These muffins are best stored in an airtight container in the fridge for up to 4 days or in the freezer for up to 3 months.*

Other Flavors

Not a fan of jalapeño and bacon? Consider this savory muffin recipe to be a base for any flavor combinations you prefer, such as basil and sun-dried tomatoes, olives and thyme, ham, or rosemary and black pepper.

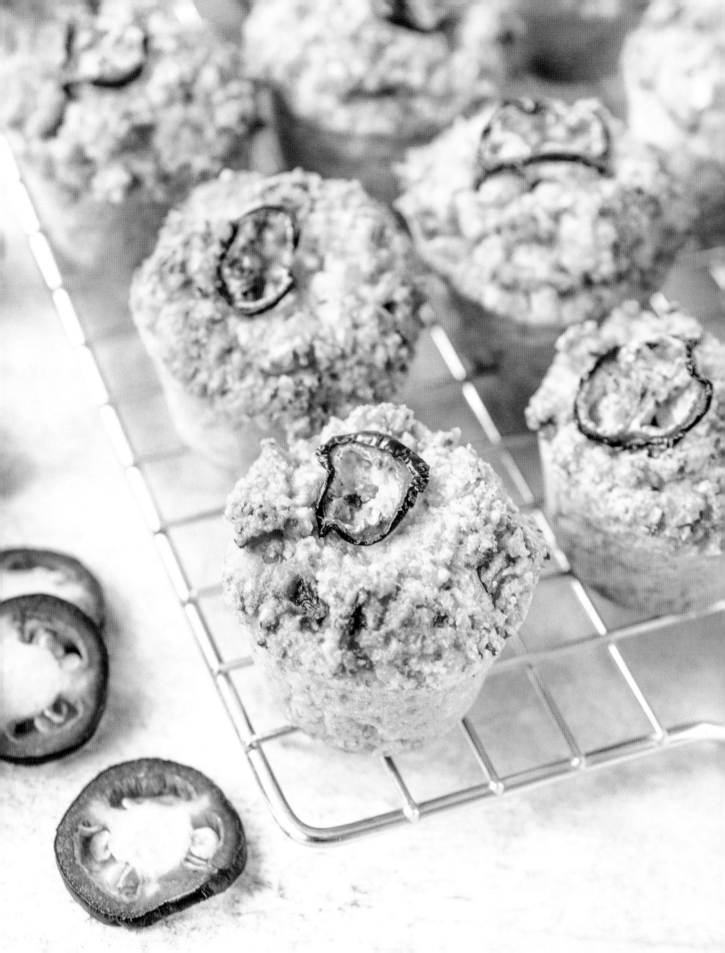

Lemon Blueberry
MUG CAKE

Yield: 1 serving **Prep Time:** 5 minutes **Cook Time:** 3 minutes

Mug cakes are an easy fix for those days when you're craving something sweet but don't have time to bake. Start to finish, this recipe takes less than 8 minutes to make; you only need a mug, a spoon, and a microwave. Flip the mug upside down to remove the cake so you can eat it on the go.

1½ tablespoons coconut oil

2 tablespoons blanched almond flour

2 tablespoons coconut flour

¼ teaspoon baking soda

1½ teaspoons grated lemon zest, plus more for optional garnish

2½ tablespoons freshly squeezed lemon juice

1 teaspoon honey

1 medium egg

1 teaspoon vanilla extract

¼ cup fresh blueberries

1 tablespoon coconut whipped cream (see tip, page 324), or 1 scoop ice cream (page 334), for serving (optional)

1. Put the coconut oil in a mug and microwave for 15 seconds until melted.

2. Add the remaining ingredients, except for the blueberries, in the order listed and mix well with a fork. Once everything is well mixed together, stir in the blueberries.

3. Microwave for 2½ to 3 minutes, until the cake has risen and the top is no longer wet to the touch.

4. Serve warm on its own or top it with a dollop of coconut whipped cream or ice cream and lemon zest (if using) or a scoop of ice cream.

STORAGE: *The cake can be removed from the mug and stored in the freezer for up to 1 month.*

Flavor Variations

Feel free to switch up the flavor of this cake by using raspberries, dried fruit, or cherries in place of the blueberries and orange or lime in place of the lemon zest and juice. Just keep in mind that you need an acidic juice to activate the baking soda; otherwise, you'll end up with a hockey puck.

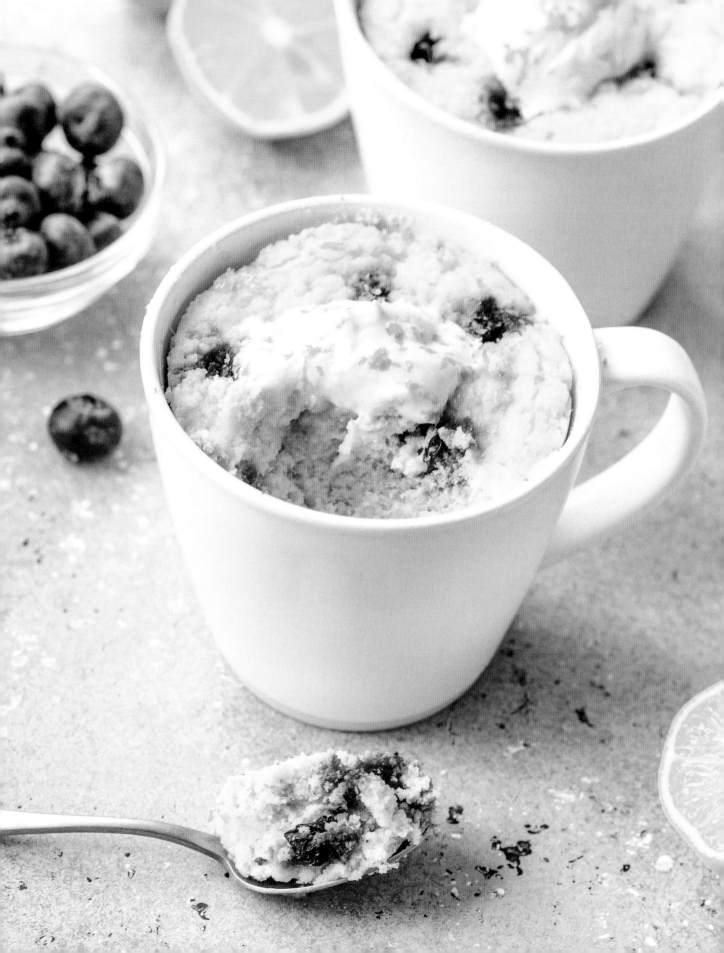

Orange, Cranberry &
PECAN ENERGY BALLS

Yield: 20 balls **Prep Time:** 20 minutes **Cook Time:** —

The combination of orange, cranberries, and pecans always reminds me of Christmas, which—even in July—is never a bad thing. These make a great quick snack, and they're delicious straight from the freezer! If you can't find sugar-free dried cranberries in your store, I've included easy instructions for making them at home in less than 40 minutes. They'll be quite tart to eat on their own, but they're fantastic when added into these energy balls or used for baking.

¾ cup raw pecans

⅔ cup Medjool dates, pitted

⅔ cup sugar-free dried cranberries

1 tablespoon honey

1 tablespoon unsweetened shredded coconut

1½ teaspoons grated orange zest

½ teaspoon ground cinnamon

1. Place the pecans and dates in a food processor and blend until the dates have broken into small pieces.

2. Add the cranberries, honey, coconut, orange zest, and cinnamon and pulse 2 or 3 times, until the mixture is combined.

3. Remove the blade from the food processor and use your hands to roll the mixture into 20 small balls about 1 inch in diameter. If the mixture becomes sticky, wet your hands as you roll. Place the balls in an airtight container and store in the fridge or freezer.

SUBSTITUTIONS: *Swap the honey for maple syrup to make these vegan.*

STORAGE: *These energy balls will last in an airtight container or zip-top bag in the fridge for up to 1 month or in the freezer for up to 3 months.*

Dried Cranberries

The first ingredient listed on the packaging of most store-bought dried cranberries is sugar (meaning the package contains more sugar than dried fruit!). Make your own dried cranberries by drizzling 1½ teaspoons of olive oil over ¾ cup of fresh cranberries and baking in a preheated 350°F oven for 35 minutes, until dry and chewy.

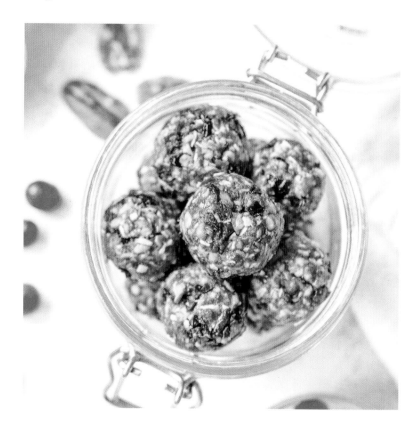

Hazelnut & Coffee
ENERGY BALLS

PALEO
VEGAN
VEGETARIAN
DAIRY-FREE
EGG-FREE

Yield: 24 balls **Prep Time:** 25 minutes **Cook Time:** —

These energy balls are the perfect mid-afternoon pick-me-up thanks to their subtle coffee flavor. I prefer eating them straight from the freezer when they are firm and crunchy.

1 cup toasted hazelnuts

1 cup Medjool dates, pitted

⅓ cup plus ¼ cup shredded unsweetened coconut

1 tablespoon finely ground coffee

1 tablespoon honey

1. Place the hazelnuts and dates in a food processor and pulse until the hazelnuts are broken into small pieces.

2. Add ⅓ cup of the shredded coconut, the coffee, and honey and pulse for another 20 seconds until well combined.

3. Remove the blade from the food processor and use your hands to roll the mixture into 24 balls about 1 inch in diameter. Then roll the balls in the remaining ¼ cup of shredded coconut to evenly coat them. Place the rolled balls in an airtight container and store in the fridge or freezer.

SUBSTITUTIONS: *Swap the honey for maple syrup to make these vegan.*

STORAGE: *These energy balls will last in an airtight container or zip-top bag in the fridge for up to 1 month or in the freezer for up to 3 months.*

Ice Cream Topping
Another great way to enjoy these energy balls is to break them into pieces and sprinkle them over vanilla ice cream (see page 334 for a recipe).

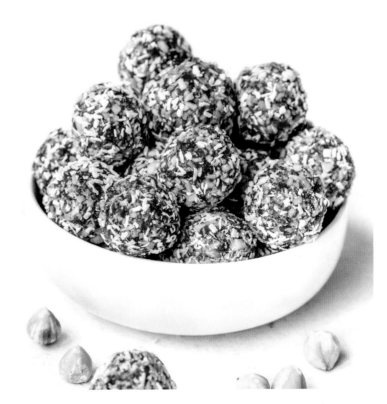

Sweet & Spicy
ALMONDS

Yield: 2 cups **Prep Time:** 5 minutes **Cook Time:** 50 minutes

The first time I made these almonds, they were on the counter all of 10 minutes before "mysteriously" disappearing. Since then, I have learned to hide them as soon as they come out of the oven. They are crunchy, salty, spicy, slightly sweet, and highly addicting. Although you don't have to, soaking the nuts gives them a nice plumpness and makes them easier to digest. If you skip soaking the almonds, reduce the baking time by 15 minutes.

2 cups raw almonds, soaked in water overnight and drained

3 tablespoons unsalted butter, ghee, or coconut oil

2 tablespoons honey

2 teaspoons ground cumin

1 teaspoon paprika

½ teaspoon cayenne pepper

1 teaspoon salt

1. Preheat the oven to 350°F and line a sheet pan with parchment paper.

2. Melt the butter in a small saucepan over medium heat. Stir in the honey, cumin, paprika, and cayenne pepper and whisk until the honey has fully dissolved and the mixture is bubbling, about 5 minutes.

3. Place the almonds on the prepared sheet pan and pour the butter mixture over them. Toss with a spoon to ensure the almonds are all well coated, then sprinkle with the salt.

4. Bake for 25 minutes, stirring every 10 minutes to ensure the almonds don't burn. After 25 minutes, remove the pan from the oven and test one almond to see if it's crunchy. If it isn't, return the pan to the oven and bake for up to 15 minutes more.

5. Allow the almonds to cool completely before serving or storing in an airtight container.

SUBSTITUTIONS: *Use maple syrup in place of honey to make these vegan.*

STORAGE: *The almonds will last in an airtight container in the fridge for up to 3 weeks.*

TIP: *Toss the almonds into salads for extra crunch.*

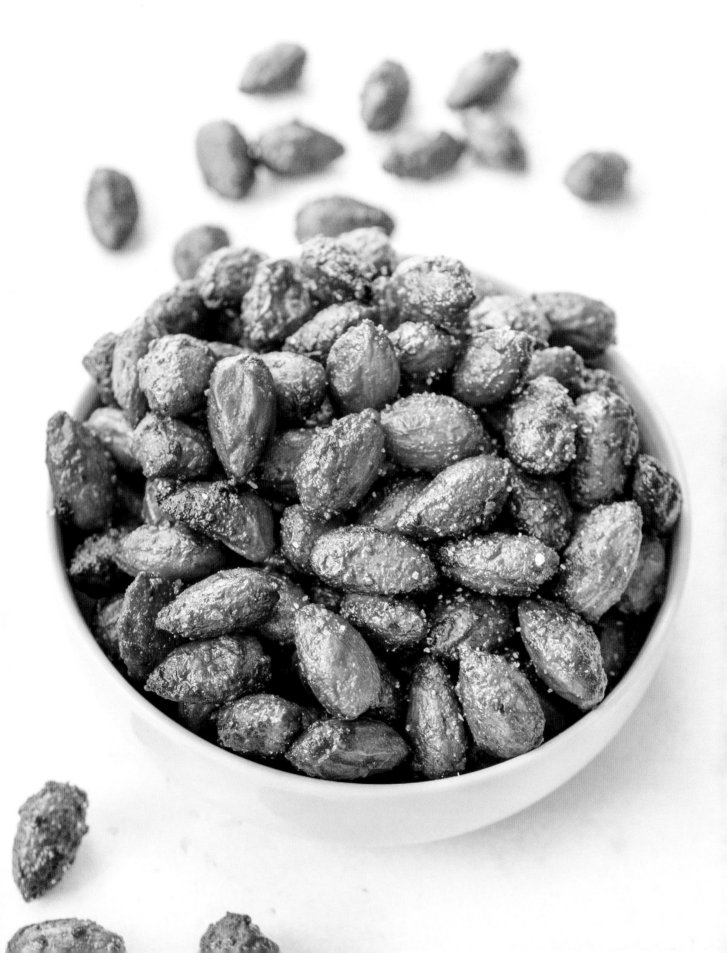

Crunchy NUT BARS

Yield: 12 bars   **Prep Time:** 15 minutes, plus at least 4 hours to chill   **Cook Time:** —

These bars are heftier than energy balls, and they have more of a crunch to them. They are a great kid-friendly snack or afternoon energy booster, and I find they really hit the spot when I'm craving something healthy yet sweet. Feel free to play around with the flavors by adding spices such as cinnamon and ginger, mixing in some dried fruit, or using other nuts.

1 cup Medjool dates, pitted

¾ cup raw cashews

¾ cup raw pecans

½ cup unsweetened, unsalted almond or peanut butter

½ cup coconut flour

⅓ cup unsweetened shredded coconut

⅓ cup raw hulled sunflower seeds

2 tablespoons honey

1 teaspoon vanilla extract

½ teaspoon salt

1. Place the dates, cashews, and pecans in a food processor and pulse until they are broken into small bits. Add the remaining ingredients and pulse until the mixture forms a ball.

2. Line an 8-inch square baking dish with a 10 by 10-inch piece of parchment paper, so the edges overhang the sides of the dish. Spoon the mixture into the dish and pack it firmly into a 1-inch-thick base. Place in the fridge to chill for a minimum of 4 hours but ideally overnight.

3. Use the parchment to lift the slab out of the baking dish, then cut the slab into 12 bars.

SUBSTITUTIONS: *Use maple syrup in place of the honey to make these vegan.*

STORAGE: *The bars are best stored in an airtight container in the fridge for up to 2 weeks or in the freezer for up to 3 months. Keep refrigerated until ready to serve; if left out at room temperature for too long, the bars can become crumbly.*

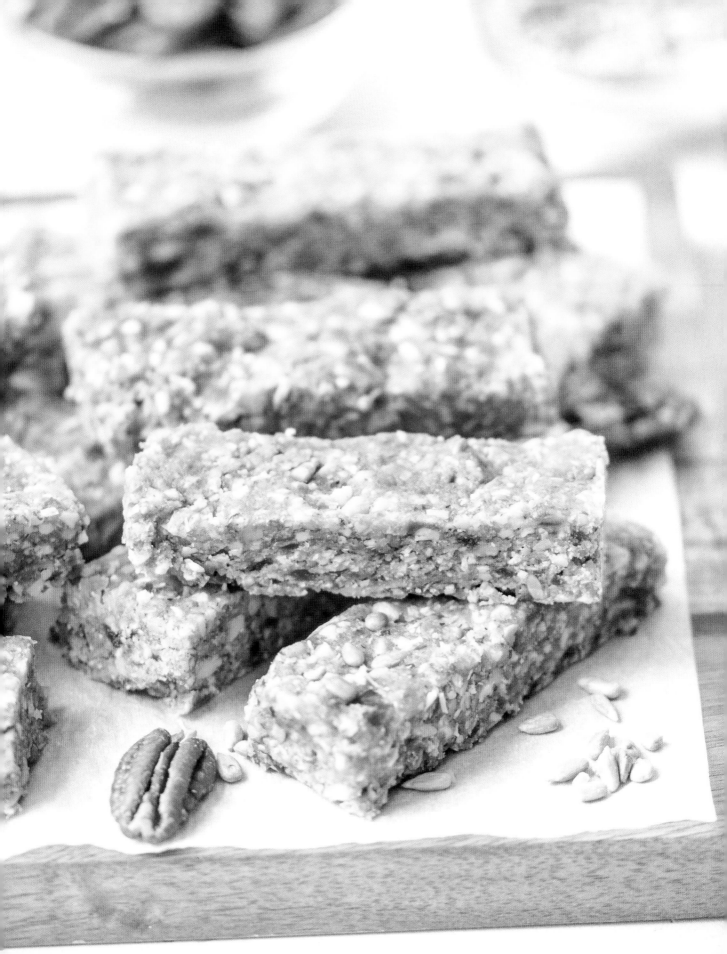

AIP
LOW-FODMAP
PALEO
VEGAN
VEGETARIAN
DAIRY-FREE
EGG-FREE
NUT-FREE

Mango Chili
FRUIT ROLL-UPS

Yield: 10 to 12 rolls   **Prep Time:** 10 minutes   **Cook Time:** 3 hours

This is my spin on Mango con Chile y Limon (mango sprinkled with cayenne pepper and lime juice), a popular street food in Mexico. It's a simple snack, but the combination of sweet and spicy can be highly addicting. You don't need a dehydrator to make these easy no-sugar-added fruit roll-ups. If you want to make a more kid-friendly version, skip the cayenne pepper; it will still be delicious.

2 large mangoes

1 tablespoon freshly squeezed lime juice

¼ teaspoon cayenne pepper

SPECIAL EQUIPMENT
1 silicone baking mat

1. Preheat the oven to 170°F and line a half sheet pan (11½ by 16½-inches) with a silicone baking mat.

2. Peel the mangoes and cut them into cubes (you should have about 4 cups). Place the cubed mango in a blender and add the lime juice. Blend until completely smooth.

3. Pour the puree onto the prepared sheet pan and use a rubber spatula to spread it out evenly to about a ⅛-inch thickness.

4. Sprinkle the cayenne pepper over the puree, then bake for 3 hours, until the middle is dry to the touch. You may need more bake time depending on the thickness of the puree.

5. Remove the pan from the oven and allow to cool slightly. Use kitchen shears to cut the fruit leather into long strips about 2 inches wide, then roll them up.

SUBSTITUTIONS: *Omit the cayenne pepper to make this snack AIP. For low-FODMAP, replace the mangoes with 3 cups of a combination of raspberries, strawberries, and blueberries.*

STORAGE: *The rolls will last in an airtight container in the fridge for up to 10 days.*

Silicone Baking Mats

For this recipe, a silicone baking mat works far better than parchment paper. Parchment paper becomes moist and creates wrinkles in the mango puree as it dries, whereas the puree stays smooth on the silicone mat

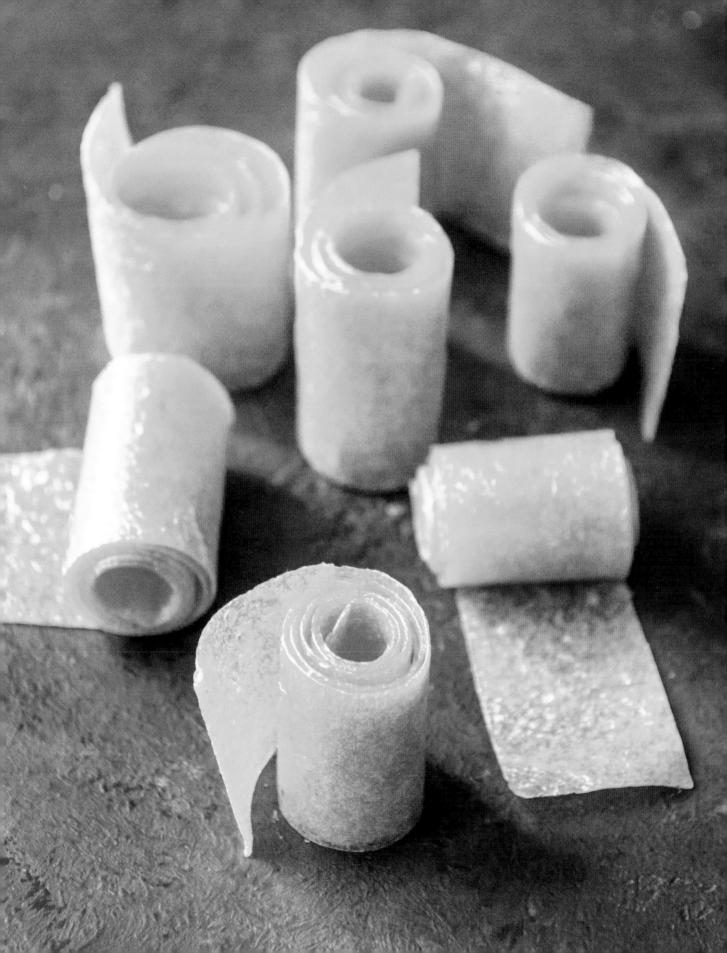

AIP
LOW-FODMAP
PALEO
DAIRY-FREE
EGG-FREE
NUT-FREE

Apple Ginger
GUMMY BEARS

Yield: about 150 gummy bears   **Prep Time:** 5 minutes, plus 20 minutes to chill   **Cook Time:** 5 minutes

My husband, SA, has a sweet tooth that can be tamed only by the candy jar that we have on our kitchen counter, which always seems to be directly in my sight line. No matter where I am in the room, it's trying to lure me over to have "just one" candy. Rather than give in, I started experimenting with homemade gummies and couldn't believe how easy and fast they are to make. Of all of the flavors I've made, this apple ginger variety is my favorite—the perfect blend of sweet apple juice, zingy ginger, and sour lemon. I now keep the candy jar filled with these gummies, and everyone is happy. They really hit the spot when we're craving sweets but offer the added bonus of being healthy.

1 (2-inch) piece ginger, peeled

1 cup unsweetened apple juice

1 teaspoon freshly squeezed lemon juice

3 tablespoons unsweetened unflavored gelatin

1. Using a box grater placed on top of a plate, grate the ginger with the largest holes. Place the grated ginger in a piece of cheesecloth (or a paper towel) and squeeze over a bowl to extract the juice.

2. Measure 1 tablespoon of the ginger juice (or more if you like the gummies very gingery) and place it along with the apple juice and lemon juice in a small saucepan over medium heat. Once the liquid is hot (but not boiling), add the gelatin and whisk. When the gelatin has dissolved (about 1 minute), remove the pan from the heat.

3. Pour the liquid into the silicone candy molds. (I like to use the dropper that came with the candy molds I bought from Amazon.) Alternatively, if you don't have silicone candy molds, pour the liquid into an 8½ by 4½-inch loaf pan lined with parchment paper.

4. Place the molds or pan in the fridge for 15 to 20 minutes, until the gummies have set.

5. Flip the candy molds over and push out the gummy bears. If you used a pan, use small cookie cutters to cut out shapes, or use a knife to cut small squares or triangles.

SUBSTITUTIONS: *For low-FODMAP, use carrot juice in place of the apple juice.*

STORAGE: *The gummies will last in an airtight container in the fridge for up to 2 weeks.*

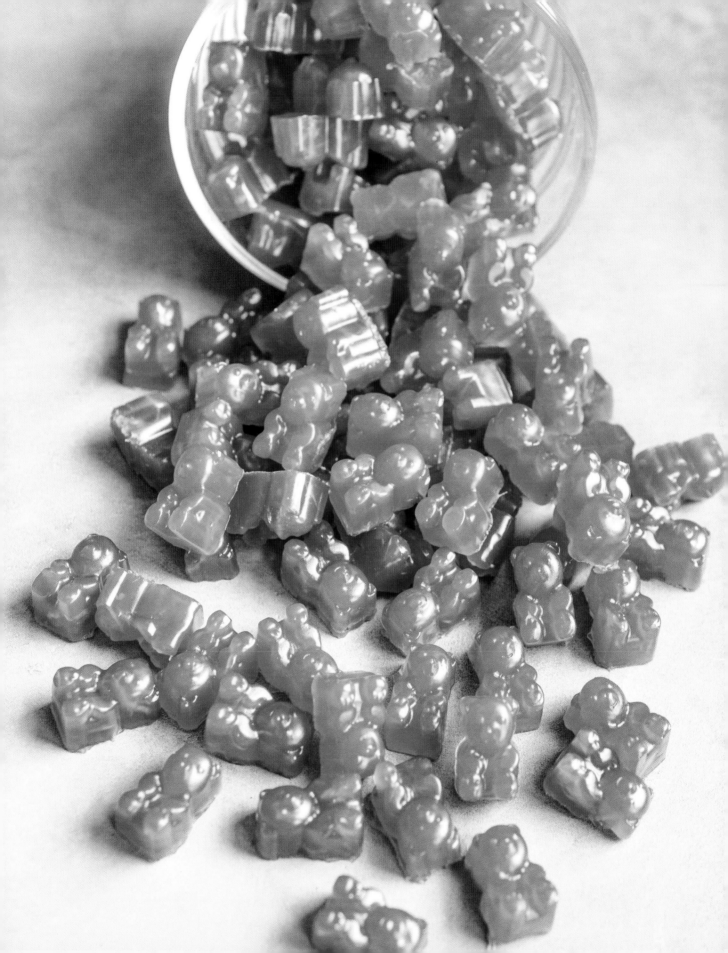

LOW-FODMAP
PALEO
VEGAN
VEGETARIAN
DAIRY-FREE
EGG-FREE

Vanilla-Coated FROZEN BANANA BITES

Yield: 25 bites   **Prep Time:** 20 minutes, plus 2 hours to freeze   **Cook Time:** —

We aren't a big sweets house, but you can always find a bag of these banana bites in the freezer, and SA loves this treat. I used to make these with a dark chocolate coating, which is not allowed on SCD. I was craving them so much, I knew I had to make an SCD-legal version, and it quickly became a hit on my blog. The frozen banana slices are topped with hazelnut and almond butter and then coated in a creamy vanilla-flavored sauce that tastes like white chocolate once frozen. These bites are a great little treat when you're in need of something sweet.

2 ripe bananas

3 tablespoons unsweetened, unsalted hazelnut butter or other nut butter of choice, divided

¾ cup raw macadamia nuts

¼ cup water

2 tablespoons coconut oil

1 tablespoon honey

2 teaspoons vanilla extract

For Garnish

3 tablespoons chopped toasted nuts, such as almonds, hazelnuts, and/or pecans

2 tablespoons unsweetened shredded coconut

½ teaspoon flaked sea salt (see tip, page 122)

1. Cut the bananas into slices about ¼ inch in width. Spoon about a teaspoon of nut butter onto half of the banana slices. Place all of the banana slices on a parchment paper–lined sheet pan and place in the freezer for a minimum of 1 hour.

2. Place the macadamia nuts in a food processor and blend until they resemble a crumbled mixture, then add the water, coconut oil, honey, and vanilla extract and continue to blend until a creamy puree has formed.

3. Remove the sheet pan from the freezer and dip each banana slice in the pureed mixture; spoon some of the nut puree over the top to ensure all sides are coated. Place back on the sheet pan and sprinkle about two-thirds of the bites with the chopped nuts and the other one-third with shredded coconut, then sprinkle all of them with the sea salt.

4. Place the sheet pan back into the freezer and leave for a minimum of 1 hour or until the coating has fully hardened.

SUBSTITUTIONS: *Use maple syrup in place of the honey to make the bites low-FODMAP or vegan.*

STORAGE: *The banana bites will last in an airtight container or zip-top bag in the freezer for up to 2 months.*

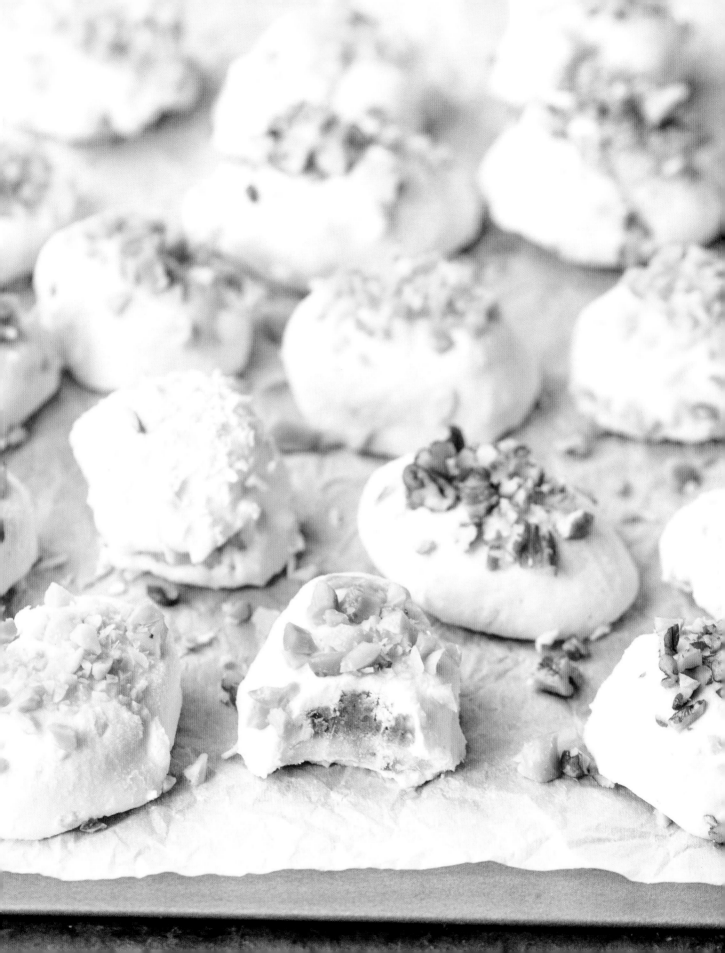

PALEO
VEGAN
VEGETARIAN
DAIRY-FREE
EGG-FREE
NUT-FREE

Three Hidden-Veggie
SMOOTHIES

Yield: 2 servings (1½ cups per serving) **Prep Time:** 5 minutes **Cook Time:** —

Smoothies are a great way to sneak veggies into your diet. With the addition of fruit, ginger, or almond butter, any signs of a vegetable are completely hidden—I promise! I keep portioned bags of cauliflower, zucchini, and even spinach in my freezer so that I can easily add them to my smoothie each morning. The more you drink these smoothies, the more comfortable you will get with decreasing the amount of sugar and adding more veggies like kale, celery, cucumber, or steamed broccoli. This is also a great way to trick kids into eating more veggies.

CAULIFLOWER

2 cups cauliflower florets, steamed and frozen

1 tablespoon unsweetened almond butter

½ teaspoon ground cinnamon, plus more for garnish if desired

1 cup unsweetened almond milk

1½ teaspoons honey (optional)

SPINACH

5 cups spinach

½ banana, frozen

1 (1-inch) piece ginger, chopped

⅓ cup apple juice

½ cup water

ZUCCHINI

1 zucchini, grated and then frozen

1 cup frozen mixed berries (strawberries, blackberries, blueberries, or raspberries)

¼ cup water

½ cup freshly squeezed orange juice

Combine all of the ingredients for the smoothie of your choice in a blender and blend until completely smooth.

STORAGE: *Each recipe makes two servings, so you can drink one immediately and store the other portion in the freezer. Allow the frozen smoothie to thaw for 20 minutes before drinking; alternatively, place the frozen smoothie in a blender with a splash of almond milk or juice and blend until smooth. These smoothies will last in the freezer for 2 months.*

Freezing Bananas
Freeze bananas whole with the peel still on. When you need to use one, run it under hot water for 5 seconds. Then you can easily twist off the peel.

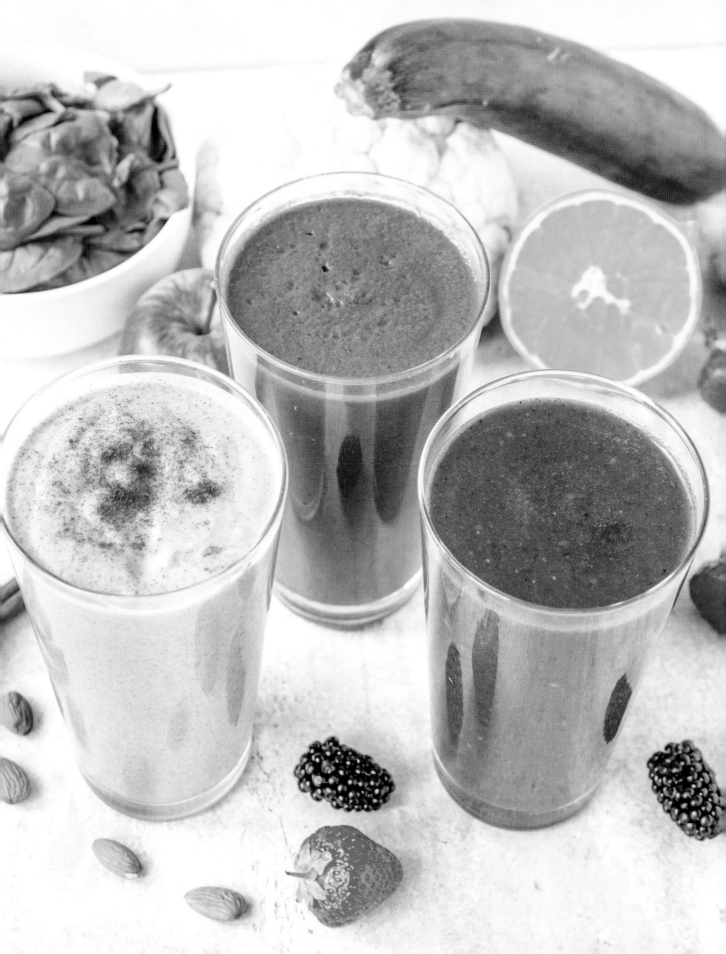

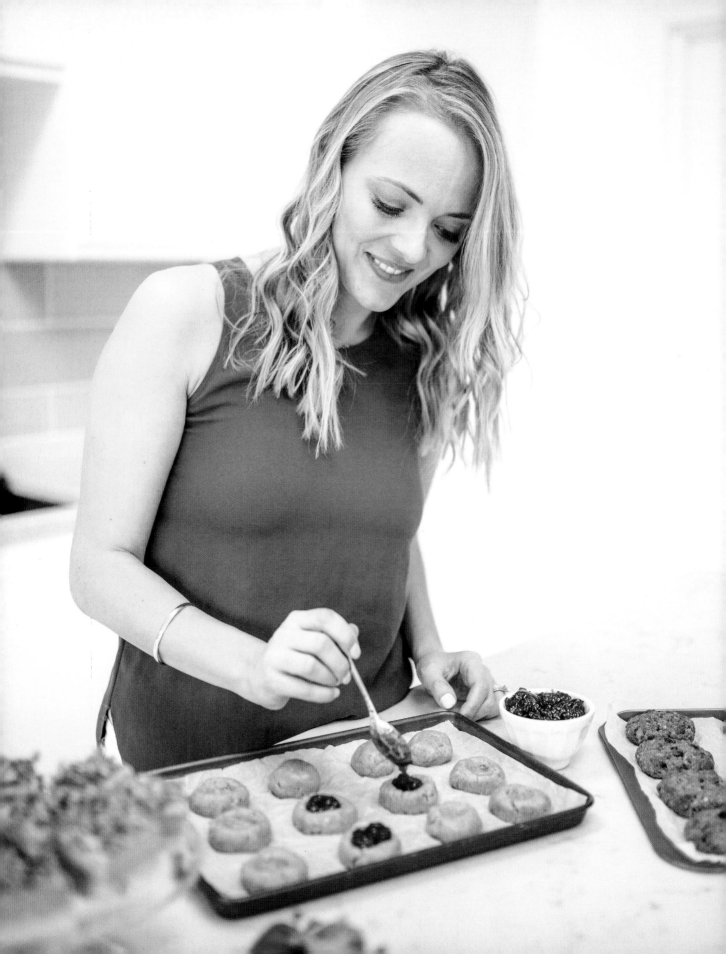

Desserts

LOW-FODMAP
PALEO
VEGAN
VEGETARIAN
DAIRY-FREE
EGG-FREE

Chewy Almond &
ORANGE COOKIES

Yield: 20 cookies   **Prep Time:** 10 minutes   **Cook Time:** 10 minutes

My all-time favorite cookies are florentines. This healthier version has a chewy texture, and the orange zest and a sprinkle of flaked sea salt really help cut through the sweetness and give them a light and fresh flavor. Once refrigerated, they become even chewier.

1½ cups sliced blanched almonds, divided

½ cup raw pecans

1 cup blanched almond flour

⅓ cup honey

¼ cup melted coconut oil

1 teaspoon grated orange zest

½ teaspoon flaked sea salt (see tip, page 122)

1. Preheat the oven to 325°F and line a sheet pan with parchment paper.

2. Place 1 cup of the almonds and the pecans in a food processor and pulse for about 5 seconds, until the nuts have broken down into small pieces. Don't over-pulse; you want them to be chunky rather than a powder.

3. Transfer the chopped nuts to a bowl and add the almond flour, remaining ½ cup of almonds, honey, coconut oil, and orange zest and stir until well mixed.

4. Use your hands to form the dough into 20 small balls about 1½ inches in diameter and place on the prepared sheet pan, about 2 inches apart. Gently press down on each ball to make it as flat as possible. It may help to wet your hands so that the cookie mixture doesn't stick to your fingers as you flatten the balls.

5. Sprinkle with the flaked salt and bake for 8 to 10 minutes, until golden brown. Keep an eye on the cookies because they can brown very quickly.

6. Allow the cookies to cool on the sheet pan for 10 minutes before removing them to a cooling rack. They will become firmer and chewier as they cool.

SUBSTITUTIONS: *Use maple syrup in place of the honey to make the cookies low-FODMAP or vegan.*

STORAGE: *The cookies will last in an airtight container in the fridge for up to 2 weeks (if you have enough self-control).*

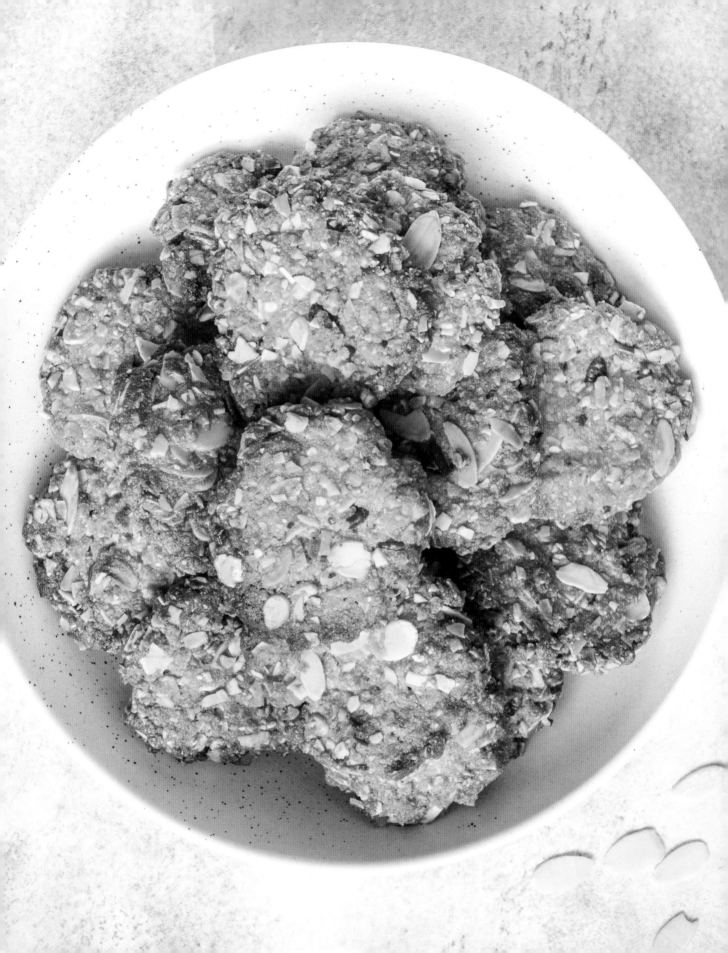

Peanut Butter & Jam THUMBPRINT COOKIES

Yield: 12 cookies   **Prep Time:** 15 minutes, plus 20 minutes to chill   **Cook Time:** 27 minutes

These cookies are a fun spin on a favorite combination: peanut butter and jam. I love raspberry jam, but feel free to swap the raspberries for strawberries, blueberries, cranberries, or even a mix depending on what's available.

Jam

2 cups fresh or frozen raspberries

1 tablespoon honey

1 teaspoon freshly squeezed lemon juice

⅓ cup crunchy unsweetened, unsalted peanut or almond butter

¼ cup melted coconut oil

¼ cup honey

1 teaspoon vanilla extract

1 cup blanched almond flour

¼ cup coconut flour

½ teaspoon baking soda

¼ teaspoon salt

1. To make the jam, place the raspberries, honey, and lemon juice in a small saucepan over medium heat and simmer for 15 minutes, stirring occasionally, until the raspberries have taken on a pureed consistency. Remove the pan from the heat and set aside; the mixture will thicken to the consistency of jam as it cools.

2. Preheat the oven to 350°F and line a sheet pan with parchment paper.

3. Using an electric mixer, cream together the peanut butter, coconut oil, honey, and vanilla extract until the mixture is well mixed. Add the flours, baking soda, and salt and mix for about 1 minute more until well combined. Put the bowl in the fridge to chill the cookie dough for 15 to 20 minutes. (This will make it easier to shape the cookies.)

4. Use your hands to form the dough into 12 balls about 1 inch in diameter and place them on the prepared sheet pan, about 2 inches apart. Flatten the balls slightly, then use your thumb to make an indentation in the center of each cookie. If the dough becomes crumbly or hard to shape, return it to the fridge for a few minutes. Place about 2 teaspoons of the jam into the center of each cookie.

5. Bake for 12 minutes, until the cookies are evenly golden. Keep an eye on them to ensure that they do not brown or burn.

6. Remove from the oven and allow the cookies to cool on the pan for 8 to 10 minutes, then transfer to a wire rack to cool further. If you handle the cookies too quickly after taking them out of the oven, they will be crumbly and fall apart.

TIP: *Make extra jam to enjoy as a condiment. Stir it into Pear & Chai Spiced Porridge (page 86) or spread it between the layers of the Lemon & Berry Layer Cake (page 328) in place of icing.*

SUBSTITUTIONS: *For Paleo, use almond butter in place of the peanut butter. Swap the honey for maple syrup to make these vegan.*

STORAGE: *The cookies will last in an airtight container in the fridge for up to a week or in the freezer for up to 2 months.*

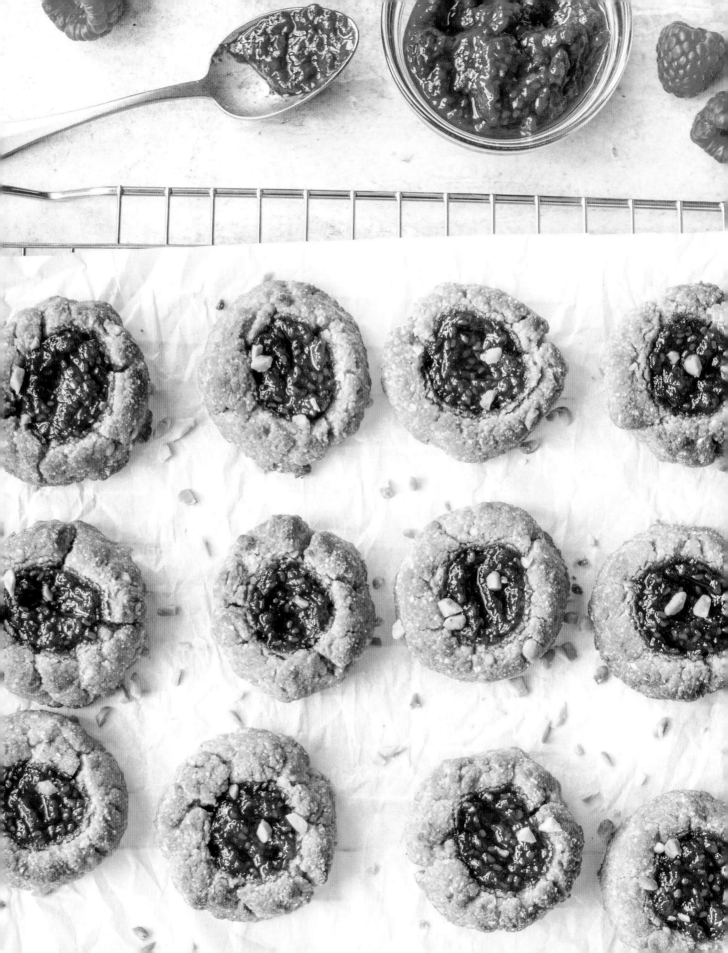

N'oatmeal
RAISIN COOKIES

Yield: 12 cookies **Prep Time:** 10 minutes **Cook Time:** 12 minutes

Although these cookies are missing the star ingredient of traditional oatmeal cookies (oatmeal), they still have a deliciously soft and chewy texture and are highly addictive. My husband, SA, loves that they aren't overly sweet; I regularly bust him stealing one (or two!) from the freezer on his way out the door. Not a fan of raisins? Swap them for another type of dried fruit, such as cherries or blueberries, or leave out the fruit altogether.

⅓ cup honey

¼ cup melted coconut oil

1 medium egg

1 teaspoon vanilla extract

1½ cups blanched almond flour

⅔ cup unsweetened shredded coconut

1 tablespoon ground cinnamon

½ teaspoon ground nutmeg

½ teaspoon baking soda

¼ teaspoon salt

⅔ cup raisins

1. Preheat the oven to 350°F and line a sheet pan with parchment paper.

2. Place the honey, coconut oil, egg, and vanilla extract in a large bowl and beat well with an electric mixer until the mixture becomes light and frothy.

3. Add the almond flour, coconut, cinnamon, nutmeg, baking soda, and salt, and mix for 10 seconds to combine; then add the raisins.

4. Use your hands to form the dough into 12 balls, about 1 inch in diameter, and place on the prepared sheet pan about 2 inches apart. Press gently on the dough to flatten each ball.

5. Bake for 10 to 12 minutes, until golden. Allow the cookies to cool for 10 minutes on the pan before transferring them to a cooling rack to cool completely before storing.

STORAGE: *The cookies will last in an airtight container in the fridge for up to 5 days or in the freezer for up to 2 months.*

Revitalizing Raisins

Raisins have a shelf life of about 1 month, although they last closer to 6 months in the fridge. After that time, they begin to dry out and harden. To plump up old raisins, soak them in a bowl of hot water for 10 minutes, then dry them and mix them into the cookie batter.

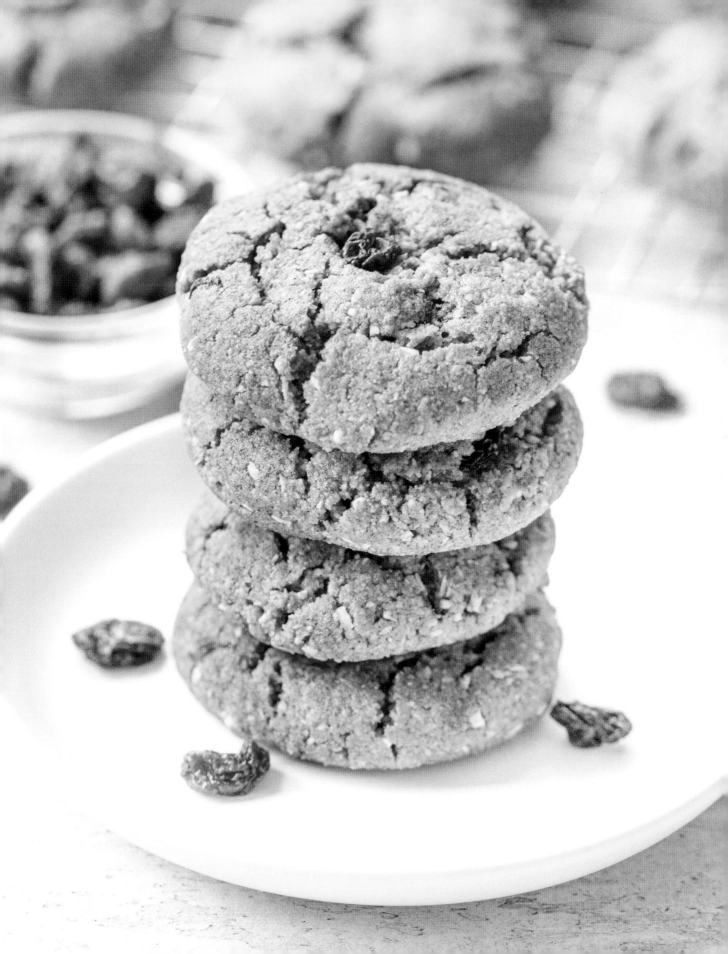

Nut Butter COOKIES

Yield: 12 cookies   **Prep Time:** 10 minutes   **Cook Time:** 10 minutes

These one-bowl cookies are dangerously quick to whip up whenever a cookie craving strikes. I love making them with crunchy peanut butter, but crunchy hazelnut butter is a very close second.

¾ cup unsweetened, unsalted crunchy peanut butter, hazelnut butter, or almond butter

⅓ cup melted coconut oil

⅓ cup honey

1 medium egg

1 teaspoon vanilla extract

1½ cups blanched almond flour

2 tablespoons coconut flour

½ teaspoon baking soda

½ teaspoon salt

1. Preheat the oven to 350°F and line a sheet pan with parchment paper.

2. Using an electric mixer, cream together the peanut butter, coconut oil, honey, egg, and vanilla extract until well mixed. Add the flours, baking soda, and salt and mix until well combined.

3. Place 12 large spoonfuls of the dough on the lined pan about 2 inches apart, then use a fork dipped in water to gently flatten the cookies in a criss-cross pattern. (The water will help prevent the dough from sticking to the fork.)

4. Bake for 10 minutes, until golden. Allow to cool before removing from the sheet pan and storing.

STORAGE: *The cookies will last in an airtight container in the fridge for up to a week or in the freezer for up to 3 months.*

Ice Cream Sandwiches

To make 6 cookie sandwiches, place 2 frozen bananas and 2 tablespoons unsweetened almond milk in a blender and blend until smooth. Sandwich large spoonfuls of the banana puree between two cookies and put them in the freezer for an hour. The ice cream sandwiches will last in an airtight container or wrapped tightly with plastic wrap in the freezer for up to 2 months.

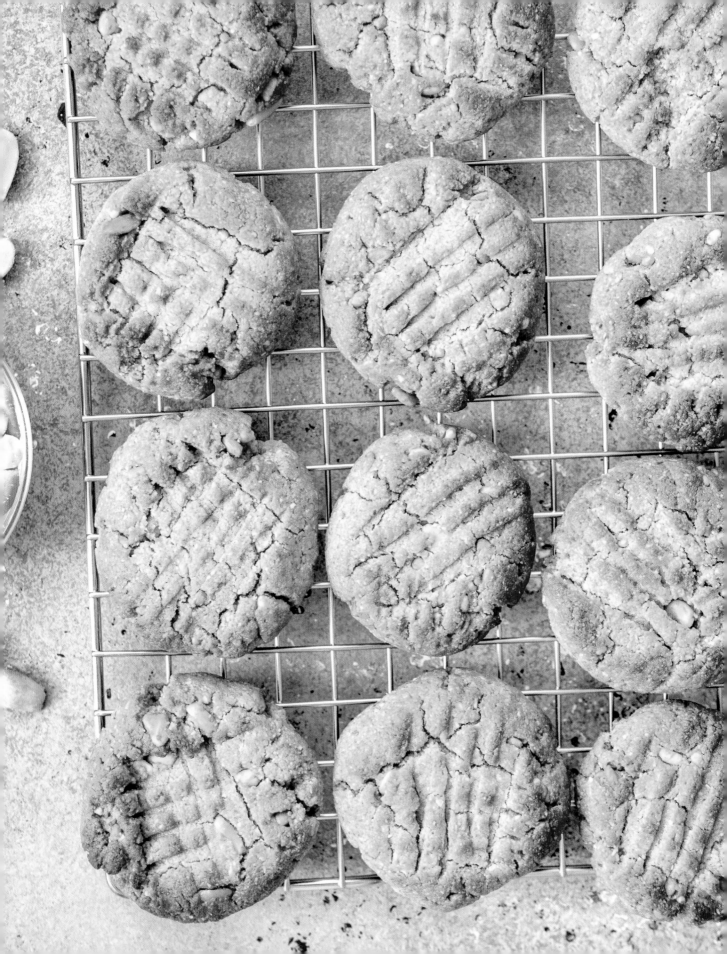

Pecan & Salted Caramel
SHORTBREAD BARS

Yield: 15 bars   **Prep Time:** 20 minutes, plus 20 minutes to chill   **Cook Time:** 12 minutes

With a crumbly shortbread base, a smooth and creamy caramel layer, and chopped pecan topping, these bars are very rich. These bars are a reader favorite on my blog, and many people say that this is the most decadent SCD treat they've ever had! Don't skip the flaked salt; it helps cut through the sweetness and really makes the flavors pop.

Shortbread Base

1½ cups blanched almond flour

⅓ cup coconut flour

⅓ cup melted coconut oil or unsalted butter

3 tablespoons honey

½ teaspoon baking soda

Caramel

1½ cups Medjool dates, pitted and soaked in hot water for 10 minutes to soften

1 cup coconut cream

¼ cup coconut oil

½ teaspoon vanilla extract

½ teaspoon salt

Topping

1¼ cups toasted pecans, chopped

½ teaspoon flaked sea salt (see tip, page 122)

1. Preheat the oven to 350°F and line a 9-inch square baking dish with aluminum foil, allowing about 1 inch of foil to hang over the edges of the dish.

2. Place all of the shortbread base ingredients in a medium-sized bowl and use a wooden spoon to stir until well combined.

3. Place the dough into the baking dish and pat down to form a ½-inch-thick base. Bake for 10 to 12 minutes, until it begins to turn golden brown. Remove from the oven and allow to cool.

4. To make the caramel, place the dates in a food processor and blend until they form a thick paste. Add the coconut cream (make sure you add only cream and not coconut water), coconut oil, vanilla extract, and salt. Blend until smooth.

5. Once the shortbread has cooled, pour the caramel on top and use a spoon to evenly distribute it across the base.

6. Toss the pecans with the flaked sea salt in a bowl, then sprinkle the salted nuts over the bars.

7. Place the baking dish in the fridge for about 20 minutes to allow the caramel to become firm. Use the aluminum foil to lift the slab out of the baking dish and move it to a cutting board. Cut the slab into 15 small bars and serve.

SUBSTITUTIONS: *Use maple syrup in place of the honey to make the bars vegan.*

STORAGE: *The bars will last in the fridge for up to 5 days or in the freezer for up to 2 months.*

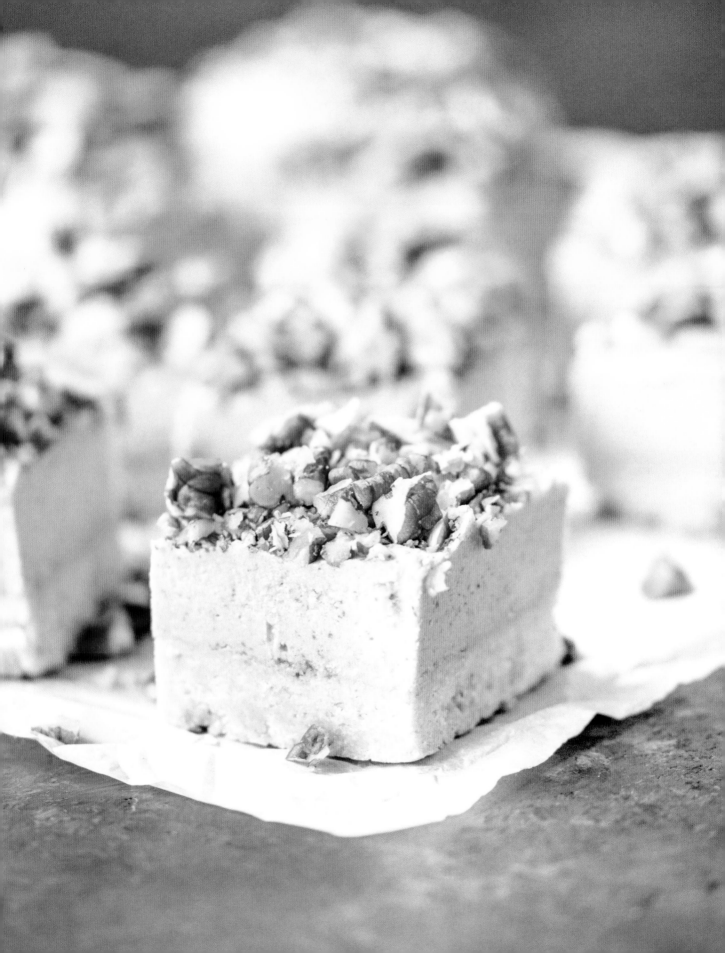

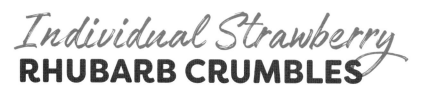

Individual Strawberry RHUBARB CRUMBLES

Yield: 4 servings **Prep Time:** 15 minutes **Cook Time:** 30 minutes

These individual crumbles are a great dessert to serve in the spring when rhubarb is in season. The tart rhubarb and sweet strawberries really balance each other out and reduce the need for a lot of added sugar. Although I love serving these in individual ramekins, you could also bake this crumble in an 8-inch square baking dish.

Filling

4 cups chopped rhubarb (about 6 large stalks)

1 cup chopped fresh strawberries

1 teaspoon grated orange zest

¼ cup no-sugar-added orange juice

2 tablespoons honey

1 tablespoon coconut oil

½ teaspoon ginger powder

Crumble Topping

⅓ cup raw pecans, roughly chopped

¼ cup blanched almond flour

3 tablespoons melted coconut oil

2 tablespoons unsweetened shredded coconut

2 tablespoons honey

½ teaspoon ground cinnamon

¼ teaspoon salt

Coconut whipped cream, for serving (optional; see tip)

SPECIAL EQUIPMENT
4 (5-ounce) ovenproof ramekins

1. Preheat the oven to 350°F.

2. Place all of the filling ingredients in a medium-sized saucepan over medium heat and simmer for 20 minutes, until the rhubarb has softened to a stewed consistency.

3. While the filling is cooking, place all of the crumble topping ingredients in a bowl and stir until well combined.

4. Place four 5-ounce ramekins on a sheet pan. Divide the filling among the ramekins, then spoon the crumble topping over the top.

5. Bake for 10 minutes, until the crumble topping is golden. Serve warm and top with coconut whipped cream, if desired.

SUBSTITUTIONS: *Use maple syrup in place of the honey to make these vegan.*

MAKE AHEAD/STORAGE: *The filling and topping can be made up to 2 days in advance and stored separately in the fridge. Assemble in the ramekins and bake before serving. The filling can be frozen for up to 3 months. The baked crumbles will last in the fridge for up to 3 days.*

Coconut Whipped Cream
To make coconut whipped cream, refrigerate a can of full-fat coconut milk for at least 12 hours, and then scoop the thick cream that has collected at the top into a tall container, such as a 3-quart spouted mixing bowl. Add ½ teaspoon of vanilla extract and 1 tablespoon of honey. Use an electric mixer with a whisk attachment to beat the mixture until it has a fluffy consistency like whipped cream.

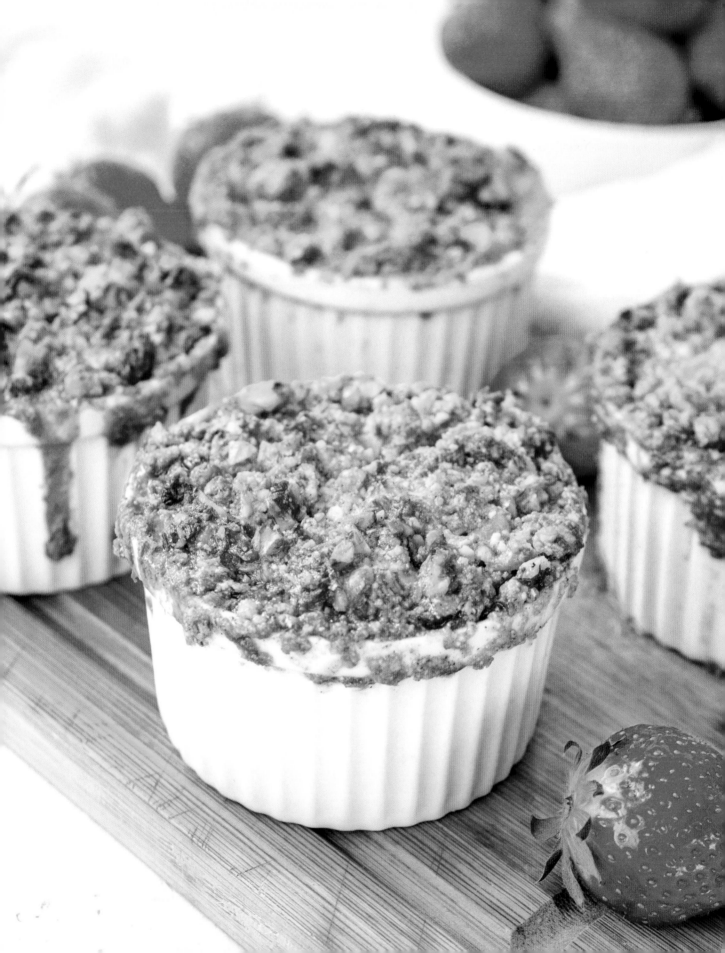

Carrot
CUPCAKES

Yield: 9 cupcakes   **Prep Time:** 30 minutes, plus 30 minutes to chill   **Cook Time:** 25 minutes

I will admit that 99.99 percent of the reason why carrot cake is my favorite flavor of cake is because of the cream cheese icing, which in the past I have been known to eat with a spoon. Re-creating that slightly tart, slightly sweet flavor in a dairy-free icing was no easy feat, but I am so happy with how these cupcakes turned out! The icing swirled on top is thick and creamy and has the delicious tang of cream cheese, which pairs perfectly with the moist carrot cupcakes.

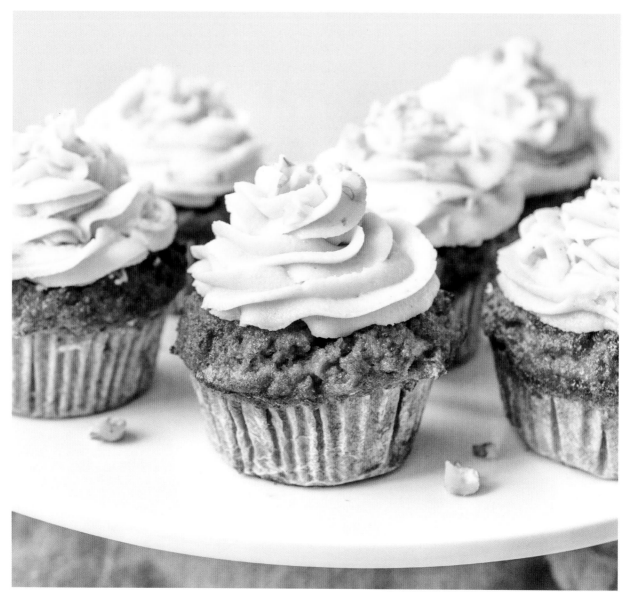

"Cream Cheese" Icing

1 cup raw cashews, soaked in boiling water for 10 minutes and drained

⅓ cup coconut cream

3 tablespoons melted coconut oil

2 tablespoons honey, plus more if needed

2 teaspoons apple cider vinegar, plus more if needed

1 teaspoon vanilla extract

½ teaspoon salt

Cupcakes

½ cup blanched almond flour

¼ cup coconut flour

½ teaspoon baking soda

1 teaspoon ground cinnamon

½ teaspoon ginger powder

½ teaspoon salt

¼ teaspoon ground nutmeg

4 medium eggs

¼ cup melted coconut oil

1 tablespoon grated orange zest

¼ cup freshly squeezed orange juice

½ teaspoon freshly squeezed lemon juice

2 tablespoons honey

1 teaspoon vanilla extract

¾ cup grated carrot (about 1 large carrot)

2 tablespoons chopped roasted walnuts, for garnish

SPECIAL EQUIPMENT
High-powered blender

Piping Icing

Don't have a piping bag? Use a small zip-top plastic bag instead! Spoon the icing into the bag and snip off a corner. If you have a metal icing tip, you can fit it into the hole in the bag to create icing designs.

To make the "cream cheese" icing:

1. Place all of the icing ingredients in a high-powered blender and blend until completely smooth. Taste and adjust by adding more honey or vinegar depending on how tart or sweet you like the icing.

2. Transfer the icing to a tall container, such as a 3-quart spouted mixing bowl, and place in the freezer for 30 minutes to firm up. After 30 minutes, remove from the freezer and use an electric mixer to whip the icing into a light and fluffy consistency. Set aside in the fridge while you prepare the cupcakes.

To make the cupcakes:

1. Preheat the oven to 350°F and line 9 wells of a standard-size 12-well muffin pan with liners.

2. Place the flours, baking soda, cinnamon, ginger powder, salt, and nutmeg in a medium-sized bowl and stir to combine. Once well mixed, stir in the eggs, coconut oil, orange zest and juice, lemon juice, honey, and vanilla extract. Then, mix in the carrots.

3. Fill each prepared muffin cup to the very top with batter and bake for 20 to 25 minutes, until a toothpick inserted in the center of a cupcake comes out clean. If the cupcakes appear to be browning too quickly on the top, place a piece of aluminum foil over the top to prevent them from burning. Allow the cupcakes to cool in the pan for 5 minutes, then transfer them to a cooling rack and allow them to cool to room temperature.

4. Use an electric mixer to whip the icing one more time, then spoon it into a piping bag and frost the cupcakes. Sprinkle with the chopped walnuts and serve.

STORAGE: *The icing and cupcakes can be stored separately in the fridge for up to 3 days. Once frosted, the cupcakes will last in the fridge for up to 2 days.*

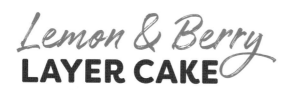

Lemon & Berry LAYER CAKE

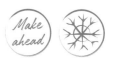

Make ahead

Yield: 8 servings   **Prep Time:** 30 minutes, plus 30 minutes to chill   **Cook Time:** 30 Minutes

I am not a baker (like AT ALL), so when I say that this cake is incredibly easy to make considering how impressive it looks, that should tell you a lot. The cake layers are light and moist with a kick of zesty lemon flavor, which helps balance out the sweet cashew-based icing. Stick with one type of berry or use a variety depending on what is in season.

Lemon Icing

1¼ cups raw cashews, soaked in boiling water for 10 minutes and drained

⅓ cup coconut cream

3 tablespoons melted coconut oil

2 tablespoons honey, plus more if needed

1 teaspoon grated lemon zest

1½ tablespoons freshly squeezed lemon juice, plus more if needed

1 teaspoon vanilla extract

¼ teaspoon salt

Lemon Cake

1 cup blanched almond flour

½ cup coconut flour

1 teaspoon baking soda

8 medium eggs

½ cup melted coconut oil

2 tablespoons grated lemon zest

⅓ cup freshly squeezed lemon juice (about 2 medium lemons)

¼ cup honey

2 teaspoons vanilla extract

2 cups fresh berries (quartered strawberries, raspberries, blueberries, and/or blackberries)

¼ cup Paleo powdered sugar, for sprinkling (optional)

SPECIAL EQUIPMENT
High-powered blender
2 (7-inch) springform pans

To make the icing:

1. Place all of the lemon icing ingredients in a high-powered blender and blend until completely smooth. Taste and adjust by adding more honey or lemon juice depending on how tart or sweet you like the icing.

2. Transfer the icing to a tall container, such as a 3-quart spouted mixing bowl, and place in the freezer for 30 minutes to firm up. After 30 minutes, remove from the freezer and use an electric mixer to whip the icing into a light and fluffy consistency. Store in the fridge while you prepare the cake.

To make the cake:

1. Preheat the oven to 350°F and grease two 7-inch springform pans.

2. Put the flours and baking soda in a medium-sized bowl and stir to combine. Add the eggs, coconut oil, lemon zest and juice, honey, and vanilla extract and stir well.

3. Pour the batter evenly into the prepared pans, using 1⅔ cups of batter per pan.

4. Bake the cakes for 25 to 30 minutes, until a toothpick inserted in the middle comes out clean. If the cakes begin to brown too quickly on top, cover the pans with aluminum foil while they bake. Allow the cakes to cool completely before removing from the pans and icing.

5. Whip the icing one more time with an electric mixer before using an offset spatula to evenly spread half of the icing on the top of one cake in a ½-inch layer. Repeat with the remaining icing and cake. Arrange half of the berries over the icing on one of the cakes, then stack the second cake on top. Decorate the top of the cake with the remaining berries. Store the cake in the fridge until ready to serve. Sprinkle with Paleo powdered sugar before serving, if desired.

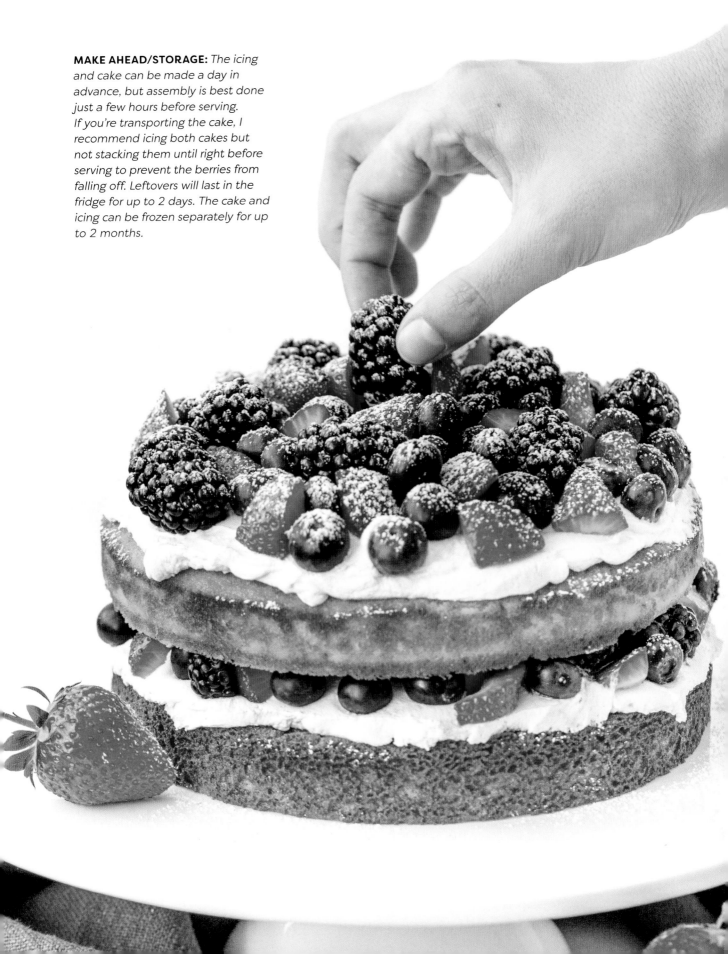

MAKE AHEAD/STORAGE: *The icing and cake can be made a day in advance, but assembly is best done just a few hours before serving. If you're transporting the cake, I recommend icing both cakes but not stacking them until right before serving to prevent the berries from falling off. Leftovers will last in the fridge for up to 2 days. The cake and icing can be frozen separately for up to 2 months.*

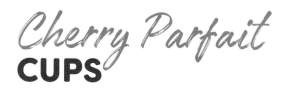

CUPS

Make ahead

Yield: 4 servings   **Prep Time:** 25 minutes   **Cook Time:** 22 minutes

These individual parfaits are a great make-ahead dessert for entertaining. With each spoonful, you get the delicious combination of crumbly shortbread, creamy coconut whip, and stewed cherries. I recommend serving them in small glass cups so that everyone can appreciate how pretty the layers are.

Coconut Whip Layer

2 cups coconut cream

2 tablespoons honey

1 teaspoon vanilla extract

Shortbread Base

1½ cups blanched almond flour

⅓ cup coconut flour

⅓ cup melted coconut oil

3 tablespoons honey

½ teaspoon baking soda

Cherry Layer

3 cups halved and pitted fresh cherries, plus 4 whole cherries for garnish

1 tablespoon honey

2 tablespoons toasted sliced almonds, for garnish

SPECIAL EQUIPMENT
4 (8-ounce) glass cups

1. Preheat the oven to 350°F and line a sheet pan with parchment paper.

2. To make the coconut whip layer, place the coconut cream, honey, and vanilla extract in a bowl and use an electric mixer to beat until the cream is well mixed and has a smooth whipped consistency. Store in the fridge until ready to assemble the cups.

3. Place the shortbread base ingredients in a medium-sized bowl and mix with a wooden spoon until the mixture has formed into a ball of dough. Put the dough on the lined sheet pan and pat it down evenly until it's ¼ to ½ inch thick. Bake for 12 minutes, until golden.

4. While the shortbread base is baking, make the cherry layer. Place the halved cherries and honey in a small saucepan over medium heat and simmer for 10 minutes, until the cherries have begun to shrivel. Remove from the heat and allow to slightly cool.

5. When the shortbread is done baking, remove it from the oven and allow it to cool before breaking it into small pieces. Place some of the shortbread pieces in four 8-ounce glass cups to form a thick base layer in each. Next, spoon a layer of the stewed cherries over the shortbread, followed by a layer of the coconut whip. Follow with layers of shortbread and cherries and finish with a layer of coconut whip. Top with a cherry and sprinkle with the almonds.

SUBSTITUTIONS: *Use maple syrup in place of the honey to make these cups vegan.*

MAKE AHEAD/STORAGE: *Each layer can be made up to 2 days in advance, and the parfaits can be assembled and stored in the fridge up to a day before serving, though they're best when eaten within a few hours of assembly. Leftover parfaits will last for up to 2 days in the fridge, although the shortbread base may become slightly soft and crumbly.*

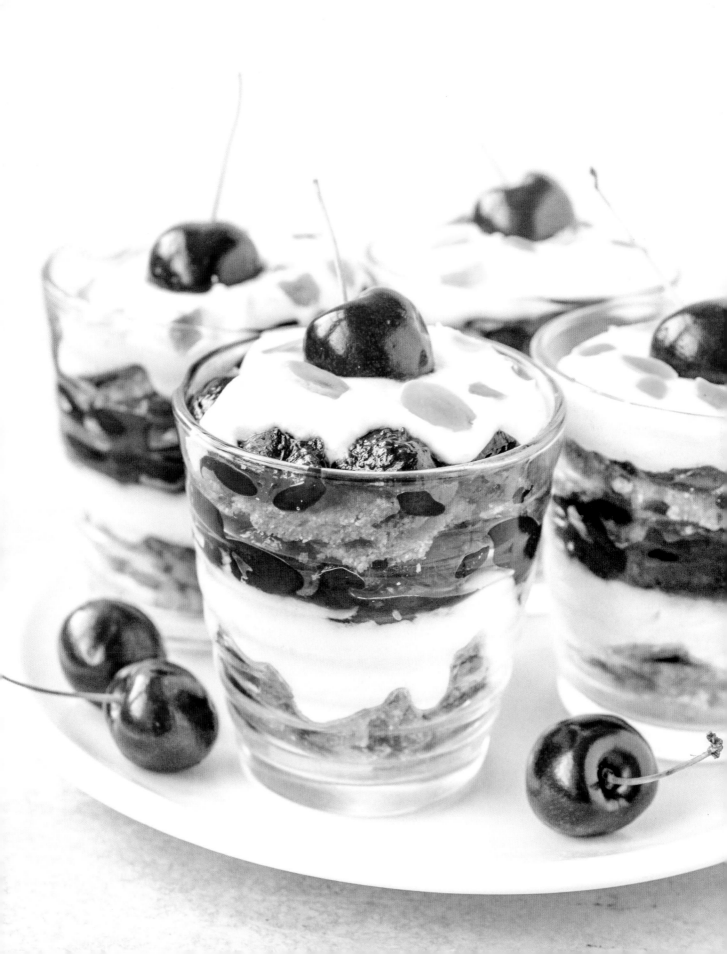

PALEO
VEGAN
VEGETARIAN
DAIRY-FREE
EGG-FREE
NUT-FREE

Caramelized Peach
SKILLET CRISP

Yield: 4 servings **Prep Time:** 7 minutes **Cook Time:** 18 minutes

My mom used to make our family fruit crisp as a special treat on Sunday nights. It took an entire hour to bake, and I always preferred to eat the crumbly topping over the dry fruit filling. This is my new and improved spin on fruit crisp, and it's become a favorite with friends and family. The peaches are caramelized in a delicious sticky sauce before being topped with crumble and quickly baked for just 10 minutes.

Caramelized Peach Filling

5 large ripe peaches

2 tablespoons coconut oil

1½ tablespoons honey

1 teaspoon vanilla extract

1 teaspoon ginger powder

Topping

⅓ cup raw pecans

⅓ cup melted coconut oil

⅔ cup blanched almond flour

⅓ cup unsweetened shredded coconut

2 tablespoons honey

1 teaspoon almond extract

1 teaspoon ginger powder

¼ teaspoon salt

For Serving (Optional)

Coconut whipped cream (see tip, page 324)

Sprinkle of ground cinnamon

In-Season Fruits

You can use different in-season fruits to make this crisp all year round. In place of peaches, use about 5 cups of chopped nectarines, plums, blackberries, cherries, or sliced apples or pears.

1. Preheat the oven to 350°F.

2. To make the filling, place the peaches in a bowl and pour boiling water over them. Leave them in the water for 30 seconds before removing them from the bowl. The skins of the peaches should easily peel off using just your fingers. Remove the pits from the peeled peaches and slice the fruit into thin wedges.

3. Heat the coconut oil, honey, and vanilla extract in a 7-inch cast-iron skillet over medium-high heat. Once the liquid begins to bubble gently, add the sliced peaches and ginger powder and stir to coat the peaches in the sauce. Cook for 8 minutes, stirring frequently, until the peaches are soft and caramelized.

4. To make the topping, pulse the pecans in a food processor until finely chopped but not powdery. Transfer the chopped nuts to a bowl and stir in the remaining topping ingredients. Spoon the mixture evenly over the peaches in the skillet, making sure to cover all the way to the edges.

5. Place the skillet in the oven and bake for 10 minutes, until the topping is golden and the peaches are bubbling. Serve topped with coconut whipped cream and a sprinkle of cinnamon, if desired.

SUBSTITUTIONS: *Make this vegan by swapping maple syrup for honey. To make this nut-free, replace the almond flour with ½ cup coconut flour, the pecans with ⅓ cup raw hulled sunflower seeds, and the almond extract with vanilla extract.*

MAKE AHEAD/STORAGE: *You can prepare both the filling and topping a day in advance and then bake it before serving. The crisp will last in the fridge for up to 3 days.*

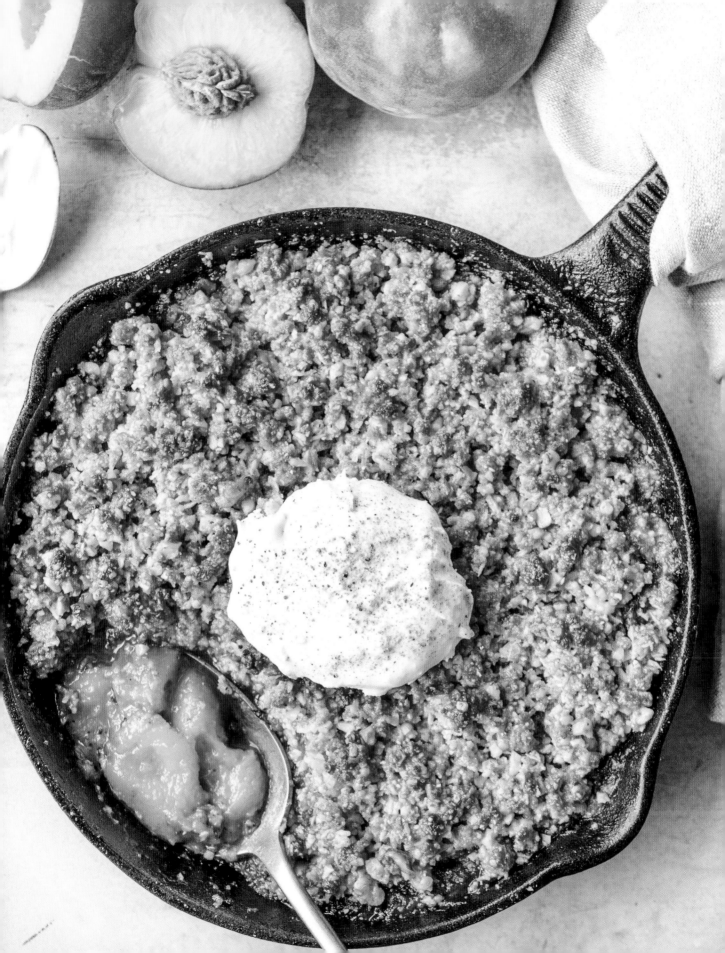

Vanilla Ice Cream with
CRUNCHY CARAMEL PECANS

Yield: 1½ pints (about 6 servings) **Prep Time:** 13 minutes, plus at least 2 hours to freeze
Cook Time: 10 minutes

This dairy-free ice cream has a deliciously creamy consistency thanks to the combination of cashews and coconut milk. The caramelized pecans are highly addicting, so be warned: You may find yourself polishing off a batch before the ice cream is even made!

Crunchy Caramel Pecans

½ cup raw pecans

1½ teaspoons coconut oil

2 tablespoons honey

¼ teaspoon salt

Vanilla Ice Cream Base

2 cups raw cashews, soaked in boiling water for 10 minutes and drained

1 (14-ounce) can full-fat coconut milk

2 tablespoons honey

½ teaspoon salt

Seeds scraped from 2 vanilla beans (about 6 inches long)

SPECIAL EQUIPMENT
High-powered blender
Ice cream maker (optional)

1. If using an ice cream maker, the night before, place the bowl of your ice cream maker in the freezer.

2. Preheat the oven to 350°F. Line a sheet pan with parchment paper.

3. To prepare the pecans, roughly chop them into pieces. In a small skillet over medium-high heat, melt the coconut oil and honey until bubbling. Add the pecans and stir to coat in the oil and honey; then pour the nuts onto the prepared sheet pan and sprinkle with the salt. Bake in the oven for 10 to 12 minutes, until the pecans begin to turn a golden color. Allow the pecans to cool while you prepare the ice cream base.

4. To prepare the vanilla ice cream base, put the cashews, coconut milk, honey, and salt in a high-powered blender and blend and until smooth.

5. Add the vanilla seeds to the cashew mixture and blend for another 10 seconds.

6. Pour the mixture into the ice cream maker and churn according to the manufacturer's instructions. (Churning usually takes about 20 minutes.) If you don't have an ice cream maker, you can skip this step and go right to Step 7; however, the result won't have the same consistency as churned ice cream.

7. Pour the ice cream into an airtight container and stir in the pecan pieces. Place in the freezer for 2 to 3 hours, until firm.

SUBSTITUTIONS: *Replace the honey with maple syrup to make the ice cream vegan.*

STORAGE: *The ice cream will last in an airtight container in the freezer for up to 1 month.*

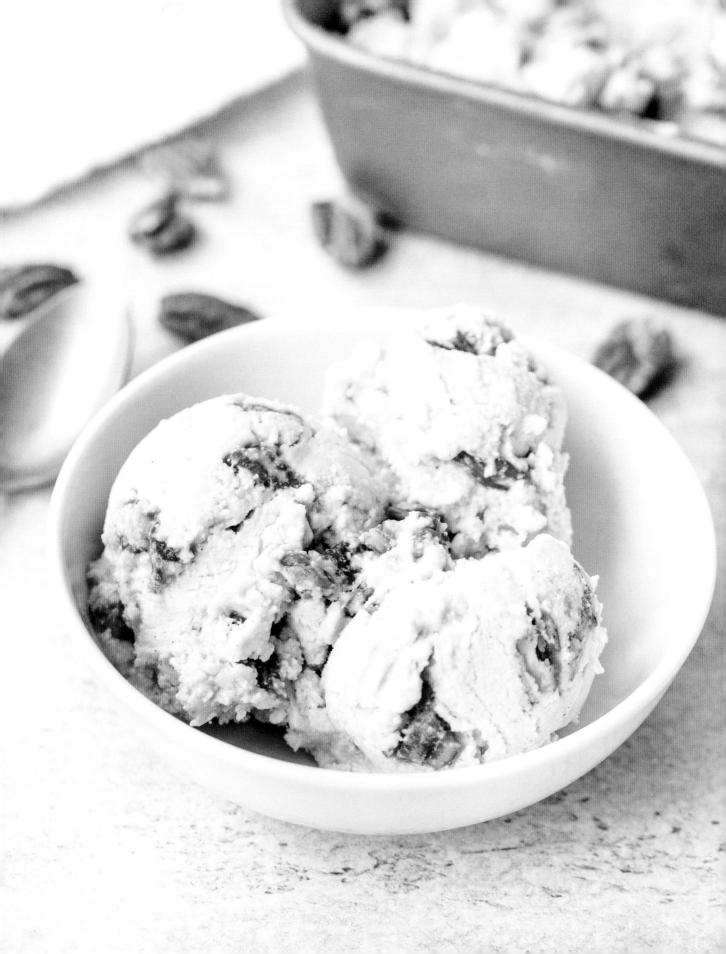

Blackberry, Lemon, or Coconut & Lime
GRANITA

Yield: 4 servings (each flavor) **Prep Time:** 20 minutes, plus 3 hours to freeze **Cook Time:** 15 minutes

I first discovered granita on a 2015 trip to Sicily (the home of granita), and since then I've made it my mission to try every flavor I can find. Granita is lighter and more refreshing than sorbet or gelato, making it the perfect summertime frozen treat. I've created three flavors, each made with a honey-sweetened simple syrup base. You can play around with the flavors; for example, try swapping the lemons for grapefruit in the lemon granita or the blackberries for raspberries, strawberries, or cherries in the blackberry granita.

Honey-Based Simple Syrup

¾ cup water

½ cup honey

BLACKBERRY GRANITA

1 batch Honey-Based Simple Syrup (from above)

2 cups fresh or frozen blackberries

¼ cup soda water

1½ tablespoons freshly squeezed lemon juice

LEMON GRANITA

1 batch Honey-Based Simple Syrup (from above)

1 cup freshly squeezed lemon juice (about 5 medium lemons)

½ cup soda water

2 teaspoons grated lemon zest

COCONUT & LIME GRANITA

1 batch Honey-Based Simple Syrup (from above)

1½ cups full-fat canned coconut milk

1 tablespoon grated lime zest

⅓ cup freshly squeezed lime juice (about 3 limes)

1. To make the simple syrup, place the water and honey in a small saucepan over medium heat and bring to a gentle simmer. Stir for about 1 minute, until the honey has dissolved, then remove the pan from the heat.

2. To make the Blackberry Granita, transfer the simple syrup to a blender along with the blackberries, soda water, and lemon juice and blend until smooth.

To make the Lemon Granita, transfer the simple syrup to a large bowl and add the lemon juice, soda water, and lemon zest. Stir until well mixed.

To make the Coconut & Lime Granita, transfer the simple syrup to a large bowl and add the coconut milk, lime zest, and lime juice. Stir until well mixed,

3. Pour the granita mixture of your choice into an 8-inch square baking dish. Place the dish in the freezer for 1 hour.

4. Remove the dish from the freezer and use a fork to scrape the surface to break up any large pieces that have frozen. Return to the freezer; after 2 more hours, scrape the surface again to break the granita into a coarse texture. Serve the granita in small glasses.

SUBSTITUTIONS: *To make the granita vegan, you can substitute maple syrup for the honey.*

STORAGE: *The granita will last in a covered container in the freezer for up to 2 weeks.*

TIPS: The honey-based simple syrup made in Step 1 is a great staple to have on hand. It will last for up to a month in the fridge and can be added to cocktails or used to make lemonade or sweeten iced tea.

If you'd like to speed up the freezing time, you can use a larger glass baking dish, up to 13 by 9 inches in size.

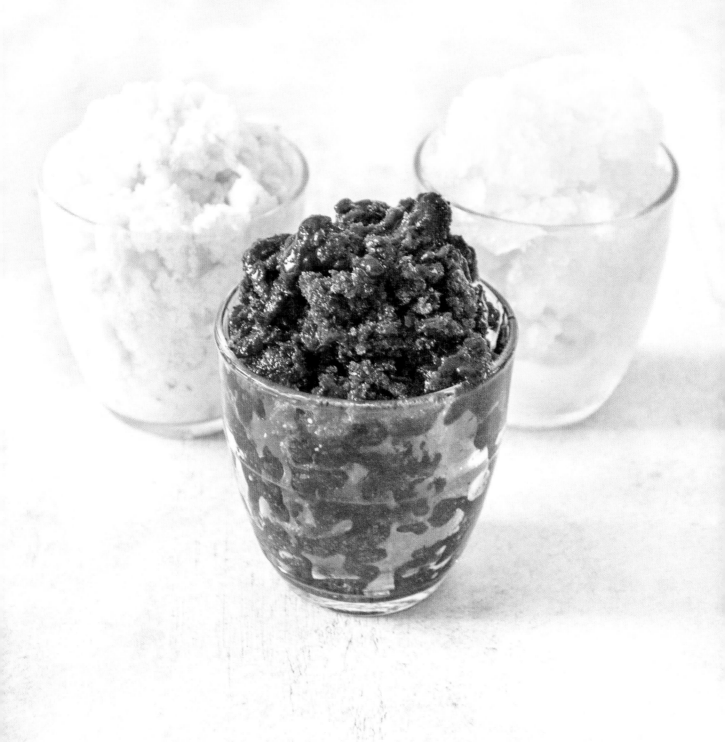

AIP
PALEO
VEGAN
VEGETARIAN
DAIRY-FREE
EGG-FREE
NUT-FREE

Strawberry Lemonade
ICE POPS

Yield: 8 ice pops **Prep Time:** 15 minutes, plus 3 hours to freeze **Cook Time:** —

These ice pops are slightly sweet, slightly tart, and so refreshing! They are one of my favorite snacks to enjoy on a hot summer day and are pretty enough to serve at a backyard cookout.

2 cups water

2 teaspoons grated lemon zest

⅔ cup freshly squeezed lemon juice (about 4 medium lemons)

¼ cup honey

5 fresh strawberries, divided

SPECIAL EQUIPMENT
1 (8-well) ice pop mold

1. Place the water, lemon zest and juice, honey, and 1 strawberry in a blender and blend until smooth.

2. Pour the mixture into an 8-well ice pop mold and place in the freezer for 1 hour.

3. Cut the remaining strawberries into thin slices. After about an hour, the ice pops should be slightly slushy but not completely frozen. Using a knife, push 3 or 4 strawberry slices into each of the molds, then return to the freezer until completely frozen, about 2 hours.

SUBSTITUTIONS: *Use maple syrup in place of the honey to make vegan ice pops.*

STORAGE: *The ice pops will last for up to 2 months in the freezer.*

TIP: *Use whole raspberries or blueberries in place of strawberries or swap the lemon zest and juice for lime zest and juice.*

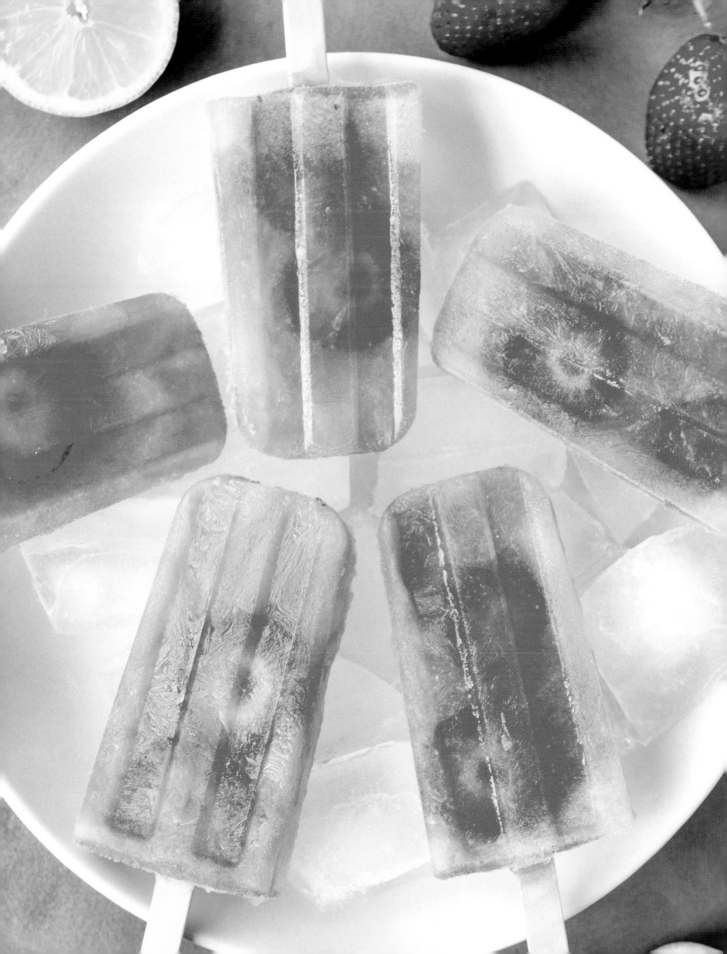

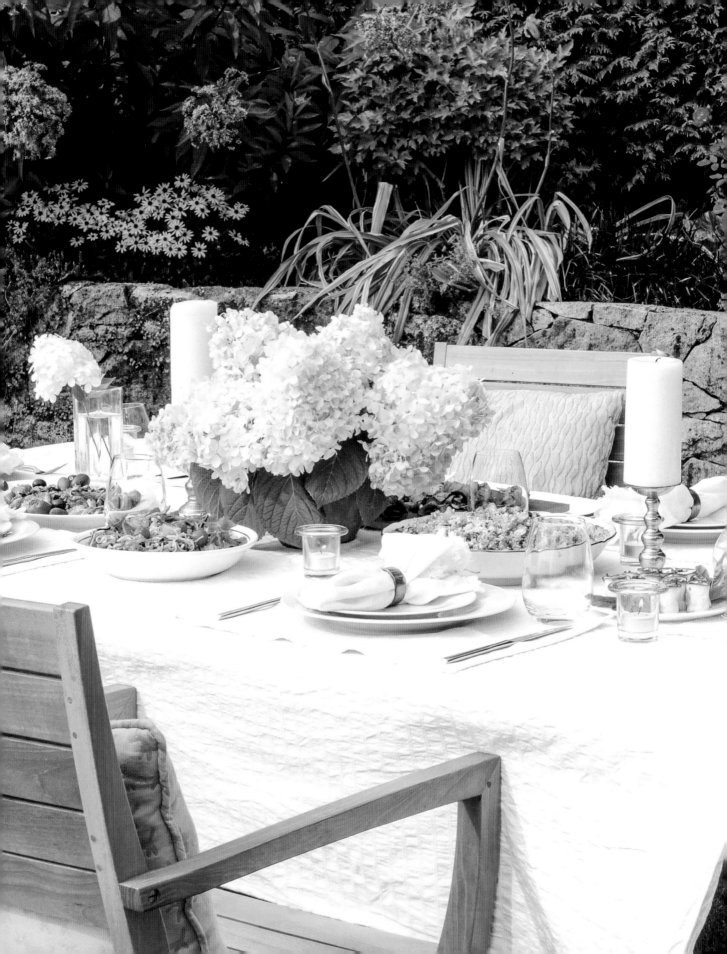

Menu PLANNER

Backyard BBQ

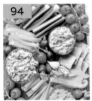
94
Roasted Cauliflower Hummus with veggies

102
Grilled Prosciutto-Wrapped Peaches Stuffed with Honey Thyme "Cheese"

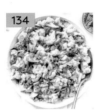
134
Sun-Dried Tomato, Chicken & Cauliflower Salad with Creamy Balsamic Dressing

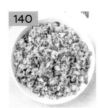
140
Moroccan "Couscous" Salad

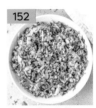
152
Crunchy Asian Slaw

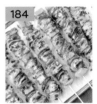
184
Hawaiian Chicken Skewers

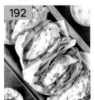
192
Italian Chicken Burgers

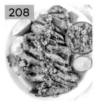
208
Grilled Skirt Steak with Asian Salsa Verde

270
Grilled Veggie Platter with Green Goddess Sauce

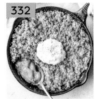
332
Caramelized Peach Skillet Crisp

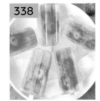
338
Strawberry Lemonade Ice Pops

Game Day Spread

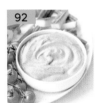
92
Jalapeño Cashew Dip

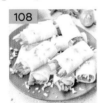
108
Vietnamese Summer Rolls

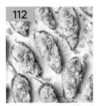
112
Chicken-Stuffed Jalapeño Poppers

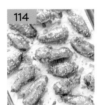
114
Spicy Orange Chicken Wings

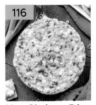
116
Hot Shrimp Dip

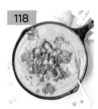
118
Queso Dip

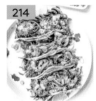
214
Korean Beef Tacos

224
Slow Cooker Honey Balsamic Ribs

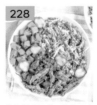
228
BBQ Pulled Pork & Coleslaw Bowl

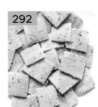
292
Seeded Crackers

Cocktail Party

 104
Zucchini Roll-Ups with Sun-Dried Tomatoes & Black Pepper "Cheese"

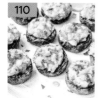 110
Crab & Shrimp–Stuffed Mushrooms

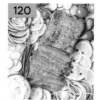 120
Salmon Gravlax & "Cream Cheese" Platter

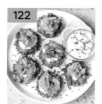 122
Celery Root Latkes with Gravlax

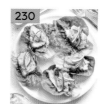 230
Pork Belly, Applesauce & Pickled Onion Lettuce Cups

Sunday Brunch

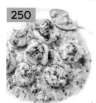 50
Chorizo

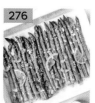 62
Salmon, Asparagus & Caper Quiche

 72
Mexican Eggs Benedict

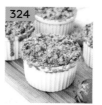 80
Raspberry Orange Muffins

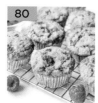 84
Tahini Cherry Granola

Date Night

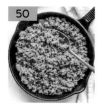 250
Bacon & Garlic Herb Butter Seared Scallops

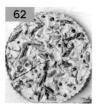 276
Lemon & Garlic Roasted Asparagus

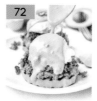 282
The BEST Cauliflower Mash

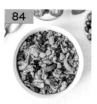 324
Individual Strawberry Rhubarb Crumbles

Fancy Dinner Party

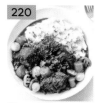 220
Short Rib Beef Bourguignonne

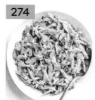 274
Patty's Melt-in-Your-Mouth Fennel & Leeks

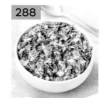 282
The BEST Cauliflower Mash

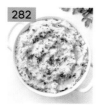 288
Creamed Spinach & Kale

 330
Cherry Parfait Cups

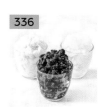 336
Blackberry, Lemon, or Coconut & Lime Granita

Vegan Dinner Party

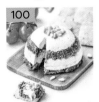
100
"Goat Cheese," Sun-Dried Tomato & Pesto Tower

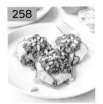
258
Butternut Squash Ravioli with Kale Pesto

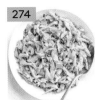
274
Patty's Melt-in-Your-Mouth Fennel & Leeks

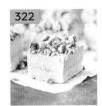
322
Pecan & Salted Caramel Shortbread Bars

Mexican Fiesta

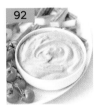
92
Jalapeño Cashew Dip

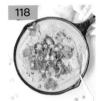
118
Queso Dip

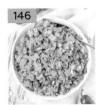
146
Chipotle Butternut Squash Salad

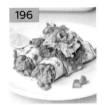
196
Chicken Enchiladas

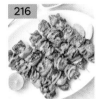
216
Steak Fajita Skewers with Cilantro Chimichurri

240
Spicy Fish Tacos

Takeout Fakeout

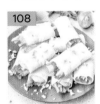
108
Vietnamese Summer Rolls

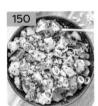
150
Smashed Cucumber Salad

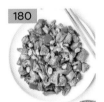
180
Kung Pao Chicken

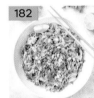
182
Peanut Chicken Noodle Bowl

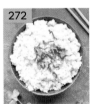
272
Coconut Cauliflower Rice

ACKNOWLEDGMENTS

Thank you to my dad, Lisa, and Mitch (aka the Fockers) for being my biggest cheerleaders from day one. Your unwavering enthusiasm for celebrating every new milestone has kept me motivated and brought me so much joy. From your threats of sky writing and billboards to talking about my blog with every person you meet, you are the best publicity team I could ever ask for. You really are a crazy bunch, but I am so lucky to be able to call you my family.

To SA, thank you for your unwavering support in everything I do and for always pushing me that little bit further. When it comes to taste-testing, you are a hard one to please, but I always value your brutally honest opinion. Thank you for keeping me sane during this whole book-writing process by putting things in perspective and always making me laugh. I can't wait for what our next chapter has in store.

To Lance and the entire Victory Belt team, your support and patience through this whole process has been so much more than I ever expected. Thank you for making my lifelong dream of writing a cookbook come to fruition.

To my agent, Coleen, thank you for helping me through the publishing process and for all the guidance you have provided.

To my recipe testers, including JA, Sam, Pam, and Jamie, thank you for taking the time to try these recipes and for all the feedback you provided.

To all my amazing friends in London, Vancouver, New York, Berlin, Los Angeles, and Arizona, thank you for your regular sanity check-ins over the past year and for all your encouragement. You guys know who you are, and I'm so thankful to have each and every one of you in my life.

And, finally, to every single follower and blog reader, THANK YOU! This book wouldn't be possible without you. Because of your support, I am lucky enough to get to do what I'm passionate about every single day. You guys are truly the best, and I am so lucky to be a part of such an amazing community of fellow foodies.

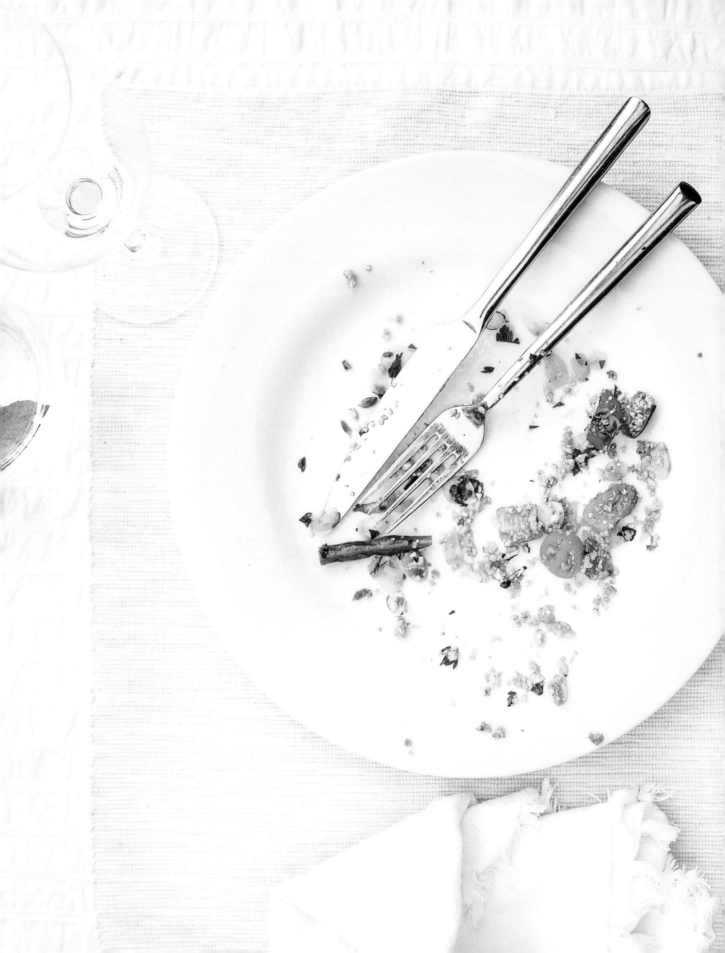

DIET & ALLERGEN INDEX

+ indicates the recipe is compliant

+ indicates the recipe is compliant with modification

RECIPE	Page	AIP	KETO	LOW-FODMAP	PALEO	VEGAN	VEGETARIAN	DAIRY-FREE	EGG-FREE	NUT-FREE
Harissa	33		+		+	+	+	+	+	+
Chipotle Paste	34		+		+	+	+	+	+	+
Tomato Paste	35		+	+	+	+	+	+	+	+
Tomato Sauce	36		+	+	+	+	+	+	+	+
Sun-Dried Tomatoes	38		+	+	+	+	+	+	+	+
Egg-Free Mayonnaise (Toum)	40	+	+		+	+	+	+	+	+
Easy 3-Minute Mayonnaise	42		+	+	+		+	+		+
Celery Root Tortillas	44	+	+	+	+	+	+	+	+	+
SCD Balsamic Vinegar	46	+			+	+	+	+	+	+
Coco-not Aminos	47				+			+	+	+
Quick Pickled Veggies	48		+			+	+	+	+	+
Chorizo	50		+	+	+			+	+	+
Beef Stock	52		+		+			+	+	+
Chicken Stock	53		+		+			+	+	+
Vegetable Stock	53		+		+	+	+	+	+	+
Butternut Squash Toast Four Ways	56				+		+	+	+	+
Avocado, Bacon & Egg Breakfast Sandwiches	58		+	+	+		+	+		+
Mexican Breakfast Casserole	60		+		+			+		+
Salmon, Asparagus & Caper Quiche	62		+		+		+	+		+
Eggplant & Harissa Shakshuka	64				+		+	+		+
Portobello Baked Eggs with Chimichurri	66		+		+		+	+		+
Asparagus Soldiers & Eggs	68		+	+	+			+		+
Roasted Vegetable Sheet Pan Frittata	70		+	+	+		+	+		+
Mexican Eggs Benedict	72		+	+	+		+	+		+
Broccoli & Bacon Egg Muffins	74		+	+	+		+	+		+
Chunky Banana & Pecan Muffins	76				+		+	+		
Apple Cinnamon Breakfast Cookies	78				+		+	+		
Raspberry Orange Muffins	80				+		+	+		
Pancakes with Berry Compote	82				+		+	+		
Tahini Cherry Granola	84				+	+	+	+	+	
Pear & Chai Spiced Porridge	86				+	+	+	+	+	+
Muhammara	90		+	+	+	+	+	+	+	
Jalapeño Cashew Dip	92		+		+	+	+	+	+	

RECIPE	Page	AIP	KETO	LOW-FODMAP	PALEO	VEGAN	VEGETARIAN	DAIRY-FREE	EGG-FREE	NUT-FREE
Roasted Cauliflower Hummus	94		+		+	+	+	+	+	+
Tzatziki	98		+		+	+	+	+	+	
"Goat Cheese," Sun-Dried Tomato & Pesto Tower	100		+	+	+	+	+	+	+	
Grilled Prosciutto-Wrapped Peaches Stuffed with Honey Thyme "Cheese"	102				+			+	+	
Zucchini Roll-Ups with Sun-Dried Tomatoes & Black Pepper "Cheese"	104		+	+	+	+	+	+	+	
Bacon & Scallion Spaghetti Squash Fritters	106		+		+		+	+		
Vietnamese Summer Rolls	108		+		+	+	+	+	+	+
Crab & Shrimp–Stuffed Mushrooms	110		+		+			+		+
Chicken-Stuffed Jalapeño Poppers	112		+	+	+			+		+
Spicy Orange Chicken Wings	114	+			+			+	+	+
Hot Shrimp Dip	116		+	+	+			+		+
Queso Dip	118		+		+	+	+	+	+	
Salmon Gravlax & "Cream Cheese" Platter	120		+	+	+			+	+	
Celery Root Latkes with Gravlax	122		+		+			+		
Charred Snap Pea & Bacon Salad with Creamy Herb Dressing	126				+	+	+	+	+	+
Roasted Broccoli, Butternut Squash & Kale Salad with Creamy Garlic Dressing	128		+		+	+	+	+	+	+
Cajun Shrimp Caesar Salad	130		+	+	+	+	+	+	+	+
Spicy Shrimp, Avocado & Peach Salad	132				+			+	+	+
Sun-Dried Tomato, Chicken & Cauliflower Salad with Creamy Balsamic Dressing	134		+		+	+	+	+	+	+
Chicken, Avocado & Bacon Salad with Ranch Dressing	136		+	+	+			+	+	+
Vietnamese Beef Salad	138	+	+		+			+	+	+
Moroccan "Couscous" Salad	140	+	+		+	+	+	+	+	+
Roasted Cauliflower, Date, Red Onion & Parsley Salad	142		+		+	+	+	+	+	+
Roasted Butternut Squash & Red Onion Salad with Orange Cinnamon Dressing	144	+			+	+	+	+	+	
Chipotle Butternut Squash Salad	146			+	+		+	+		+
Roasted Pepper, Tomato & Basil Salad	148		+	+	+	+	+	+	+	+
Smashed Cucumber Salad	150		+		+	+	+	+	+	+
Crunchy Asian Slaw	152		+		+	+	+	+	+	+
Quick Vietnamese Beef Pho	156	+	+	+	+			+	+	+
Wonton Meatball Soup	158	+	+	+	+			+	+	+
Hot & Sour Soup	160	+	+		+		+	+	+	+
Zuppa Toscana	162		+	+	+			+	+	+
Southwest Chicken & Bacon Chowder	164		+		+			+	+	+
Mom's Feel-Better Chicken & Rice Soup	166	+	+		+	+	+	+	+	+
Chicken Pot Pie Soup	168	+	+		+			+	+	+
Greek Avgolemono Soup	170		+		+		+	+		+
Cheesy Broccoli Soup	172		+	+	+	+	+	+	+	
Butternut Squash, Leek & Apple Soup	174	+			+	+	+	+	+	+

RECIPE	Page	AIP	KETO	LOW-FODMAP	PALEO	VEGAN	VEGETARIAN	DAIRY-FREE	EGG-FREE	NUT-FREE
Kung Pao Chicken	180		+		+			+	+	+
Peanut Chicken Noodle Bowl	182			+	+	+	+	+	+	
Hawaiian Chicken Skewers	184				+			+	+	+
Harissa & Orange Spatchcock Roast Chicken	186				+			+	+	+
Balsamic Chicken & Grapes	188	+	+		+			+	+	+
Spicy Honey Un-Fried Chicken	190		+	+	+			+	+	+
Italian Chicken Burgers	192		+	+	+			+		+
Sun-Dried Tomato, Basil & "Goat Cheese" Stuffed Chicken Breasts	194		+		+			+	+	
Chicken Enchiladas	196		+	+	+			+		+
One-Pan Spanish Chicken & Rice	198		+		+			+	+	+
Sheet Pan Greek Chicken	200		+	+	+			+	+	+
Butter Chicken Meatballs	202		+	+	+			+	+	+
Creamy Chicken & Spinach Cannelloni	204		+		+			+	+	
Grilled Skirt Steak with Asian Salsa Verde	208		+		+			+	+	+
The Most Epic Grain-Free Beef Lasagna	210				+			+	+	
Shredded Beef Ragu	212		+	+	+			+	+	+
Korean Beef Tacos	214		+		+			+		+
Steak Fajita Skewers with Cilantro Chimichurri	216		+	+	+			+	+	+
Beef Stroganoff	218		+		+			+	+	
Short Rib Beef Bourguignonne	220		+		+			+	+	+
Greek 7-Layer Lamb Dip	222		+	+	+			+	+	
Slow Cooker Honey Balsamic Ribs	224	+	+		+			+	+	+
Dan Dan Noodles	226		+	+	+			+	+	+
BBQ Pulled Pork & Coleslaw Bowl	228		+	+	+			+		+
Pork Belly, Applesauce & Pickled Onion Lettuce Cups	230	+			+			+	+	+
Sweet Chili Salmon	234				+			+	+	+
Creamy Honey Mustard Baked Salmon	236		+		+			+		+
Easy Canned Tuna Cakes	238	+	+	+	+			+		
Spicy Fish Tacos	240		+		+			+		+
Sheet Pan Roasted Cod with Fennel, Olives, Red Onion & Tomatoes	242		+	+	+			+	+	+
Chili Mayo Shrimp Lettuce Cups	244		+	+	+			+		+
Ginger & Black Pepper Shrimp Stir-Fry	246	+	+		+			+	+	+
Creamy Lemon Dill Shrimp	248		+		+			+	+	
Bacon & Garlic Herb Butter Seared Scallops	250		+	+	+			+	+	+
Cashew e Pepe	254				+	+	+	+	+	
Creamy Spring Risotto	256				+	+	+	+	+	+
Butternut Squash Ravioli with Kale Pesto	258		+	+	+	+	+	+	+	
Eggplant Ragu	260		+	+	+	+	+	+	+	+

RECIPE	Page	AIP	KETO	LOW-FODMAP	PALEO	VEGAN	VEGETARIAN	DAIRY-FREE	EGG-FREE	NUT-FREE
Eggplant Meatless Meatballs	262		+	+	+		+	+		
Tandoori Grilled Cauliflower Steaks	264				+	+	+	+	+	
Mushroom & Onion Risotto	266		+		+	+	+	+	+	+
Grilled Veggie Platter with Green Goddess Sauce	270		+		+	+	+	+	+	+
Coconut Cauliflower Rice	272	+	+		+	+	+	+	+	+
Spicy Rice	273		+		+	+	+	+	+	+
Patty's Melt-in-Your-Mouth Fennel & Leeks	274	+	+	+	+	+	+	+	+	+
Lemon & Garlic Roasted Asparagus	276	+	+		+	+	+	+	+	+
Green Beans with Hazelnuts & Tahini Lemon Sauce	278		+		+	+	+	+	+	
Garlic Roasted Mushrooms	280	+	+		+	+	+	+	+	+
The BEST Cauliflower Mash	282		+		+	+	+	+	+	+
Roasted Brussels Sprouts & Bacon	284	+	+		+	+	+	+	+	+
Loaded Cauliflower Casserole	286		+		+		+	+	+	
Creamed Spinach & Kale	288		+		+	+	+	+	+	
Seeded Crackers	292		+	+	+		+	+		
Jalapeño, Bacon & Cauliflower Muffins	294		+		+		+	+		
Lemon Blueberry Mug Cake	296				+		+	+		
Orange, Cranberry & Pecan Energy Balls	298				+	+	+	+	+	
Hazelnut & Coffee Energy Balls	299				+	+	+	+	+	
Sweet & Spicy Almonds	300				+	+	+	+	+	
Crunchy Nut Bars	302				+	+	+	+	+	
Mango Chili Fruit Roll-Ups	304	+		+	+	+	+	+	+	+
Apple Ginger Gummy Bears	306	+		+	+			+	+	+
Vanilla-Coated Frozen Banana Bites	308			+	+	+	+	+	+	
Three Hidden-Veggie Smoothies	310				+	+	+	+	+	+
Chewy Almond & Orange Cookies	314			+	+	+	+	+	+	
Peanut Butter & Jam Thumbprint Cookies	316				+	+	+	+	+	
N'oatmeal Raisin Cookies	318				+		+	+		
Nut Butter Cookies	320				+		+	+		
Pecan & Salted Caramel Shortbread Bars	322				+	+	+	+	+	
Individual Strawberry Rhubarb Crumbles	324				+	+	+	+	+	
Carrot Cupcakes	326				+		+	+		
Lemon & Berry Layer Cake	328				+		+	+		
Cherry Parfait Cups	330				+	+	+	+	+	
Caramelized Peach Skillet Crisp	332				+	+	+	+	+	+
Vanilla Ice Cream with Crunchy Caramel Pecans	334				+	+	+	+	+	
Blackberry, Lemon, or Coconut & Lime Granita	336	+			+	+	+	+	+	+
Strawberry Lemonade Ice Pops	338	+			+	+	+	+	+	+

RECITE INDEX

Basics

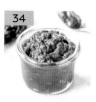
33
Harissa

34
Chipotle Paste

35
Tomato Paste

36
Tomato Sauce

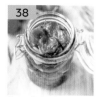
38
Sun-Dried Tomatoes

40
Egg-Free Mayonnaise (Toum)

42
Easy 3-Minute Mayonnaise

44
Celery Root Tortillas

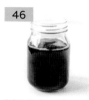
46
SCD Balsamic Vinegar

47
Coco-not Aminos

48
Quick Pickled Veggies

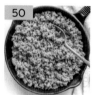
50
Chorizo

52
Stocks

Breakfast

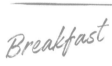
56
Butternut Squash Toast Four Ways

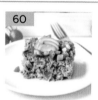
58
Avocado, Bacon & Egg Breakfast Sandwiches

60
Mexican Breakfast Casserole

62
Salmon, Asparagus & Caper Quiche

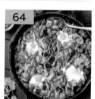
64
Eggplant & Harissa Shakshuka

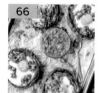
66
Portobello Baked Eggs with Chimichurri

68
Asparagus Soldiers & Eggs

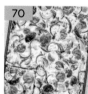
70
Roasted Vegetable Sheet Pan Frittata

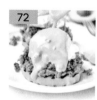
72
Mexican Eggs Benedict

74
Broccoli & Bacon Egg Muffins

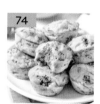
76
Chunky Banana & Pecan Muffins

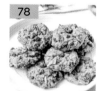
78
Apple Cinnamon Breakfast Cookies

80
Raspberry Orange Muffins

82
Pancakes with Berry Compote

84
Tahini Cherry Granola

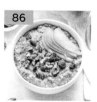
86
Pear & Chai Spiced Porridge

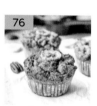
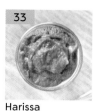

Appetizers

 90
Muhammara

 92
Jalapeño Cashew Dip

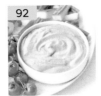 94
Roasted Cauliflower Hummus

 98
Tzatziki

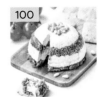 100
"Goat Cheese," Sun-Dried Tomato & Pesto Tower

 102
Grilled Prosciutto-Wrapped Peaches Stuffed with Honey Thyme "Cheese"

 104
Zucchini Roll-Ups with Sun-Dried Tomatoes & Black Pepper "Cheese"

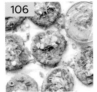 106
Bacon & Scallion Spaghetti Squash Fritters

 108
Vietnamese Summer Rolls

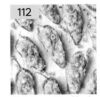 110
Crab & Shrimp-Stuffed Mushrooms

 112
Chicken-Stuffed Jalapeño Poppers

 114
Spicy Orange Chicken Wings

 116
Hot Shrimp Dip

 118
Queso Dip

 120
Salmon Gravlax & "Cream Cheese" Platter

 122
Celery Root Latkes

Salads

 126
Charred Snap Pea & Bacon Salad with Creamy Herb Dressing

 128
Roasted Broccoli, Butternut Squash & Kale Salad with Creamy Garlic Dressing

 130
Cajun Shrimp Caesar Salad

 132
Spicy Shrimp, Avocado & Peach Salad

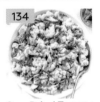 134
Sun-Dried Tomato, Chicken & Cauliflower Salad with Creamy Balsamic Dressing

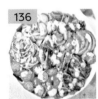 136
Chicken, Avocado & Bacon Salad with Ranch Dressing

 138
Vietnamese Beef Salad

 140
Moroccan "Couscous" Salad

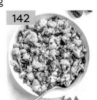 142
Roasted Cauliflower, Date, Red Onion & Parsley Salad

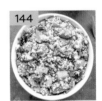 144
Roasted Butternut Squash & Red Onion Salad with Orange Cinnamon Dressing

 146
Chipotle Butternut Squash Salad

 148
Roasted Pepper, Tomato & Basil Salad

 150
Smashed Cucumber Salad

 152
Crunchy Asian Slaw

Soups

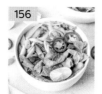
156
Quick Vietnamese Beef Pho

158
Wonton Meatball Soup

160
Hot & Sour Soup

162
Zuppa Toscana

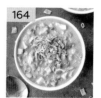
164
Southwest Chicken & Bacon Chowder

166
Mom's Feel-Better Chicken & Rice Soup

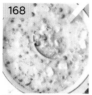
168
Chicken Pot Pie Soup

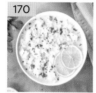
170
Greek Avgolemono Soup

172
Cheesy Broccoli Soup

174
Butternut Squash, Leek & Apple Soup

Mains/ Chicken

180
Kung Pao Chicken

182
Peanut Chicken Noodle Bowl

184
Hawaiian Chicken Skewers

186
Harissa & Orange Spatchcock Roast Chicken

188
Balsamic Chicken & Grapes

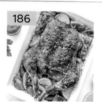
190
Spicy Honey Un-Fried Chicken

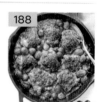
192
Italian Chicken Burgers

194
Sun-Dried Tomato, Basil & "Goat Cheese" Stuffed Chicken Breasts

196
Chicken Enchiladas

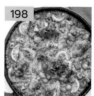
198
One-Pan Spanish Chicken & Rice

200
Sheet Pan Greek Chicken

202
Butter Chicken Meatballs

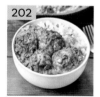
204
Creamy Chicken & Spinach Cannelloni

Mains/Meat

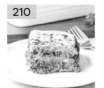
208 Grilled Skirt Steak with Asian Salsa Verde

210 The Most Epic Grain-Free Beef Lasagna

212 Shredded Beef Ragu

214 Korean Beef Tacos

216 Steak Fajita Skewers with Cilantro Chimichurri

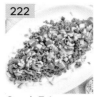

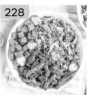

218 Beef Stroganoff

220 Short Rib Beef Bourguignonne

222 Greek 7-Layer Lamb Dip

224 Slow Cooker Honey Balsamic Ribs

226 Dan Dan Noodles

228 BBQ Pulled Pork & Coleslaw Bowl

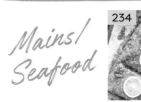

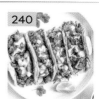

230 Pork Belly, Applesauce & Pickled Onion Lettuce Cups

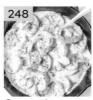
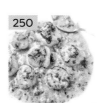

Mains/Seafood

234 Sweet Chili Salmon

236 Creamy Honey Mustard Baked Salmon

238 Easy Canned Tuna Cakes

240 Spicy Fish Tacos

242 Sheet Pan Roasted Cod with Fennel, Olives, Red Onion & Tomatoes

244 Chili Mayo Shrimp Lettuce Cups

246 Ginger & Black Pepper Shrimp Stir-Fry

248 Creamy Lemon Dill Shrimp

250 Bacon & Garlic Herb Butter Seared Scallops

Mains/ Vegetarian

 254
Cashew e Pepe

 256
Creamy Spring Risotto

 258
Butternut Squash Ravioli with Kale Pesto

 260
Eggplant Ragu

 262
Eggplant Meatless Meatballs

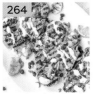 264
Tandoori Grilled Cauliflower Steaks

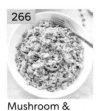 266
Mushroom & Onion Risotto

Side Dishes

 270
Grilled Veggie Platter with Green Goddess Sauce

 272
Coconut Cauliflower Rice

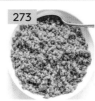 273
Spicy Rice

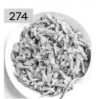 274
Patty's Melt-in-Your-Mouth Fennel & Leeks

 276
Lemon & Garlic Roasted Asparagus

 278
Green Beans with Hazelnuts & Tahini Lemon Sauce

 280
Garlic Roasted Mushrooms

 282
The BEST Cauliflower Mash

 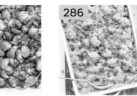 284
Roasted Brussels Sprouts & Bacon

286
Loaded Cauliflower Casserole

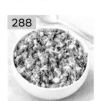 288
Creamed Spinach & Kale

Snacks

292 Seeded Crackers

294 Jalapeño, Bacon & Cauliflower Muffins

296 Lemon Blueberry Mug Cake

298 Orange, Cranberry & Pecan Energy Balls

299 Hazelnut & Coffee Energy Balls

300 Sweet & Spicy Almonds

302 Crunchy Nut Bars

304 Mango Chili Fruit Roll-Ups

306 Apple Ginger Gummy Bears

308 Vanilla-Coated Frozen Banana Bites

310 Three Hidden-Veggie Smoothies

Desserts

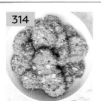
314 Chewy Almond & Orange Cookies

316 Peanut Butter & Jam Thumbprint Cookies

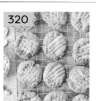
318 N'oatmeal Raisin Cookies

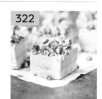
320 Nut Butter Cookies

322 Pecan & Salted Caramel Shortbread Bars

324 Individual Strawberry Rhubarb Crumbles

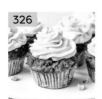
326 Carrot Cupcakes

328 Lemon & Berry Layer Cake

330 Cherry Parfait Cups

332 Caramelized Peach Skillet Crisp

334 Vanilla Ice Cream with Crunchy Caramel Pecans

336 Blackberry, Lemon, or Coconut & Lime Granita

338 Strawberry Lemonade Ice Pops

GENERAL INDEX